MOLECULAR AND CELLULAR REPAIR PROCESSES

MOLECULAR AND CELLULAR REPAIR PROCESSES

FIFTH INTERNATIONAL SYMPOSIUM ON MOLECULAR BIOLOGY

Sponsored by Miles Laboratories, Inc.

The Thomas B. Turner Auditorium
The Johns Hopkins Medical Institutions
Baltimore, Maryland
June 3-4, 1971

Edited by

Roland F. Beers, Jr., Roger M. Herriott and R. Carmichael Tilghman

Supplement Number 1
of
The Johns Hopkins Medical Journal
by
The Johns Hopkins University Press
Baltimore

The Johns Hopkins University Press, Baltimore, Maryland 21218

The Johns Hopkins University Press Ltd., London

Library of Congress Catalog Card Number 78-184199

ISBN 0-8018-1376-X

The following figures are reprinted by permission of *Mutation Research:* in Chapter 6, Fig. 2, p. 57 (Mutat. Res. 6:359, 374), Fig. 3, p. 58 (Mutat. Res. 6:374), Fig. 4, p. 59 (Mutat. Res. 6:361), Fig. 5, p. 60 (Mutat. Res. 8:413, Fig. 6, p. 61 (Mutat. Res. 8:414), and Fig. 7, p. 61 (Mutat. Res. 6:366); and in Chapter 7, Fig. 1B, p. 66 (Mutat. Res. 10:281), Fig. 2, p. 69 (Mutat. Res. 10:287, 296, 299), and Fig. 6, p. 76 (Mutat. Res. 7:267).

Academic Press has granted permission to reprint the following figures, for which they hold copyright: in Chapter 6, Fig. 1, p. 55 (*Photophysiology,* ed. A. C. Giese [New York, 1971], p. 287), and in Chapter 13, Fig. 8, p. 135 (*Radiation Research* 37 [1969] : 93).

The acceleration in the investigation and understanding of molecular repair mechanisms, particularly from the enzymatic viewpoint, and growing appreciation of the nature of cellular repair processes in response to acute and chronic injury from a variety of environmental agents, including chemical, ultraviolet and ionizing radiation, make timely the correlation of those disciplines concerned with mechanisms of repair processes. The knowledge may be applied to such matters as the induction of selective injury to malignant cells and the establishment of standards of maximum permissible levels of exposure to toxic, mutagenic and carcinogenic agents. Under the sponsorship of Miles Laboratories, Inc., chaired by Professors Roland F. Beers, Jr. and Roger M. Herriott, of The Johns Hopkins University School of Hygiene and Public Health, this Symposium was arranged and the record of the proceedings constitutes Supplement Number 1 of The Johns Hopkins Medical Journal.

THE JOHNS HOPKINS MEDICAL JOURNAL

Established in 1889 as The Johns Hopkins Hospital Bulletin

Published monthly under the sponsorship of
The Johns Hopkins University School of Medicine, The Johns Hopkins Hospital
and The Johns Hopkins Medical and Surgical Association

The Johns Hopkins Medical Journal, established in 1889 as The Johns Hopkins Hospital Bulletin, is dedicated to the publication of results of original research and reviews, especially of interdisciplinary interest to those working in the biomedical sciences, and to those in the broadest sense involved in the practice of medicine. It is designed particularly to reflect the contributions of present and former faculty, staff and students of The Johns Hopkins Medical Institutions. In addition, contributions from others are welcome. The circulation of The Journal includes libraries and individuals throughout the world.

THE JOHNS HOPKINS UNIVERSITY PRESS

BALTIMORE, MARYLAND 21218

LIST OF AUTHORS

CONTENTS

AUTHORS, CO-AUTHORS AND DISCUSSANTS

P. V. N. Acharya, Bjorkstan Research Foundation, Madison, Wisconsin

Max L. Baker, University of Arkansas Medical Center and Veterans Administration Hospital, Little Rock, Arkansas

James A. Belli, Harvard Medical School, Boston, Massachusetts

John M. Boyle, Christie Hospital and Holt Radium Institute, Manchester, England

Neal Brown, University of Maryland, College Park, Maryland

Alan K. Bruce, State University of New York at Buffalo, Buffalo, New York

Peter Ceruitti, University of Florida, Gainesville, Florida

A. Chiling, Ohio State University, Columbus, Ohio

John S. Cook, Oak Ridge National Laboratories, Oak Ridge, Tennessee

James E. Cleaver, University of California School of Medicine, San Francisco, California

Ronald Cole, Yale University, New Haven, Connecticut

M. Coyle, University of Chicago, Chicago, Illinois

Glenn V. Dalrymple, University of Arkansas Medical Center and Veterans Administration Hospital, Little Rock, Arkansas

M. Dolyniuk, University of Chicago, Chicago, Illinois

Franz-Josef Ferdinand, Friedrich-Miescher-Laboratorium der Max-Planck-Gesellschaft, Tubingen, Germany

Brian Fox, Christie Hospital and Holt Radium Institute, Manchester, England

Helga Harm, University of Texas at Dallas, Dallas, Texas

Walter Harm, University of Texas at Dallas, Dallas, Texas

Paul Howard-Flanders, Yale University, New Haven, Connecticut

P. C. Huang, The Johns Hopkins University School of Hygiene and Public Health, Baltimore, Maryland

Ronald M. Humphrey, M. D. Anderson Hospital and Tumor Institute, Houston, Texas

F. Hutchinson, Yale University, New Haven, Connecticut

Eugene Jackim, National Marine Water Quality Laboratory, Narragansett, Rhode Island

K. Kato, University of Chicago, Chicago, Illinois

Albert Kelner, Brandies University, Waltham, Massachusetts

Rolf Knippers, Friedrich-Miescher-Laboratorium der Max-Planck-Gesellschaft, Tubingen, Germany

John T. Lett, Colorado State University, Fort Collins, Colorado

Tomas Lindahl, Karolinska Institutet, Stockholm, Sweden

M. McMahon, University of Chicago, Chicago, Illinois

Timothy Merz, The Johns Hopkins University School of Hygiene and Public Health, Baltimore, Maryland

R. E. Meyn, M. D. Anderson Hospital and Tumor Institute, Houston, Texas

Osayuki Morita, Temple University School of Medicine, Philadelphia, Pennsylvania

A. J. Moss, Jr., University of Arkansas Medical Center and Veterans Administration Hospital, Little Rock, Arkansas

John C. Nash, University of Arkansas Medical Center and Veterans Administration Hospital, Little Rock, Arkansas

Robert B. Painter, University of California, San Francisco, California

Bibek Ray, North Carolina State University, Raleigh, North Carolina

John Roberts, Chester Beatty Research Institute, Buckinghamshire, England

D. M. Robinson, American Red Cross Blood Research Laboratory, Bethesda, Maryland

Claud S. Rupert, University of Texas at Dallas, Dallas, Texas

William L. Russell, Oak Ridge National Laboratories, Oak Ridge, Tennessee

J. L. Sanders, University of Arkansas Medical Center and Veterans Administration Hospital, Little Rock, Arkansas

Tsuigo Satoh, Temple University School of Medicine, Philadelphia, Pennsylvania

James Schaeffer, The Johns Hopkins University School of Hygiene and Public Health, Baltimore, Maryland

Robert Stoller, Bureau of Radiological Health, Rockville, Maryland

Bernard S. Strauss, University of Chicago, Chicago, Illinois

Wolf Strätling, Friedrich-Miescher-Laboratorium der Max-Planck-Gesellschaft, Tubingen, Germany

R. W. Tuveson, University of Illinois, Urbana, Illinois

K. T. Wheeler, Jr., Colorado State University, Fort Collins, Colorado

K. P. Wilkinson, University of Arkansas Medical Center and Veterans Administration Hospital, Little Rock, Arkansas

Nobuto Yamamoto, Temple University School of Medicine, Philadelphia, Pennsylvania

K. Lemone Yielding, University of Alabama, Birmingham, Alabama

INTRODUCTION

Roland F. Beers, Jr.

The Johns Hopkins University School of Hygiene and Public Health
Baltimore, Maryland

Among the properties assigned to living organisms are the capacities to grow differentially and to replicate. The former frequently leads to overspecialization with its attendant high risks against survival of the species; the latter, depending upon its relative efficiency, compensates for those risks.

There is a third property of life to which we are addressing ourselves during the next two days, namely the capacity for self-repair. It is a subject which is as broad as the life sciences themselves and can be said to be the basis for most biomedical research motivated by clinical needs. The capacity of an organism to repair by replacement or restoration of a damaged component is vital to its functional survival but the success of the repair process is dependent upon the magnitude and duration of the stress load and resultant damage.

We are living in an era noted for its concern for the biological consequences of environmental stresses which range from ionizing radiation to chemical carcinogens to sonic radiation. Every conceivable product of our technological civilization is coming under close scrutiny for its potential damaging effects on living organisms. The emergence of a no-risk criterion of acceptability of any product, as embodied in the Delaney amendment to the Food and Drug Act and expressed by many crusaders for the public welfare today, reflects an underestimate of the capacity of living organisms to cope with stresses.

Indeed, living organisms survive and evolve precisely because of and not in spite of stresses imposed upon them. At our stage of ignorance about biological repair processes it is probably of equal folly to claim that some stresses, such as radiation, are permanently damaging at all dose levels or to make the counterclaim that all stresses are beneficial at proper dose levels. Depending upon the circumstances both claims may be right or wrong. Critical for any such assessment is a knowledge of the role of repair processes.

The subjects that have been chosen for this Symposium are concerned with repair processes at the molecular (or enzymatic) level and at the cellular (or subcellular) level. I would hope that during the discussions the speakers will have time to reflect and comment on several issues relevant to the initiation and consequences of repair processes.

For example, consider the relationships between dose response and repair processes. To what extent are threshold or pseudothreshold levels of toxic agents a function of repair? What factors, such as time or post exposure conditions, modify repair processes? What consideration should be given to repair processes by public officials in reaching decisions about maximum permissible levels of exposure.

Another issue is the experimental rationale for detecting threshold phenomena. The extensive and extremely tedious methods of evaluation employed by the Russells and Bentley Glass, who utilized mice and Drosophila, respectively, to study low levels of radiation, have reached a point of costly diminishing returns. Where threshold phenomena are a function of repair processes, it may be important to consider an experimental model in which the repair processes are blocked. What information can we gleam from such a model?

This problem of tolerance levels is equally important in evaluating the biological effects of drugs, food additives, pesticides and other exotic chemicals. The massive long-term screening programs required for approval of new and old drugs suffers from the inherent impossibility of proving a negative. The politically expedient solution implicit in the Delaney amendment reflects that imponderable problem. History indicates that the search for absolutes in safety and in risks and their implementation through legal processes is as difficult a task as any attempted by a civilization expecting to govern itself on the basis of absolutes.

The validity of extrapolating to man results obtained with bacteria, insects or lower mammals, when it is very likely that many of the mechanisms and efficiencies of repair processes differ widely from species to species and possibly from strain to strain of a given species, is questioned with increasing frequency.

A question which is just beginning to gain attention is the role of repair processes in maintaining genetic stability. The popularity and beauty of the Watson-Crick model of DNA lies in part in its stability because of its structural configuration, a stability that persists during the replication process. If repair processes are important in maintaining genetic stability, then the evolutionary development of repair mechanism becomes of critical importance.

Permanent mutation in an organism may depend upon the absence of an effective repair process that can reverse the mutation, although a repair process might well perpetuate the mutation through its incorporation into the functioning DNA. The role of repair processes and their manipulation in genetic "engineering" are parameters that must be included in evaluating any feasible objective in this rapidly developing field of applied genetics. Reverse mutations, translocations and hybridization are among some of the phenomena which are influenced by repair processes.

Finally, there remains the important relationship between aging and repair processes. If aging results in part from a failure of repair mechanisms, this failure can occur either because the lesions produced with age are not reparable by existing systems of repair or because the systems themselves may become deficient. Since aging is also a function of stress on the organism, clearly the apparent accelerated aging process brought about by such stressful agents as radiation and toxic compounds, hormonal and genetic factors, and diet must be examined in terms of their relationship to repair processes.

Although this Symposium is only indirectly concerned with the specific biochemical lesions susceptible to repair, it is obvious that an understanding of the mechanisms of repair must include a knowledge of the lesions involved. The meaning of "sensitivity" of an organism to a particular stress is a function of both parameters, although until recently repair mechanisms have not been consistently identified as such. It is quite clear that some "repair processes" may lead to severe or lethal abnormalities, depending upon the kind of lesion produced. Thus, repair processes should not be judged to be unusually beneficial for the survival of the individual organism or of the species. Like stress, repair mechanisms of the cell may be a two-edged sword.

Part I

ENZYMATIC DARK REPAIR PROCESSES

MAMMALIAN DEOXYRIBONUCLEASES ACTING ON DAMAGED DNA

Tomas Lindahl[1]

Department of Chemistry II, Karolinska Institutet
Stockholm, Sweden

Both microorganisms and mammalian cells have the ability to remove various types of damaged nucleotide residues from their DNA. One mechanism of repair apparently involves the consecutive action of at least four different enzymes: an endonuclease that recognizes a particular type of DNA damage and catalyzes the formation of a single-strand break close to the damaged nucleotide(s), an exonuclease that excises this residue and a number of additional nucleotides, a DNA polymerase responsible for repair replication and a DNA ligase that rejoins the remaining strand interruption. Enzymes of all four types have been found in microorganisms, and their function in DNA repair has been confirmed by the isolation of radiation-sensitive mutant strains with defective enzymes (1-3).

As mammalian cells are also known to respond to radiation damage by DNA excision, repair replication and joining of interrupted DNA strands (4-6), it appears likely that similar repair enzymes are present in higher organisms. A DNA ligase (7) and a DNA polymerase (8) have in fact been found in the nucleoplasm of mammalian cells.[2] Because of the lack of radiation sensitive mutant cell types, it is not possible to prove directly whether these mammalian enzymes function in DNA repair in vivo. However, as the purified mammalian DNA ligase and DNA polymerase have biochemical properties similar to the corresponding microbial enzymes, it is a reasonable working hypothesis to assume that the mammalian enzymes are indeed involved in DNA repair. This indirect approach of comparing the biochemical properties of mammalian enzymes potentially functioning in DNA repair with microbial enzymes of known function has now been extended to several nucleases.

ENZYMATIC EXCISION OF PYRIMIDINE DIMERS

Two exonucleases, referred to as DNase III and DNase IV, have been found in the nucleoplasm of rabbit cells and have been partly purified (9,10). Both enzymes have an alkaline pH optimum, require Mg^{++} and lack DNA polymerase activity in vitro. They release $5'$-mononucleotides as the main degradation product, but also liberate a minor part (15% - 20%) of the products in the form of small oligonucleotides (9,11). The DNase III attacks at $3'$-ends and degrades denatured DNA and single-stranded poly-deoxynucleotides four times more rapidly than double-stranded substrates. In contrast, DNase IV attacks at $5'$-ends (with either a P- or an OH- end group) and degrades the

[1]The author's work was supported by the Swedish Natural Research Council and the Swedish Cancer Society.
[2]Proteins in the "nucleoplasm" or "nuclear sap" are not firmly associated with the chromatin and leach out on extraction of cell nuclei with an isotonic salt solution.

3

double-stranded synthetic polydeoxynucleotide poly (d(A-T)) much more rapidly than single-stranded polydeoxynucleotides or native or denatured DNA from natural sources. The relative ability of the enzymes to degrade UV-irradiated DNA is shown in Figure 1. DNase IV was not detectably inhibited by the presence of pyrimidine dimers in native DNA exposed to high doses of UV irradiation (Fig 1A) though a small inhibitory effect due to irradiation has been noted of the relatively much more rapid degradation of poly (dA · dT) (11). The unusual ability of this exonuclease to hydrolyze effectively

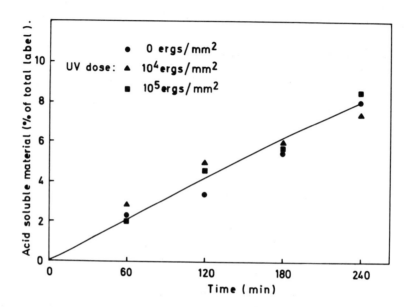

Fig 1A. Enzymatic degradation of unirradiated- and UV-irradiated native E. coli [^{32}P] DNA at 37°. Hydrolysis by DNase IV. The DNA (20 μM in nucleotide equivalents, mol wt 10^7) was incubated with the enzyme (2 units/ml) in 0.07 M Tris-HCl, pH 8.3, 0.004 M MgCl$_2$, 0.001 M EDTA, 0.001 M 2-mercaptoethanol, 0.01% bovine serum albumin. Aliquots were removed at times indicated, chilled, precipitated with an equal volume of 0.8 M HClO$_4$ and the amount of acid-soluble radioactive material was determined.

UV-irradiated substrates suggests that the enzyme may be responsible for the excision of damaged residues during DNA repair in vivo. In contrast, DNase III was strongly inhibited by the presence of pyrimidine dimers in DNA (Fig 1B). It, therefore, seems unlikely that the in vivo function of the latter enzyme involves excision of radiation products from DNA.

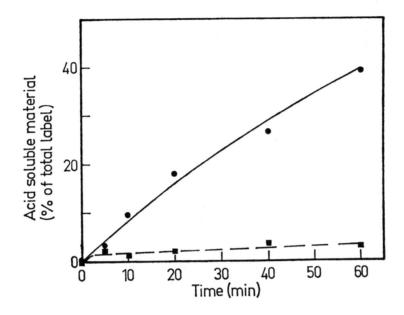

Fig 1B. Enzymatic degradation of unirradiated- and UV-irradiated native E. coli $[^{32}P]$ DNA at 37°. Hydrolysis by DNase III. The DNA (20 μM) was incubated with the enzyme (10 units/ml) in 0.05 M Tris-HCl, pH 8.5, 0.005 M $MgCl_2$, 0.001 M EDTA, 0.01 M 2-mercaptoethanol, 0.01% bovine serum albumin.

●————————●   non-irradiated substrate

■— — — —■   irradiated substrate (exposed to 4 x 10^3 ergs/mm^2).

DNase IV releases pyrimidine dimers from DNA as parts of small oligonucleotides (11). The enzyme has two properties in common with exonuclease activities from bacteria that appear to be involved in DNA repair: the rate of hydrolysis is not markedly reduced when pyrimidine dimers are present in the substrate, and the enzyme degrades its substrate in the $5' \rightarrow 3'$-direction.

Of the bacterial activities of this type, the $5' \rightarrow 3'$-nuclease function of E. coli DNA polymerase (12) shows a strong preference for double-stranded substrates, while the M. luteus UV exonuclease prefers single-stranded DNA (13). These observations indicate that the relative rates of attack on double-stranded vs single-stranded substrates may be of little importance for exonucleases involved in DNA repair. The mammalian DNase IV, purified from rabbit tissues, was originally thought to be specific for double-stranded substrates (10), but recently also has been found to degrade denatured DNA at a slow rate. Moreover, an apparently very similar enzyme has been obtained from rat tissue (lungs) by the same purification procedure; the rat enzyme again degrades poly (d(A-T)) much more rapidly than DNA, but hydrolyzes denatured DNA four times faster than native DNA.

As DNase IV may function in the excision of pyrimidine dimers, it was of interest to determine if this enzyme also had intrinsic UV endonuclease activity, so that it could introduce single-strand breaks near radiation-damaged residues. Transforming DNA from B. subtilis is inactivated by single-strand scissions (14), but retains most of its transforming activity after exposure to low doses of UV-irradiation. Such irradiated DNA, but not unirradiated DNA, is rendered inactive by a bacterial UV endonuclease that catalyzes

TABLE I

Release of Pyrimidine Dimers from UV-irradiated DNA by Treatment with
UV Endonuclease (from M. luteus) and Mammalian DNase IV

10 μg native B. subtilis DNA, labelled with [^{14}C] thymine (8000 cpm/μg DNA), was exposed to UV-irradiation (10^5 ergs/mm^2) and then incubated with 50 μg UV endonuclease in 1 ml of 0.05 M potassium phosphate, pH 7.0, 0.001 M EDTA, 0.001 M 2-mercaptoethanol for 4 hours at 37°. (The M. luteus UV endonuclease, which introduces single-strand scissons at the 5$'$-side of pyrimidine dimers (18), was purified 100-fold by phase partition, DEAE cellulose chromatography and phosphocellulose chromatography (17) before use.) The reaction was stopped by extraction with one volume of redistilled phenol, followed by three ether extractions and dialysis against 0.07 M Tris-HCl, pH 8.3, 0.001 M EDTA. A control sample (A.) was treated in the same fashion, except that no UV endonuclease was added.

The treated DNA preparations were subsequently incubated in 0.07 M Tris-HCl, pH 8.3, 0.004 M MgCl$_2$, 0.001 M EDTA, 0.001 M 2-mercaptoethanol for 4 hours at 37°, with (A. and C.) or without (B.) DNase IV. The reaction was stopped by addition of one volume of 0.8 M HClO$_4$ at 0°, and the supernatant solutions were recovered after centrifugation. After hydrolysis with 6 M HClO$_4$ at 100° for 3 hours, reneutralization with KOH, and concentration, the pyrimidine dimers were separated from monomeric thymine by paper chromatography (11) and the radioactivity of the different fractions was determined.

The DNA in each reaction mixture contained 8 500 pmoles thymine as monomer and 530 pmoles at dimer.

	[^{14}C] thymine, p-moles released	
	Dimer fraction	Monomer fraction
A. DNase IV treatment, no previous UV endonuclease treatment	12	220
B. UV endonuclease treatment, not followed by DNase IV treatment	28	58
C. UV endonuclease treatment, followed by DNase IV treatment	74	260
Material released from nicked DNA by DNase IV (C-B)	46	202

the formation of single-strand interruptions next to pyrimidine dimers in the DNA (15). However, UV-irradiated transforming DNA was found to be inactivated at essentially the same rate as unirradiated DNA by DNase IV. Therefore it may be concluded that DNase IV has no intrinsic UV endonuclease activity, but would have to act in concert with a separate enzyme that could create a strand interruption on the $5'$-side of a damaged residue. After appropriate endonuclease action, DNase IV would presumably be able to excise the damaged residue, as this exonuclease can initiate hydrolysis at both single-strand and double-strand breaks in DNA (16).

A mammalian UV endonuclease activity has not yet been found in cell extracts. A model experiment to test the hypothesis that DNase IV may have a physiological role in the excision of damaged residues from DNA therefore was performed with M. luteus UV endonuclease (13,17) in combination with the mammalian enzyme. UV-irradiated DNA, labelled in the thymine residues and containing 6% of these residues in the form of pyrimidine dimers, was treated with the microbial UV endonuclease. To exclude any contribution of the M. luteus UV exonuclease activity (13), this step was performed in an EDTA-containing buffer without Mg^{++} and was followed by phenol treatment and dialysis of the DNA. A small amount of acid-soluble material was released from the DNA by the UV endonuclease (1% of the total radioactivity, as seen in Table I) and presumably resulted from breaks at closely located pyrimidine dimers. When the pretreated DNA was subsequently incubated with mammalian DNase IV, a significantly increased proportion of pyrimidine dimers (19%) was found in the material released by this enzyme. On the other hand, if the UV endonuclease treatment was excluded, DNase IV did not by itself release pyrimidine dimers selectively from the irradiated DNA (Table I). Thus it appears that DNase IV can attack at a single-strand interruption in DNA on the $5'$-side of a pyrimidine dimer and release the dimer. However, even after very limited hydrolysis, more monomeric thymine residues than pyrimidine dimers were released by the enzyme. The data indicate that DNase IV liberated 20-60 monomeric nucleotide residues simultaneously with the pyrimidine dimer at each damaged site.

PARTLY PROCESSIVE DNA DEGRADATION

After removal of a damaged residue and a few adjacent mononucleotides in DNA by an exonuclease, further nuclease action in some way must be prevented in order to avoid extensive degradation of the DNA. It is presently not clear how exonuclease action is controlled. The presence of DNA exonuclease inhibitors has been postulated, but no such inhibitors have yet been found, nor is it obvious how an inhibitor would act to interrupt hydrolysis some fifty nucleotides away from a damaged residue. A different possibility is that the physical mode of action of the exonuclease itself would account for the limited hydrolysis. For this reason, a more detailed study of the mode of substrate attack by DNase IV was made, employing poly (d(A-T)) and DNA labelled both uniformly throughout the chains (with $[^3H]$) and in the $5'$-terminal residue (with $[^{32}P]$). The kinetics of release of the two kinds of labelled residues were followed separately. As expected, the nucleotides at the $5'$-ends were released more rapidly than the rest of the material. However, the rate of release of these terminal residues was not as fast as anticipated: from a poly (d(A-T)) chain 10^4 nucleotides long, the first residue was only released at a 7- to 10-fold greater rate than an internal residue (16). In separate experiments, no selective release of labelled residues at the $3'$-ends was observed and no endonuclease activity was detected in alkaline sucrose gradient centrifugation experiments with partly digested poly (d(A-T)) (10).

These results are consistent with a kinetic theory for the enzymatic degradation of polymers from one end proposed by Bailey and French (19). It is suggested that the polymer and the enzyme may remain associated and just move relative to each other during hydrolysis, but that the complex can dissociate at any time

$$E + S_1 \underset{k_{-1}}{\overset{k_1}{\rightleftarrows}} ES_1 \overset{k_2 \uparrow^P}{\longrightarrow} ES_2 \overset{k_2 \uparrow^P}{\longrightarrow} ES_3 \longrightarrow etc.$$

$$k_1 \Updownarrow k_{-1} \qquad k_1 \Updownarrow k_{-1}$$

$$E + S_2 \qquad E + S_3$$

In this modified Michaelis expression, the kinetic constants k_1, k_{-1} and k_2 govern the rate of formation of an enzyme-substrate complex, its lifetime and the rate of product formation, respectively. Thus, if the rate constant k_2 is ten times larger than k_{-1}, a "multiple" (19) or "partly processive" (16) mode of attack will occur, in that on

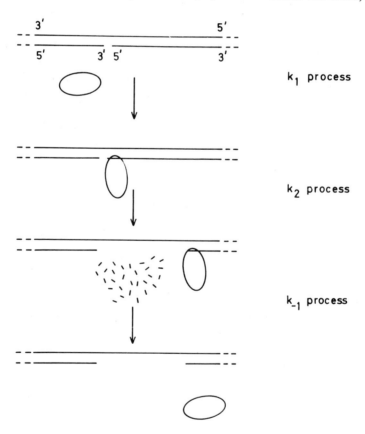

Fig 2. Possible action pattern of mammalian DNase IV. A single attack by the enzyme on a DNA molecule is shown.

the average ten monomeric residues will be released as the result of a single enzyme-substrate encounter. The proposed action pattern of DNase IV is illustrated in Figure 2. The kinetics of hydrolysis of native DNA at 37° indicate that 50-200 nucleotides are released in each encounter with DNase IV (16).

For an exonuclease involved in DNA repair, an action pattern of this type appears advantageous because separate exonuclease inhibitors might not be necessary to limit the extent of hydrolysis in vivo. As exonuclease action on the DNA would take place in "bursts" of activity rather than in an even fashion, repair replication and joining of DNA could presumably occur between two attacks by the exonuclease.

AN ACTIVITY ATTACKING DNA WITH HEAT-INDUCED LESIONS

As DNase IV apparently would have to work in concert with an endonuclease in DNA repair, a search for mammalian endonucleases that attack at damaged residues was undertaken, using extracts from both whole cells and cell nuclei. The method employed was the selective further inactivation of transforming B. subtilis DNA containing lesions. The same technique was used earlier by Strauss in his discoveries of an UV endonuclease and an endonuclease that attacks alkylated DNA in M. luteus (15,20). A study of this kind on mammalian cells is facilitated by the fact that the nucleoplasm contains very little, if any, endonuclease activity against "intact" native DNA. At least one DNA endonuclease is present in cell nuclei, but this enzyme appears to be associated firmly with the chromatin (21,22). Extranuclear DNases also do not interfere greatly in many mammalian tissue extracts: the lysosomal enzymes have an acid pH optimum and show very little

TABLE II

Selective Inactivation of Preheated B. subtilis DNA by a Cell Extract from Rabbit Thymus

Transforming DNA was heated at 70° for 40 min in 0.1 M NaCl, 0.01 M sodium citrate, pH 5.0, at a DNA concentration of 10 μg/ml. An equal volume of 0.1 M Hepes-KOH, pH 8.0, containing 0.001 M dithiothreitol, was then added, followed by a 0.005 volume of a crude cell extract from rabbit thymus (12 mg/ml protein in 0.1 M NaCl, 0.05 M Hepes-KOH, pH 7.4, 0.001 M dithiothreitol, 0.001 M EDTA). After 20 min at 37°, the reaction mixtures were chilled, agitated with chloroform and assayed for transforming activity (25) at a final DNA concentration of 0.05 μg/ml on a highly competent derivative of B. subtilis strain 168-2.

	Number of trp[+]-transformants/ml x 10^{-3}	
	No extract added	+ extract
Preheated DNA	100	4
Unheated DNA	220	230
Unheated DNA, treated with 0.03 volume of cell extract	–	185

activity at alkaline pH values, a mitochondrial endonuclease requires solvents containing a neutral detergent for efficient extraction (23) and a DNA endonuclease inhibitor is present in high concentrations in the cytoplasm (24).

In a survey with transforming DNA preparations containing various types of lesions, an activity was found in cell extracts from rabbit and calf thymus, and from rabbit spleen, bone marrow and lung, that selectively would inactivate DNA exposed to high temperatures below the T_m (Table II). Such heat treatment of DNA does not disrupt the secondary structure of the molecule, but leads to a slow and irreversible chemical degradation according to pseudo first-order kinetics (Fig 3). This degradation is an acid-catalyzed process and mainly depends on depurination of the DNA (26,27).

The activity present in mammalian cell extracts was due to a macromolecule, as it eluted before a lysozyme marker on gel filtration on Sephadex G-75 or G-150. Its elution position would indicate a molecular weight of $\sim$ 35000 for a globular protein.

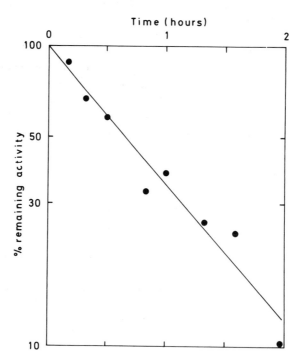

Fig 3. Heat degradation of double-stranded B. subtilis transforming DNA. The DNA (5 μg/ml) was incubated for various times at 70^0 in 0.1 M NaCl, 0.01 M sodium citrate, pH 5.0, and then assayed for trp[+]-transforming activity at a final DNA concentration of 0.05 μg/ml. No increase ($<$ 3%) in the A_{260} of a DNA solution was detected after 4 hours of heat treatment.

Moreover, it responded well to classical methods of enzyme purification: it precipitates between 50% and 70% ammonium sulfate saturation and has been purified approximately 30-fold by adsorption to and elution from alumina Cγ gel and by hydroxyapatite chromatography. The purified activity shows a broad pH optimum between 7 and 9, does not require divalent cations for activity and is inactivated by heating at 70° for 5 minutes. The determination of the mechanism of action of the activity will have to await its further purification. However, it does not appear to be a substance that simply binds to preheated transforming DNA and interferes with its uptake by competent cells, as re-isolation of the exposed DNA by phenol treatment did not restore its transforming activity. Further, the activity does not seem to be identical with any of the known mammalian DNases, as judged from its fractionation properties and lack of Mg^{++} requirement. Conceivably the activity depends on a new type of endonuclease that attacks DNA at depurinated sites.

CHEMICAL STABILITY OF DNA

Would it be necessary to have a repair system to protect cellular DNA against spontaneous chemical degradation? This damage probably consists mainly of loss of purine residues, but chain breakage and deamination of cytosine residues (28) could also be lesions that would occur at a relevant rate. Greer and Zamenhof (29) have followed

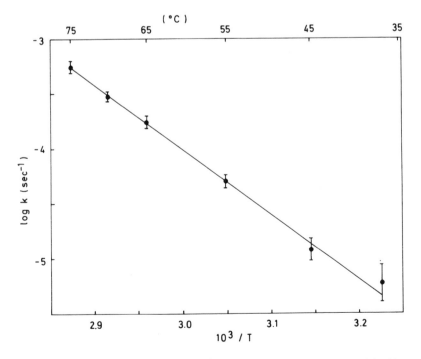

Fig 4. Arrhenius plot. Temperature dependence of the rate of heat inactivation of double-stranded transforming DNA at pH 5.0. Experimental conditions as in Figure 3.

the loss of transforming activity and the rate of depurination as determined by direct chemical analysis. Their results indicate that one inactivating hit in transforming DNA, under conditions in which the helical structure remains intact, corresponds to the loss of ~ 1 purine residue per 1000 base pairs.

As it would be technically difficult to measure directly the exceedingly slow spontaneous inactivation of transforming DNA at 37° and pH 7.4, the temperature dependence of the inactivation rate of transforming DNA was investigated at pH 5.0. Then the reaction still proceeds at an easily measurable rate down to temperatures 50° below the T_m. A linear Arrhenius plot with a slope corresponding to an activation energy of 27 kcal was obtained (Fig 4). At 70°, the rate of inactivation was found to be 30 times faster at pH 5.0 than at pH 7.4. With the reasonable assumption that the activation energy for irreversible degradation of double-stranded DNA is similar at pH 7.4 and at pH 5.0, it can be estimated that the rate of depurination at 37° and pH 7.4 would be ~ 1 purine per 10^6 base pairs per hour. For a transforming DNA molecule, this corresponds to one inactivating hit per six weeks, and for an E. coli cell to the loss of about three purine residues per genome in each generation. For a mammalian cell, with its much higher DNA content and longer generation time, on the order of 10^5 purine bases then should be lost from the DNA during one cell generation. While histones and other factors may afford some protection in vivo, it nevertheless appears necessary to postulate the existence of an efficient repair system to handle this type of cellular damage, in order to prevent a very high spontaneous mutation rate (30). Whether the activity towards heated DNA we have detected in mammalian cell extracts is a part of such a repair system, remains to be seen.

REFERENCES

1. Yasuda, S. and Sekiguchi, M.: Proc. Nat. Acad. Sci. USA, 67:1839, 1970.
2. deLucia, P. and Cairns, J.: Nature, 224:1164, 1969.
3. Gellert, M. and Bullock, M. L.: Proc. Nat. Acad. Sci. USA, 67:1580, 1970.
4. Regan, J. D., Trosko, J. E. and Carrier, W. L.: Biophys. J., 8:319, 1968.
5. Painter, R. B. and Cleaver, J. E.: Radiat. Res., 37:451, 1969.
6. Lett, J. T., Caldwell, I., Dean, C. J. and Alexander, P.: Nature, 214:790, 1967.
7. Lindahl, T. and Edelman, G. M.: Proc. Nat. Acad. Sci. USA, 61:680, 1968.
8. Smith, M. J. and Keir, H. M.: Biochim. Biophys. Acta, 68:578, 1963.
9. Lindahl, T., Gally, J. A. and Edelman, G. M.: J. Biol. Chem., 244:5014, 1969.
10. Lindahl, T., Gally, J. A. and Edelman, G. M.: Proc. Nat. Acad. Sci. USA, 62:597, 1969.
11. Lindahl, T.: Europ. J. Biochem., 18:407, 1971.
12. Kelly, R. B., Atkinson, M. R., Huberman, J. A. and Kornberg, A.: Nature, 224:495, 1969.
13. Kaplan, J. C., Kushner, S. R. and Grossman, L.: Proc. Nat. Acad. Sci. USA, 63:144, 1969.
14. Bodmer, W.: J. Gen. Physiol., 49:233, 1966.
15. Strauss, B. S.: Proc. Nat. Acad. Sci. USA, 48:1670, 1962.
16. Lindahl, T.: Europ. J. Biochem., 18:415, 1971.
17. Nakayama, H., Okubo, S. and Takagi, Y.: Biochim. Biophys. Acta, 228:67, 1971.
18. Kushner, S. R., Kaplan, J. C. and Grossman, L.: Fed. Proc., 29:405, 1970.
19. Bailey, J. M. and French, D.: J. Biol. Chem., 226:1, 1957.
20. Strauss, B. S. and Robbins, M.: Biochim. Biophys. Acta, 161:68, 1968.
21. Swingle, K. F., Cole, L. J. and Bailey, J. S.: Biochim. Biophys. Acta, 149:467, 1967.
22. O'Connor, P. J.: Biochem. Biophys. Res. Commun., 35:805, 1969.

23. Curtis, P. J., Burdon, M. G. and Smellie, R. M. S.: Biochem. J., 98:813, 1966.
24. Lindberg, U. and Skoog, L.: Europ. J. Biochem., 13:326, 1970.
25. Anagnostopoulos, C. and Spizizen, J.: J. Bact., 81:741, 1961.
26. Ginoza, W. and Zimm, B. H.: Proc. Nat. Acad. Sci. USA, 47:639, 1961.
27. Roger, M. and Hotchkiss, R. D.: Proc. Nat. Acad. Sci. USA, 47:653, 1961.
28. Shapiro, R. and Klein, R. S.: Biochemistry, 5:2358, 1966.
29. Greer, S. and Zamenhof, S.: J. Molec. Biol., 4:123, 1962.
30. Strack, H. B., Freese, E. B. and Freese, E.: Mutat. Res., 1:10, 1964.

GENETIC AND PHYSIOLOGICAL FACTORS RELATING TO EXCISION-REPAIR IN ESCHERICHIA COLI

John M. Boyle

Paterson Laboratories, Christie Hospital and Holt Radium Institute
Manchester, England

In 1964, the excision-repair hypothesis was proposed (1,2) for the repair of ultra-violet (UV) light induced damage in DNA. The following three years saw the development of techniques (3-5) which allowed the sequential steps of the process to be examined, but at the Brookhaven Symposium of 1967 (6) barely any mention was made of the enzymes involved in these reactions. Since then, however, considerable progress towards the isolation and characterization of proteins having the expected properties of repair enzymes has been made. Although the excision-repair hypothesis was developed to explain the repair of UV-damaged DNA containing cyclobutyl pyrimidine dimers, this mechanism and that of recombination repair, have been implicated in the repair of DNA damaged by a variety of other agents including ionizing radiation and radiomimetic chemicals (7,8).

The rapidity of these developments has been possible largely because of the availability and ease of genetic manipulation of mutant strains of bacteria and their viruses. Lack of these facilities until now has frequently limited the analysis of DNA repair in mammalian cells. These cells are nevertheless of prime interest because radiation is still the most extensively used tool in cancer therapy. We are, however, at the start of a period of mammalian cell genetics which perhaps is comparable to the period around 1950 when microbial genetics, as we know it today, was in its infancy. I feel, therefore, that this meeting is being held at a very opportune time for us to review the status of knowledge of DNA repair and our discussions will probably indicate many of the problems for future research.

In this paper I shall concentrate mainly on the excision-repair of pyrimidine dimers. Firstly, I shall review recent information concerning enzyme activities thought to be responsible for steps in excision-repair. Then I shall describe the results of studies in which I was involved during a postdoctoral fellowship at the Biology Division, Oak Ridge National Laboratory, and shall conclude with some remarks concerning a relatively unexplored area, the role that damage to membranes might play in excision-repair.

EXCISION-REPAIR ENZYMES

The essential features of excision-repair are shown in Figure 1. The lesions induced in DNA by UV-irradiation which have the greatest biological significance are pyrimidine dimers (9). The presence of dimers results in a localized structural distortion of the DNA helix which probably serves as a recognition site for endonuclease attack. Several laboratories (10-12) have reported the isolation and partial purification of endonuclease activities from M. luteus, an organism used in preference to E. coli because of

14

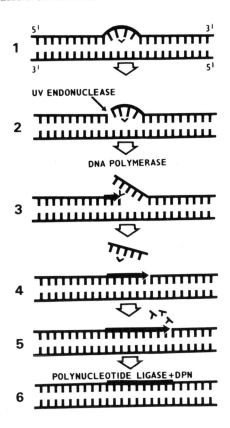

Fig 1. A model for excision-repair (after Kelly et al (17)). 1. A UV-irradiated double helix of DNA is represented containing one pyrimidine dimer. 2. The region adjacent and on the 5' side of the dimer is attacked by an endonuclease specific for UV-irradiated DNA. 3. DNA polymerase binds to DNA at the nicked site, and by addition of 5' nucleotide triphosphates starts repair polymerisation of the damaged strand using the template of the complementary strand. The dimer region becomes displaced. 4. When the 5' to 3' exonuclease site of the polymerase reaches the next hydrogen bonded base pair, the phosphodiester bond is hydrolyzed releasing the dimer in a short oligonucleotide. 5. The polymerizing and hydrolytic activities may continue in the 5' to 3' direction until 6. the polymerase is displaced by polynucleotide ligase which together with DPN restores the integrity of the phosphodiester backbone of DNA.

high nonspecific nuclease levels in the latter species. Differences in the properties of the endonuclease activities reported by different laboratories may result from differing degrees of purity which have been achieved.

The overall picture is that micrococcal endonuclease activity is associated with a protein of approximately 15,000 daltons which produces single-strand breaks only in UV-irradiated double-stranded DNA, and not in unirradiated double-stranded DNA or single-stranded DNA even when the latter contains dimers. The enzyme prepared by Grossman et al attacks DNA close to and on the 5' side of a dimer and leaves a 3'-phosphoryl group, which suggests that the additional activity of a phosphatase may be necessary before repair polymerization can occur. One phosphoryl group is cleaved per dimer and the activity requires no cofactor. Carrier and Setlow (10) using annealed DNA molecules with one strand irradiated and the other not, have shown that breaks are introduced only into the irradiated strand. Treatment of UV-irradiated Hemophilus DNA with UV-endonuclease and subsequent transformation of a Hemophilus mutant unable to perform the first step in dimer excision caused an increased survival of transformed markers compared to that of untreated DNA (14). This experiment confirmed earlier observations (15,16) that treatment of irradiated DNA with crude Micrococcal extracts initiated the recovery of biological activity. An objection to the activities of UV-endonuclease observed in vitro having anything to do with excision in vivo has been presented by Takagi et al (11). These workers obtained transformants of a UV sensitive strain of M. luteus which was shown by Grossman et al (12) to have no detectable UV-endonuclease. The transformants, although having wild type UV resistance, were shown not to have endonuclease activity. Genetic analyses of these transformants appears necessary to demonstrate the nature of their newly-acquired resistance.

The second step in excision-repair (Fig 1) is excision of the dimer in a small oligonucleotide accompanied by the release of mononucleotides. The gap left is filled by newly-synthesized DNA using the exposed template of the opposite strand. An exonuclease of M. luteus has been purified 1,500 fold. In the presence of Mg^{++} this enzyme can perform the excision step, but is devoid of polymerizing activity (12,13). The enzyme is active on denatured but not native DNA, and attacks either the $5'$ or $3'$ hydroxyl ends releasing $5'$ nucleotides. Unlike the activity of similar enzymes, such as snake venom phosphodiesterase, it is not inhibited by the presence of photoproducts in the DNA. A sequential attack by UV-endonuclease and the exonuclease upon UV-irradiated DNA release about 6 nucleotides, including the dimer in a trinucleotide fragment, per endonucleolytic break.

An exciting report by Kelly, Atkinson, Huberman and Kornberg (17) demonstrated that DNA polymerase purified to homogeneity from E. coli is able in vitro to release dimers from UV-irradiated DNA. This enzyme has a complex range of activities but for excision-repair the relevant ones are those of hydrolysis of double-stranded DNA in the $5'$ to $3'$ direction and polymerization in the same direction by addition of $5'$ mononucleotides to $3'$ hydroxyl termini (18). The hydrolytic activity, once termed exonuclease II, can occur in the absence of DNA synthesis and releases both mononucleotides and small oligonucleotides (19). Using UV-irradiated DNA in which nicks were introduced by pancreatic DNase, to mimic the action of UV-endonuclease, the $5'$ to $3'$ exonuclease activity of DNA polymerase released thymine dimers in small oligonucleotides. A comparison of the properties of the Kornberg and Grossman enzymes, suggest that Grossman's exonuclease may be a fragment of the DNA polymerase of M. luteus. The exonuclease and polymerizing activities of E. coli DNA polymerase have been separated by protease digestion (20).

The overall picture at present is that steps 2 to 5 in Figure 1 are probably mediated by the Kornberg polymerase. Since polymerization and hydrolysis of DNA both occur in the $5'$ to $3'$ direction the net result is to displace the endonuclease nick in that direction until the structural distortion caused by the dimer is reached. The absence of hydrogen bonding between the two DNA helices permits the displacement of the dimer region and the polymerase continues along the DNA until the next hydrogen-bonded base pair is reached. The 5' to 3' exonuclease activity hydrolyses the next phosphodiester bond releasing the dimer-containing oligonucleotide.

The polymerase may continue along the DNA until it is displaced by a rejoining enzyme which seals the final phosphodiester bond. The candidate for this reaction is polynucleotide ligase (22). This enzyme reacts in two stages, firstly with its cofactor, which in E. coli is diphosphopyridine nucleotide (DPN) and then with DNA thus:

1. Ligase + DPN $\longrightarrow$ ligase $\sim$ AMP + NMN.

2. Ligase $\sim$ AMP + (5'P & 3' OH adjacent termini) $\longrightarrow$ ligase + AMP + phosphodiester bond in DNA.

In mammalian cells and phage T4, the ligase receives AMP from ATP with the release of inorganic pyrophosphate. The evidence that the ligase is the rejoining enzyme in E. coli excision comes from studies with a temperature sensitive mutant (23,24). When irradiated cells of this mutant are plated and the plates held for 2 hr at the nonpermissive temperature (40°) before incubation at 25°, the survival of colony-forming units is less than when the same cells are not held at 40°. The strain is able to excise dimers and undergo repair synthesis normally and is apparently unable to perform the rejoining step at 40°. The mutant possesses low levels of ligase but the in vitro activity is not affected by temperature.

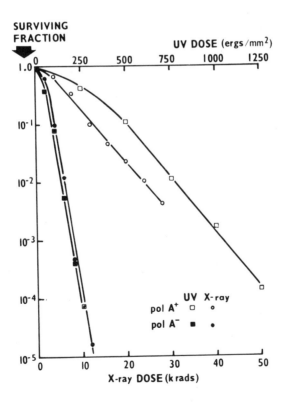

Fig 2. UV- and X-ray survival curves of pol A+ and pol A- cells. The methods used to obtain these curves are given by Boyle, Paterson and Setlow (28,29).

PROPERTIES OF MUTANTS DEFICIENT IN DNA POLYMERASE

Mutants of E. coli whose extracts are deficient in Kornberg DNA polymerase activity have been isolated. The first of these was reported by De Lucia and Cairns and designated pol A⁻. As expected for a strain lacking a putative excision enzyme the mutant was UV sensitive, but replicated with normal kinetics indicating that the Kornberg polymerase was not the enzyme responsible for DNA replication. (A second DNA polymerase activity with properties different from that of the Kornberg enzyme has been found in pol A⁻ mutants and is presumably the replicating enzyme) (26,27).

We compared pol A⁻ with its parent strain, for excision-repair associated properties after both UV- and X-irradiation (28,29). The sensitivity of colony-forming ability of pol A⁻ was 4 to 5 times greater than that of pol A⁺ for both UV- and X-rays (Fig 2). The most outstanding response of the strain to irradiation was the extent of DNA breakdown to acid soluble fragments (Fig 3). After 250 ergs/mm² at 254nm, 85% of the cellular DNA was degraded within 90 mins (cf to 20% for pol A⁺). Degradation of pol A⁻ DNA after X-rays was less extensive, a dose of 28kr resulting in 55% degradation in 90 min (cf to 30% for pol A⁺). At UV doses which gave comparable cell survivals, the extent of DNA degradation was the same for both strains, but this correlation did not hold for X-irradiated cells. In order to examine the properties of cells that would survive irradiation,

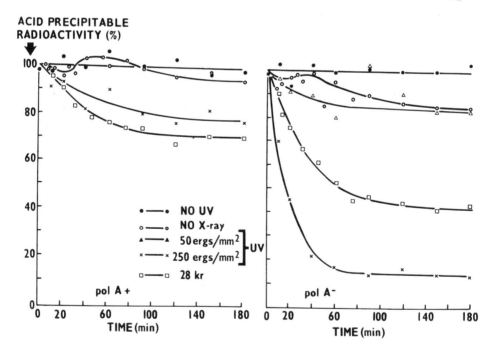

Fig 3. DNA degradation of irradiated pol A⁺ and pol A⁻ cells. Cells were labelled with ³H thymidine before irradiation with UV- or X-rays with the doses indicated. Irradiated cells were diluted into non-radioactive growth medium and incubated at 37°. At intervals degradation was measured in terms of changes in acid precipitable material by collection of samples on filter paper discs which were treated with ice cold 5% trichloracetic acid, dried and the radioactivity counted by scintillation spectrometry.

subsequent experiments were performed with UV doses of less than 100 ergs/mm^2 so as to limit the general loss of radioactive label by degradation.

Figure 4 shows the results of three experiments to determine kinetics of dimer excision. The data show that dimers are selectively excised from the pol A$^-$ mutant but possibly at a slower rate than in pol A$^+$, although the final fraction of dimers removed is

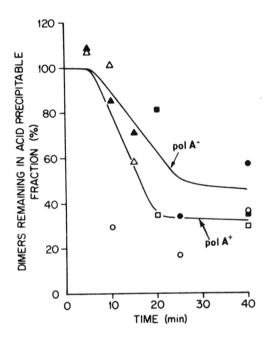

Fig 4. Excision of dimers by pol A$^+$ and pol A$^-$ cells. The results of three experiments to determine the rate of excision of thymine dimers from UV-irradiated cells is shown as a function of time of post-irradiation incubation in growth medium at 37°. The UV doses used were 70 to 180 ergs/mm^2 which produced 0.03 to 0.08% dimers. Open symbols, pol A$^+$; closed symbols, pol A$^-$.

approximately the same for both strains. Figure 5 shows the results of alkaline sucrose gradient analysis of the molecular size distribution of irradiated DNA isolated from cells incubated in growth media for varying periods after UV. It can be seen that with pol A$^+$, irradiation results in very little change in molecular distribution during 40 mins incubation, indicating that very few single-strand breaks remain open as a result of excision-repair. Those which occur are rapidly repaired. With pol A$^-$, on the other hand, there is an immediate decrease in MW on irradiation and following incubation a large fraction of the radioactivity bands at positions less than 1 x 10^{8}D. On the other hand, some repair of strand breaks is indicated by the material which sediments to a position 0.3 of the gradient length. The fraction of radioactivity banding at this position decreases from about 11.5% (No UV) to about 3.2% by 10 mins after UV, then increases slowly to about 6% by 40 minutes.

ACID PRECIPITABLE
RADIOACTIVITY
RECOVERED (%)

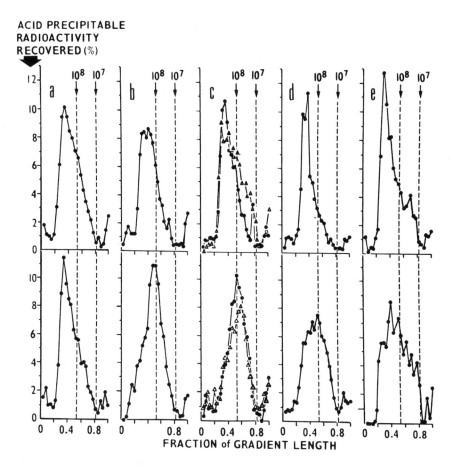

Fig 5. Alkaline sucrose gradient profiles of UV-irradiated pol A$^+$ and pol A$^-$ DNA. Cells were pre-labelled with ^{3}H thymidine and irradiated. Samples taken at various times were washed and the cells converted to protoplasts, layered onto the top of 5-20% alkaline sucrose gradients and sedimented for 90 min at 30,000 rpm (21°) in a SW-56 rotor of a Spinco model L centrifuge, essentially according to the method of McGrath and Williams (4). Fractions were collected on paper discs, treated with ice cold 5% TCA and the radioactivity counted by scintillation spectrometry. UV doses used were 50 to 85 ergs/mm^2. Upper row pol A$^+$, lower row pol A$^-$. a) Nonirradiated. b) to e) irradiated and incubated for 0, 10, 30, and 40 min respectively. Sedimentation was from right to left.

The increased UV-sensitivity of pol A$^-$ therefore appears to be due to a defect following step 4 (Fig 1) and is related to an increase in degradation of irradiated DNA. We have no information concerning the nature of the degradation. However, the simplest assumption is that it results from the polymerase mutation, in which case it could reflect either increased 5′-3′ exonuclease activity or decreased repair polymerization which allows strand breaks to remain susceptable to nonspecific nuclease attack. Similar conclusions were made by Kanner and Hanawalt (30). Witkin (31) has demonstrated that the pol A$^-$ mutation does not affect UV-induction of mutations and again concludes that the result is consistent with the cells having a defect late in the excision sequence. Kato and Kondo (32) have recently described the properties of four mutants derived from E. coli B which are UV- and X-ray sensitive. These mutants like pol A⁻ of E. coli K12 (33) map close to met E at a locus termed res. Three of the four res⁻ mutants showed no Kornberg DNA polymerase activity and, like pol A⁻, showed marked degradation of DNA after both UV- and X-rays. The double mutants hcr⁻ res⁻, that is, strains which are unable to initiate excision-repair, showed only limited degradation, but behaved the same as hcr⁺ res⁻ after X-rays, indicating that degradation after UV occurs at sites of single-strand breaks. Single-strand breaks induced by X-rays in one res⁻ mutant, R 15, were not rejoined. We have observed a similar effect with pol A⁻.

All these results imply that mutations in the gene coding for DNA polymerase (65) result in increased UV- and X-ray sensitivities that are related to extensive degradation of irradiated cellular DNA.

THE REPAIR OF PHAGE DNA BY HOST CELL ENZYMES

For many years now it has been known that following UV-irradiation, the plaque-forming ability of the majority of phage types is dependent on that particular bacterial host strain to which the irradiated phage has been absorbed. Phages are more sensitive when assayed on hcr⁻ cells, which are known to be unable to perform the initial endonuclease step on their own DNA, than when assayed on hcr⁺ cells, which are able to perform this function. This dependency of phage sensitivity on the host bacterium is called Host Cell Reactivation (HCR). Another type of reactivation phenomenon, Ultra-violet Reactivation (UVR), is observed when irradiated phage is assayed on lightly irradiated bacteria. In this case a further increase in survival may be observed over that obtained using unirradiated hosts.

We have measured (34) the kinetics of dimer excision from both phage λ and cellular DNA under conditions of either HCR (either phage or bacteria irradiated) or UVR (both phage and bacteria irradiated). Our results (Fig 6) confirmed the assumption that HCR of phage λ is due to dimer excision of phage DNA mediated by host cell enzymes. We asked the question: how is the rate of dimer excision affected by the UV dose, and is the kinetics of excision *per cell* the same for bacterial and phage dimers? In Figure 7 (upper panel) a rate (numbers of dimers excised per cell in 50 min) versus substrate (original numbers of dimers per cell) plot of the excision of bacterial dimers is shown. Initially the rate of excision at low UV doses increases in a manner which resembles first order kinetics. At about 4000 dimers per cell the kinetics become zero order suggesting a limiting enzyme concentration. This point approximates to the start of the exponential decrease in cell survival. In Figure 7 (lower panel) it can be seen that bacterial excision enzymes are able to excise more dimers from bacterial DNA than from phage DNA.

When both phage and bacteria are irradiated, the competition of dimers in the different DNAs for the excision enzymes can be investigated by measuring, for example, the effect of dimers in phage DNA on the excision of bacterial dimers, and vice versa. The results of this experiment are shown in Figure 8. It is apparent from these data and those in Figure 7 that dimers in λDNA are much better inhibitors of excision of dimers in bacterial DNA than are bacterial dimers for the excision of dimers in λ or in bacterial DNA. The lower panel of Figure 8 also demonstrates that UVR of λ does not involve an increase

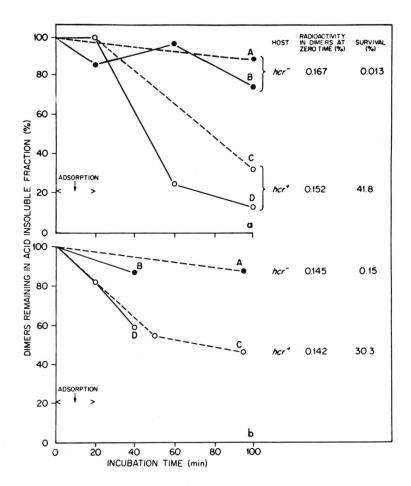

Fig 6. Excision of dimers from E. coli and phage λDNA. Upper curves: Excision from cells irradiated with 250 ergs/mm² at 254 nm. Lower curves: Excision from λirradiated with 250 ergs/mm² at 265 nm. (○) Hcr⁺ cells or complexes; (●) Hcr⁻ cells or complexes. Solid lines, curves B and D, excision in absence of chloramphenicol; dashed lines, curves A and C, excision in the presence of chloramphenicol (50 μg/ml).

in the rate of excision of phage dimers. Whilst we were doing these experiments, independent studies of UVR of λ were being conducted by Radman et al (35) and Hart and Ellison (36). These groups showed that UVR is dependent on the activity of two genes lex (exr) and rec A, thought to be involved in recombination, but not that of a third, rec C.

The role of Kornberg polymerase in the repair of UV-irradiated phage DNA has been investigated using host cells defective in DNA polymerase. Phages λ (29,37), φX174 (37) and T4 (37) all show increased sensitivity to UV when assayed on pol A⁻, compared to assays performed with pol A⁺. Phages T5 (38) and T7 (25) on the other hand show no increase in sensitivity on pol A⁻. Kato and Kondo (32) reported that HCR of infectious

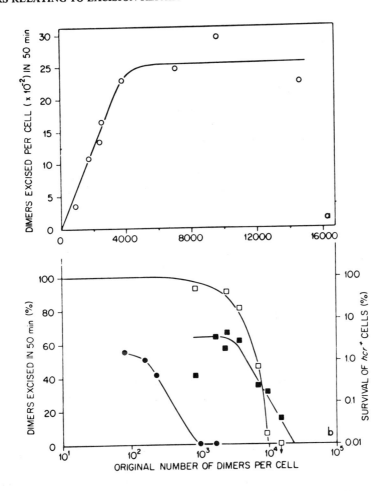

Fig 7. Inhibition of excision by large UV doses. (a) *Number* of dimers excised per cell in 50 min from bacterial DNA in hcr[+] cells is plotted as a function of the *numbers* of dimers originally present per cell. (b) The *fraction* of dimers excised per hcr[+] cell in 50 min versus *number* of dimers originally present per cell. (•) excision of dimers from λDNA; (■) excision of dimers from bacterial DNA; (□) survival curve of hcr[+] cells. The data and method of calculation of numbers of dimers per cell are given by Boyle and Setlow (34).

P1 phage DNA was unaffected by res mutations, but no HCR of transducing DNA of P1 was observed in res⁻ strains. We have shown (29) that the increased sensitivity of λ in pol A⁻ is associated with increased degradation of phage DNA in the same way that increased cell sensitivity is associated with increased degradation of cell DNA. The normal HCR observed with some phages may result from complementation of the defective cellular enzyme by a phage induced polymerase. It may be significant that the Kornberg polymerase coded by T4 DNA is lacking in 5′-3′ exonuclease activity (39) and this phage is more sensitive to UV when assayed on pol A⁻ cells.

24

JOHN M. BOYLE

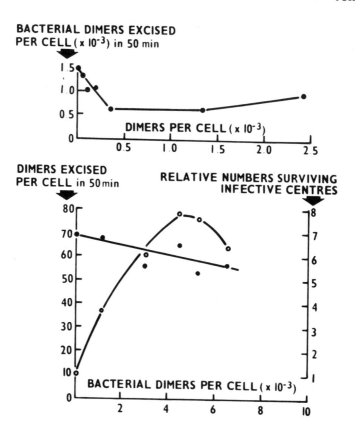

Fig 8. Competition for excision by dimers in bacterial and phage DNA. Upper curve shows the effect of the presence of dimers in λDNA on excision of dimers from bacterial DNA. A culture of ^{3}H thymidine labelled hcr$^+$ cells was irradiated to produce 0.122% dimers. Immediately after irradiation, cells were infected at a multiplicity of 5.7 with λ particles that had been irradiated with varying UV doses. The fraction of dimers excised from bacterial DNA during 50 min incubation was determined and the data converted to numbers of dimers per cell. Lower curve shows ultraviolet reactivation and excision of dimers from λDNA. Radioactively labelled λ was irradiated with UV to produce 0.8% dimers. Unlabelled hcr$^+$ cells were irradiated with varying UV doses and infected with λ at a multiplicity of 1.1. UVR was measured by plaque assay immediately after absorption and dimer excision measured after 50 min in growth medium.

We have shown (29) that UVR of phage λ occurs to a very small degree in pol A$^-$ cells irradiated with very small UV doses, but aborts at slightly higher doses. In this case, abortion of UVR is associated with a loss of the capacity of irradiated cells to support the growth of unirradiated λ.

THE PHYSIOLOGY OF UV-IRRADIATED E. COLI

Cells which possess repair enzymes are frequently killed by relatively small doses of ultraviolet irradiation. For example, 99.5% of logarithmic phase E. coli B/r cells are inactivated by a dose of 520 ergs/mm² at 254 nm. We have seen above that one factor inhibiting the repair of DNA appears to be a limiting concentration of the excision enzymes. However, given enough time, turnover of the available enzymes should result in DNA repair leading to cell survival if this were the only response of cells to irradiation. This is obviously not the case, and since nucleic acids, RNA as well as DNA, are the most sensitive UV targets, and dimers in DNA can interfere with transcription as well as DNA replication, it seems equally obvious that UV-induced changes in general cell metabolism can lead to cell death. An essential requirement for the restoration of normal metabolism is available chemical energy. During the past five years, Dr. Paul Swenson at Oak Ridge has developed a system for looking at the effects of radiation on the respiration of E. coli cells, particularly B/r. Cells are grown in M63, a mineral salts solution containing glycerol as the sole carbon source, to 2 x 10⁸/ml. The culture is washed in M63 minus glycerol and resuspended in this buffer at 8 x 10⁷/ml for irradiation at 254 nm using a germicidal lamp. After irradiation, the cells are centrifuged and resuspended at 2 x 10⁸/ml in complete M63 for use in measuring the responses of respiration, growth, viability and other aspects, during 5hr of postirradiation incubation. M63 containing glycerol as the sole carbon source was chosen for these experiments because cells grown on this medium continue to respire normally for about 40 min after irradiation, but by 90 min respiration ceases in some experiments for 3 hrs before slowly starting again (Fig 9a). With UV-irradiated cells respiration and growth (changes in optical density) remain coupled (Fig. 9b).

Cells grown in other media generally show higher levels and a more transient inhibition of respiration and are not so easy to work with. However, it should be emphasized that we believe that the underlying basis of the effects which we observe with

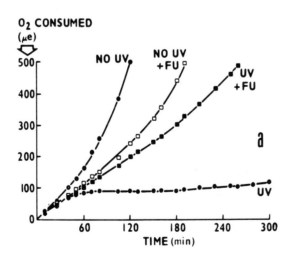

Fig 9. UV Responses of E. coli B/r to UV-irradiation. Cells were grown in logarithmic phase to 2 x 10⁸/ml in M63 solution containing 0.2% glycerol. The culture was washed, irradiated with an incident dose of 520 ergs/mm² in buffer, and returned to M63gly for postirradiation incubation at 37°. (a) Respiration responses of irradiated and nonirradiated cells measured on a Gilson respirometer.

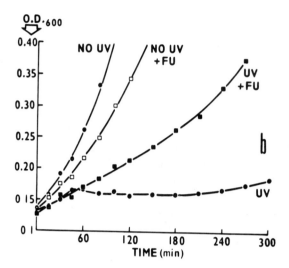

Fig 9. (b) Growth response measured as changes in optical density at 600 nm measured on a Beckman DU spectrophotometer.

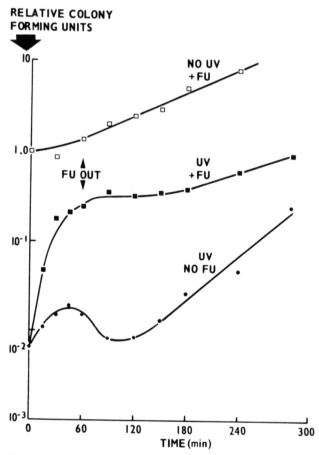

Fig 9. (c) Viability of cultures measured as colonies on M63gly agar plates incubated at 37° for 2 days. The results are expressed as a fraction of the titre of unirradiated cells at zero time.

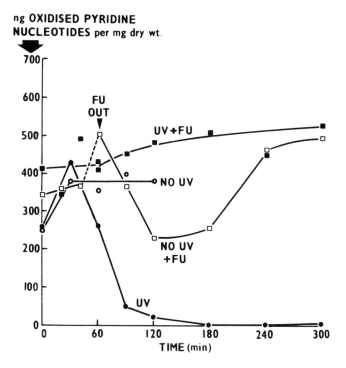

Fig 9. (d) Variation in the specific activity of pyridine nucleotides as expressed in terms of dry weight of cells. Pyridine nucleotides were determined by the methyl ethyl ketone method of Carpenter and Kodicek (63). To some cultures FU (50 μg/ml) was added to the liquid M63gly immediately after irradiation, and where indicated was removed at 60 min by centrifugation.

glycerol-grown cells is the same in cells grown on other carbon sources, but may be modified by the use of different oxidation pathways, as exemplified in the argument below.

The working hypothesis which has evolved during the study of this system is as follows:

1. Following UV-irradiation of B/r, respiration ceases at about 90 min due to the loss of pyridine nucleotides (41), the co-enzymes of many respiratory dehydrogenases. In addition glycerol kinase activity disappears and this double block probably accounts for the greater inhibition of respiration of glycerol-grown cells than that seen when other carbon sources are used which do not need glycerol kinase.

2. Cessation of respiration occurs as a result of transcription and translation of the irradiated DNA (40,41). The destruction of the DNA template by phage T4-induced nucleases prevents respiratory turnoff. Similarly, respiration continues in E. coli B_{s-1} cells whose DNA is extensively degraded after irradiation. The use of rifampicin, an inhibitor of mRNA synthesis, or 5-fluorouracil (FU) (Fig 9a) which causes erroneous coding properties in mRNA, or chloramphenicol, which inhibits protein synthesis, all permit respiration to continue. It

appears that the protein(s), or their synthesis, involved in turning off respiration, are thermolabile since incubation of irradiated cells at 42° also prevents turnoff. In each case where respiration continues pyridine nucleotide levels remain high (Fig 9d).

      3. By comparing irradiated cells treated with FU with untreated cells we have been able to correlate the effect of maintained respiratory activity with the repair of DNA and the recovery of cell viability (42). Figures 9, 10 and 11 show some of the responses we observed. A parallel series of experiments have been performed with essentially the same results, using incubation of irradiated

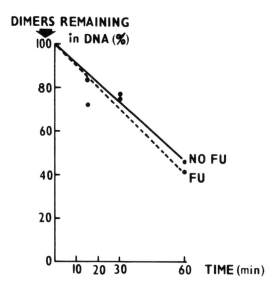

Fig 10. Effect of 5-fluorouracil on dimer excision. E. coli B/r cells were labelled with ^{3}H thymidine and irradiated as for Figure 9. Cells were returned to M63 glycerol and the suspension split in two. One half was incubated in the absence of FU and the other was incubated with 50 μg/ml FU added. Dimers were assayed at different times according to the method of Setlow and Carrier (3) and expressed as a fraction of those originally present.

cells at 42° to maintain respiration (Boyle, Schenley and Swenson, manuscript in preparation). The effect of adding FU (50 μg/ml) to irradiated cells results in a dramatic increase of viability (from 0.65% to about 30% survival) during the first 60 min incubation. Prolonging the incubation with FU beyond 60 min results in FU induced death of cells which is unrelated to respiration.[1] However, if FU is removed from the cultures at 60 min the increased viability is maintained as seen in Figure 9. Cells incubated without FU show a 2 to 3 fold increase in

[1]We have since found that lower doses of FU, namely, 0.5 μg/ml, can cause the increase in viability observed during the first 60 min incubation, without subsequently killing the cells.

viability during the first 45 min incubation which then declines by 90 min and is followed by a rise in viability starting at about 2 hr which we believe is due to the division of surviving cells and not the accumulation of freshly recovered ones.

4. During the first hour of incubation the excision of dimers in cells treated with FU is only marginally greater than that in untreated cells (Fig 10). Degradation of DNA to acid soluble material in FU treated cells is the same as that in untreated cells following 520 ergs/mm^2, although at higher UV doses rather more degradation occurs in FU treated cells than the controls. Alkaline sucrose gradient analysis of the molecular weight distribution of single strands of DNA (Fig 11) shows that the average MW of DNA of irradiated cells decreases during the first 30 min incubation and is followed by a modest but reproducible increase at 60 min. With cells incubated with FU this increased MW is maintained but in the absence of FU further lowering of the MW occurs.

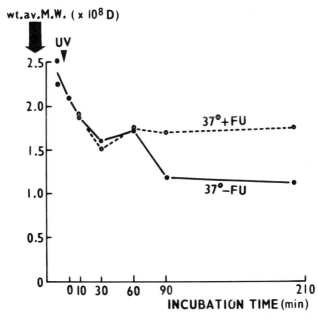

Fig 11. Molecular weight distribution of denatured DNA from UV-irradiated E. coli B/r during postirradiation incubation. Labelled E. coli B/r cells were grown and irradiated as in Figures 9 and 10. At intervals during postirradiation incubation of the cells in M63gly samples were taken, the cells converted to protoplasts and subjected to alkaline sucrose gradient analysis as described in Figure 5. From analysis of the gradient profiles weight average molecular weights were calculated as described by Regan, Setlow and Ley (64). A concentration of 50 μg/ml FU was added to the indicated culture at zero time.

5. In summary, the cessation of respiration in UV-irradiated glycerol-grown cells results from the loss of at least glycerol kinase and pyridine nucleotides. The loss of these activities is the result of postirradiation transcription and translation. Dimers are excised normally during the first hour after UV. At times later than this, excision enzymes may be inhibited by the lack of energy supply.

(Dimer excision is inhibited by cyanide (43) or by starvation (1,44).) Even when dimers have been excised, repair appears to be inhibited by the absence of diphosphopyridine nucleotide, which besides being the co-enzyme of respiratory dehydrogenases, is also the co-enzyme of polynucleotide ligase the putative rejoining enzyme of excision-repair (Fig 1).

THE ROLE OF MEMBRANES IN DNA REPAIR

Studies of DNA repair have until now been mainly concerned with establishing (a) the sequence of reactions involved in repair, (b) the nature of the enzymes performing the reactions and (c) the nature of enzymatic defects of radiation sensitive mutants. As this Symposium concerns "Cellular Repair Processes," it may not be out of place to draw attention to a cell structure which probably plays an important role in restoring normality to the irradiated cell, namely the cell membrane. A number of studies concerning the effects of ionizing irradiations on membranes have been reported, with a review by Okada (45). However, since the primary and major consequence of UV-irradiation is damage to nucleic acids, little attention has been paid so far to the effect of membrane damage that results from this type of radiation. I will try briefly to summarize a number of observations which suggest that alterations in membrane structure, resulting either from mutation or irradiation, may markedly affect the ability of cells to survive small doses of UV. For convenience, we can consider membranes in two ways, as a possible site of location of repair enzymes, and as the site of attachment of DNA and initiation of its synthesis.

1. Repair enzymes and membranes

Several lines of evidence suggest that DNA repair enzymes exist within cells in localized regions. The Kornberg polymerase has been shown to be associated with membrane components of B. subtilis (46) and phage T4 induced polymerase with the membrane of E. coli (47). One explanation of the results of our competition experiments on the excision of dimers from phage λ and E. coli DNA (Fig 8) is that the endonuclease (step 1) and the exonuclease (step 2) of the excision sequence are located differently within the cell. We have suggested (34) that the exonuclease is preferentially localized on cellular DNA and that its action is the rate limiting step for the excision of λ dimers, whereas the endonuclease is the rate limiting step for bacterial excision. Other examples suggesting the localization of repair enzymes come from the work of Setlow, Boling and Beattie (48) who have shown that irradiated Hemophilus transforming DNA is only repaired when integrated into the recipient genome. Muraoka and Kondo (49) showed that E. coli photoreactivating enzyme monomerizes four times the number of dimers in cellular DNA than in phage T1 DNA, and concluded that this enzyme is concentrated around the bacterial DNA. Each of these examples might imply equally well that the relevant repair enzymes are associated with the cell membrane near the point of DNA attachment. If this were the case, then one might expect a sequential repair of DNA lesions like that suggested for photoreactivation by Davies, Tyler and Webb (50).

Cellular dehydrogenases and their co-enzymes are well known to be localized in membranes (51). This fact and the results presented above concerning the effects of radiation on respiration and excision-repair in E. coli may be extrapolated to mean that the DPN dependent polynucleotide ligase of E. coli also acts at a cell membrane site.

2. Membranes and DNA synthesis

The synthesis of DNA in bacterial cells requires the attachment of DNA to a specific site, the mesosome (52) which is observed by electron microscopy as an infolding of the cell membrane. The mesosome is involved in the initiation of DNA synthesis and the segregation of daughter DNA molecules. The replication of viral DNA in bacterial cells requires the attachment of phage DNA to one of a small number of membrane sites that appear to have some degree of specificity for particular phages (53,54). Modification of the membrane structure following radiation may result in altered mesosome function.

A number of different classes of bacterial mutants are known in which synthesis of the DNA of specific phages is blocked very early after infection. With rep⁻ mutants (55-57) replication of the DNA of ϕX 174 and P2 is blocked at a stage following circularization of the DNA molecules. Attachment of P2 DNA to the membrane of rep⁻ cells has been observed (56). Other mutants which do not allow phage DNA replication have been described by Shapiro et al (58) (DNA A) and by Holland et al (Cet C) (59). In both the latter cases the mutant cells have altered membrane properties, and rep⁻ and cet C⁻ mutants have been shown to be UV sensitive. The UV sensitivity of lon⁻ and fil⁺ strains is well known to be associated with an impairment of the formation of cell septa following irradiation. Since most biological assays of cell survival involve some form of colony or plaque formation resulting from repeated cell and DNA replication, it is evident that if radiation modifies the role of membranes in DNA replication, biological estimates of survival can underestimate the extent of DNA repair. That this may be so is indicated by studies in which replication of repaired DNA has been observed to cease after a few rounds of replication. These considerations suggest that a study of the effects of radiation on cell membranes may contribute significantly to our understanding of the regulation of DNA repair processes and their relationship to DNA replication.

REFERENCES

1. Setlow, R. B. and Carrier, W. L.: Proc. Nat. Acad. Sci. USA, 51:226, 1964.
2. Boyce, R. P. and Howard-Flanders, P.: Proc. Nat. Acad. Sci. USA, 51:293, 1964.
3. Carrier, W. L. and Setlow, R. B.: Edited by L. Grossman and K. Moldave. In: Methods in Enzymology, vol 21, Academic Press, New York, in press. 1971.
4. McGrath, R. A. and Williams, R. W.: Nature, 212:534, 1966.
5. Pettijohn, D. and Hanawalt, P.: J. Molec. Biol., 9:395, 1964.
6. Recovery and Repair Mechanisms in Radiobiology, Brookhaven Symposia in Biology, 20: 1967.
7. Howard-Flanders, P.: Ann. Rev. Biochem., 37:175, 1968.
8. Strauss, B. S.: Curr. Topics Microbiol. Immun., 44:1, 1969.
9. Setlow, R. B. Prog. Nucl. Acid Res., 8:257, 1968.
10. Carrier, W. L. and Setlow, R. B.: J. Bact., 102:178, 1970.
11. Takagi, T., Sekiguchi, S., Okubo, H., Nakayama, H., Shimada, K., Yasuda, S., Nishimoto, T. and Yoshihara, M.: Cold Spring Harbor Symp. Quant. Biol., 33:219, 1968.
12. Grossman, L., Kaplan, J. C., Kushner, S. R. and Mahler, I.: Cold Spring Harbor Symp. Quant. Biol., 33:229, 1968.

13. Grossman, L., Kushner, S., Kaplan, J. and Mahler, I.: Biophysical Society Abstracts, Biophys. J., 10:17a, 1970.
14. Setlow, R. B., Setlow, J. K. and Carrier, W. L.: J. Bact., 102:187, 1970.
15. van Sluis, C. A. and Rörsch, A.: Int. J. Radiat. Biol., 9:596, 1965.
16. Elder, R. L. and Beers, R. F.: J. Bact., 90:681, 1965.
17. Kelly, R. B., Atkinson, M. R., Huberman, J. A. and Kornberg, A.: Nature, 224:495, 1969.
18. Kornberg, A.: Science, 163:1410, 1969.
19. Deutscher, M. P. and Kornberg, A.: J. Biol. Chem., 224:3029, 1969.
20. Bruntlag, D. A., Atkinson, M. R., Setlow, P. and Kornberg, A.: Biochem. Biophys. Res. Commun., 37:982, 1969.
21. Klenow, H. and Henningen, I.: Proc. Nat. Acad. Sci. USA, 65:168, 1970.
22. Olivera, B. M., Hall, Z. W., Anraku, Y., Chien, J. R. and Lehman, I. R.: Cold Spring Harbor Symp. Quant. Biol., 33:27, 1968.
23. Pauling, E. C. and Hamm, L.: Proc. Nat. Acad. Sci. USA, 60:1495, 1968.
24. Pauling, C. and Hamm, L.: Proc. Nat. Acad. Sci. USA, 69:1195, 1969.
25. De Lucia, P. and Cairns, J.: Nature, 224:1164, 1969.
26. Smith, D. W., Schaller, H. E. and Bonhoeffer, F. J.: Nature, 226:711, 1970.
27. Kornberg, T. and Gefter, M. L.: Biochem. Biophys. Res. Commun., 40:1348, 1970.
28. Boyle, J. M., Paterson, M. C. and Setlow, R. B.: Nature, 226:708, 1970.
29. Paterson, M. C., Boyle, J. M. and Setlow, R. B.: J. Bact., 107:61, 1971.
30. Kanner, L. and Hanawalt, P.: Biochem. Biophys. Res. Commun., 39:149, 1970.
31. Witkin, E. M.: Nature, New Biol., 229:81, 1971.
32. Kato, T. and Kondo, S.: J. Bact., 104:871, 1970.
33. Gross, J. and Gross, M.: Nature, 224:1166, 1969.
34. Boyle, J. M. and Setlow, R. B.: J. Molec. Biol., 51:131, 1970.
35. Radman, M., Cordonne, L., Krsmanovic-Simic, D. and Errera, M.: J. Molec. Biol., 49:203, 1970.
36. Hart, M. G. R. and Ellison, H.: J. Gen. Virol., 8:197, 1970.
37. Klein, A. and Niebch, U.: Nature, New Biol., 229:82, 1971.
38. Maynard-Smith, S., Symonds, N. and White, P.: J. Molec. Biol., 54:391, 1970.
39. Cozzarelli, N. R., Kelly, R. B. and Kornberg, A.: J. Molec. Biol., 45:513, 1969.
40. Swenson, P. A. and Schenley, R. L.: Mutat. Res., 9:443, 1970.
41. Swenson, P. A. and Schenley, R. L.: J. Bact., 104:1230, 1970.
42. Boyle, J. M., Schenley, R. L. and Swenson, P. A.: J. Bact., 106:896, 1971.
43. Setlow, R. B. and Carrier, W. L.: In: Replication and Recombination of Genetic Material. Edited by W. J. Peacock and R. D. Brock, p 134. Canberra: Australian Academy of Sciences, 1968.
44. Searashi, T. and Strauss, B. Mutat. Res., 4:372, 1967.
45. Okada, S.: In: Radiation Biochemistry, Vol 1. 1970. Cells. Edited by K. I. Altman, G. B. Gerber, and S. Okada, p 148. Academic Press, New York.
46. Okazaki, T. and Kornberg, A.: J. Biol. Chem., 239:259, 1964.
47. Frankel, F. R., Majumdar, C., Weintraub, S. and Frankel, D. M.: Cold Spring Harbor Symp. Quant. Biol., 33:495, 1968.
48. Setlow, J. K., Boling, M. E. and Beattie, K. A.: M. D. Anderson Symposium on Genetic and Neoplasia. Symposium on Fundamental Cancer Research, 23:555, 1970.
49. Muraoka, N. and Kondo, S.: Photochem. Photobiol., 10:295, 1969.
50. Davies, D. J. G., Tyler, S. A. and Webb, R. B.: Photochem. Photobiol., 11:371, 1970.
51. Tissieres, A.: In: Haematin Enzymes. Edited by J. Falk, R. Lembert and R. Morton, p 218, 1961. Pergamon Press, Oxford.
52. Jacob, F., Brenner, S. and Cuzin, F.: Cold Spring Harbor Symp. Quant. Biol., 28:329, 1963.
53. Salivar, W. O. and Sinsheimer, R. L.: J. Molec. Biol., 41:39, 1969.
54. Burton, A. J.: Biophysical Society Abstracts Biophys. J., 10:153a, 1970.
55. Denhardt, D. T., Dressler, D. H. and Hathaway, A.: Proc. Nat. Acad. Sci. USA, 57:813, 1967.
56. Calendar, R., Lindqvist, B., Sironi, G. and Clark, A. J.: Virology, 40:72, 1970.

57. Naha, P. M.: Virology, 36:434, 1968.
58. Shapiro, B., Siccardi, A., Hirota, Y. and Jacob, F.: J. Molec. Biol., 52:75, 1970.
59. Holland, I. B., Threlfall, E. J., Holland, E. M., Darby, V. and Samson, A. C. R.: J. Gen. Microbiol., 62:371, 1970.
60. Adler, H. I. and Hardigree, A. A.: J. Bact., 87:720, 1964.
61. Howard-Flanders, P., Simson, E. and Theriot, L.: Genetics, 49:237, 1964.
62. Billen, D. and Bruns, L. H.: Biophys. J., 10:509, 1970.
63. Carpenter, K. J. and Kodicek, E.: Biochem. J., 46:421, 1950.
64. Regan, J. D., Setlow, R. B. and Ley, R.: Proc. Nat. Acad. Sci. USA, 68:708, 1971.
65. Kelley, W. S. and Whitfield, H. J.: Nature, 230:33, 1971.

DNA POLYMERASES OF ESCHERICHIA COLI

Rolf Knippers, Franz-Josef Ferdinand and Wolf Strätling

Friedrich-Miescher-Laboratorium der Max-Planck-Gesellschaft
Tübingen, West Germany

INTRODUCTION

Recently several groups have described a deoxynucleotide polymerizing enzyme in E. coli cells which had been overlooked before (11,15,16,20). This enzyme has risen to sudden prominence due to the fact that it was the only DNA polymerase which could be purified from an E. coli strain (2) lacking the well-known DNA polymerase I, the enzyme studied extensively by Kornberg and his group (6,14). The newly-discovered DNA polymerase II, therefore, became a possible candidate for the polymerizing factor in the replicating apparatus of the bacterial cell. This conclusion, however, can be drawn only by way of exclusion. No direct proof (or disproof) for its participation in DNA replication is known so far. In this paper, some relevant biochemical properties of the known E. coli DNA polymerases will be compared, and an attempt will be made to define the biological functions of these enzymes.

SOME BIOCHEMICAL PROPERTIES OF DNA POLYMERASE II

When a nucleic-acid-free extract from E. coli cells is passed through a DNA-agarose column, about 95-97% of all proteins show apparently no affinity to DNA and run through the column or are washed off with a neutral buffer (containing 0.05-0.1 M NaCl). The remaining proteins are eluted with a salt gradient. When the extract is prepared from wild type E. coli cells, two or possibly three protein peaks with deoxynucleotide polymerizing activity are found in the eluate (Fig 1a). A smaller peak (peak B in Fig 1), appearing at 0.3-0.4 M NaCl, contains 2-6% of the total recovered deoxynucleotide polymerizing activity. The activity of this peak can be distinguished conveniently from a similar enzymatic activity in the larger peak C (eluted by 0.5-0.6 M NaCl) by its sensitivity to mercury compounds. In most of our DNA column chromatograms we find in addition to these two activities a minor peak (peak A of Fig 1a) of polymerizing activity at 0.2-0.25 M NaCl. This additional enzymatic activity is also mercury sensitive. An additional minor polymerizing activity has also been described recently by Kornberg and Gefter (16). It is not yet clear, however, whether the peak A activity of Figure 1 corresponds to their additional polymerizing enzyme.

From the chromatogram of Figure 1(a) it is apparent that the various polymerizing activities have different affinities to DNA. The binding to DNA of the two activities in peaks A and B is more sensitive to an increase in salt concentration than that of the larger activity. Consistent with this observation are the different salt concentrations required for optimal incorporating activity of the different enzymes, noted in the insert of Figure 1(a). These biochemical data and those described elsewhere (11,16,20) show

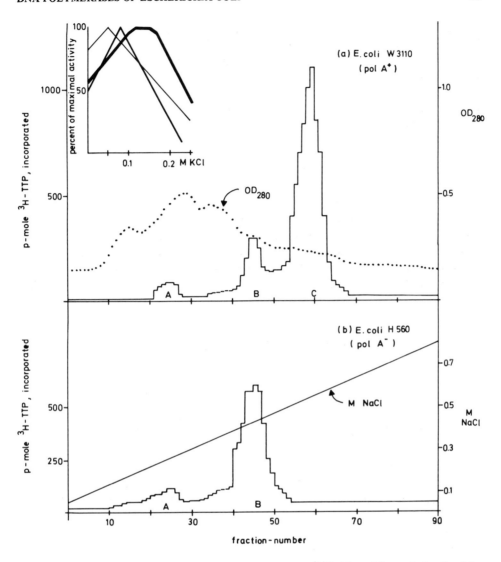

Fig 1. Chromatographic separation of DNA polymerase I and II. About 20 g packed cells of the strains E. coli W 3110 (pol A$^+$) (a) and H 560 (pol A$^-$) (b) (33) were lysed with lysozyme (20 mg) in 100 ml 0.05 M tris-0.001 M EDTA, pH 7.6. The lysate was ultrasonicated and subjected to the phase separation procedure of Okazaki and Kornberg (21) to remove nucleic acids. The protein phase was dialysed against 4 changes of 2 liters (1) standard buffer (0.005 M tris-HCl, pH 7.6, 0.005 M β-mercaptoethanol, 0.001 M EDTA) and passed through a 20 cm x 4 cm DNA-agarose column (Schaller and Bonhoeffer, personal communication). The column was washed with 0.1 M NaCl in standard buffer until no ultraviolet light absorbing material could be detected in the effluent. The remaining proteins were then eluted with a linear NaCl gradient. Fraction–volume: 6 ml. Flow rate: 0.5 ml/min. DNA-polymerizing activity was determined in a 0.2 ml volume, containing 0.05 M KCl, 0.05 M tris-HCl–pH 7.6, 0.006 M MgSO$_4$, 0.005 M mercaptoethanol; 10 μg of ultrasonicated calf thymus DNA and an 10^{-5} M of an equimolar mixture of dATP, dGTP, dCTP and dTTP containing ^{3}H-TTP in a specific activity of 1C/0.01 mole. To this mixture was added 0.01 ml of each fraction. Incubation was for 30 min at 37°C. Radioactivity was determined after trichloroacetic acid precipitation on nitrocellulose filters. The optimal KCl-concentration was determined in standard buffer (containing 0.006 M MgSO$_4$ plus increasing concentrations of KCl) with sonicated calf thymus DNA and deoxynucleoside triphosphates as specified above.

Thin line: activity of peak A   Medium line: activity of peak B   Bold line: activity of peak C

that there are at least two and possibly three deoxyribonucleoside polymerizing enzymes in wild type E. coli cells. The major activity (peak C) corresponds to the DNA polymerase of Kornberg (1969) and is absent in pol A1 mutants (2) as noted in Figure 1(b). This activity is now called DNA polymerase I. The mercury sensitive enzyme of peak B has been termed DNA polymerase II. The least active enzyme (peak A) has not yet been fully characterized. We can not exclude the possibility that it represents a modified form of DNA polymerase II.

TEMPLATE REQUIREMENTS

A functional difference between the DNA polymerases I and II becomes apparent when their template requirements are assayed in vitro after further purification (Ferdinand and Knippers, in preparation). The schematic summary, in Figure 2, shows that both enzymes are able to add deoxynucleotides to the 3'-end of a DNA strand which is hydrogen-bonded to an overlapping template strand. DNA polymerase II does not accept single-stranded DNA or endonucleolytically nicked DNA as templates (11). These DNA structures do prime the catalytic activity of DNA polymerase I (14).

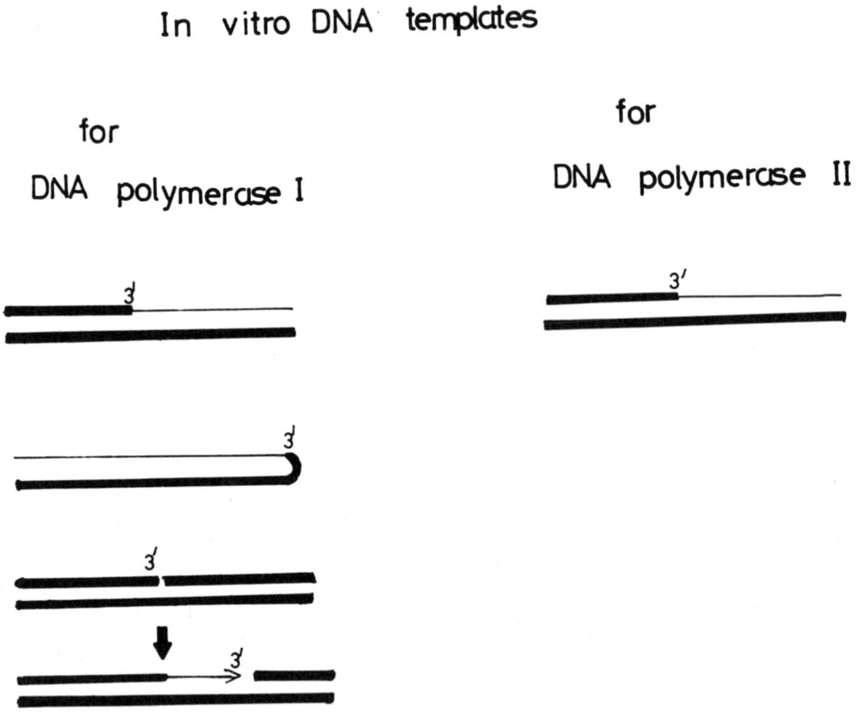

Fig 2. Template requirements for E. coli DNA polymerases. Bold lines: schematic structure of the DNA templates added to the reaction mixture in vitro. Thin lines: poly-deoxynucleotides, synthesized under the conditions of the in vitro assay.

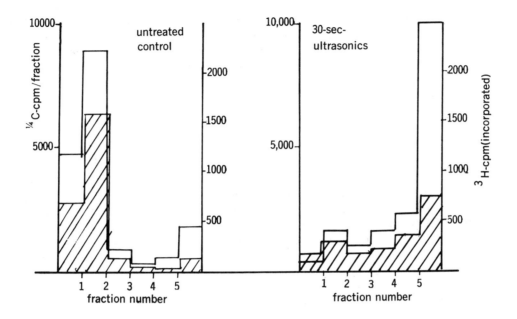

per cent of total counts

in fast sedimenting complex

length of ultrasonication (seconds)	DNA	incorporating activity
0	74	80
5	23	28
20	15	20
40	10	20

Fig 3. Location of DNA polymerase II. E. coli H560 (pol A1, endo I⁻) (from Dr. H. Hoffmann-Berling) was grown in 200 ml TPA-medium (13) in the presence of ^{14}C-thymine and deoxyadenosine. At a density of about 4×10^8 cells/ml, the bacteria were sedimented, washed and gently lysed as described by Knippers and Strätling (1970). One part of the lysate was then sedimented through a 10 ml 30% sucrose column (buffered by 0.05 M N-morpholino-3-propane-sulfonic acid, pH 7.2, in the presence of 0.008 M $MgSO_4$ and 0.05 M KCl) onto a 3 ml 60% sucrose shelf. At the end of the run (Spinco SW 27-rotor; 20,000 rpm; 2°C; 30 minutes) six samples were collected. The incorporating activity of each fraction was tested after addition of 40 μg ultrasonicated calf thymus DNA and 2×10^{-5} M of an equimolar mixture of all four deoxynucleoside triphosphates, including ^{3}H-TTP. Incubation was at 37°C for 15 minutes.

Another part of the same preparation was sonicated at 0°C-2°C using the microtip of the Branson Sonifier B12 for 30 seconds. Sedimentation and the assay for deoxynucleotide incorporating activity were performed as described above.

In Table I a summary of the data from a similar experiment is presented. Ultrasonication was performed for various lengths of time. (Redrawn after Strätling and Knippers (30).)

It must be emphasized that the artificial DNA structures which we commonly use in the in vitro assays create a situation for the enzymes which is probably quite different from the one they encounter in the living cell. The template requirements in vitro therefore do not allow any immediate conclusions as to the functions of these enzymes in the cell.

LOCATION OF THE DNA POLYMERASES

Several groups showed by different techniques that most of DNA polymerase II is not freely diffusible in gently lysed cell extracts (28), but bound to a fast sedimenting large cellular component (12,23). This fact can be demonstrated best in extracts from pol A1 cells (Fig 3). Most of the deoxynucleotide polymerizing activity in an extract from these cells sediments with an S of > 2,000. The fast sedimenting activity can be tested in the absence of an external primer-template DNA. The addition of a DNA primer does not stimulate further the deoxynucleotide incorporating activity. This shows that the enzyme is firmly associated with its authentic template.

The activity could be associated with either the bacterial chromosome (labeled with ^{14}C-thymine in Figure 3) or with the cellular envelope (labeled in a separate experiment with [14]-C-oleic acid (30)). The alternative can be decided by a simple experiment. Short ultrasonication does not disrupt the bacterial membrane. It still sediments rapidly through sucrose gradients (30). By the same treatment, the bacterial chromosome is fragmented and remains at the top of the sucrose gradient. As shown in Figure 3, the DNA synthesizing activity is released from the fast sedimenting structure with the same kinetics as the ^{14}C-labeled bacterial DNA. We propose therefore that DNA polymerase II is associated with the bacterial chromosome rather than with the cellular membrane. In Figure 4, the distribution of DNA synthesizing activity in a H560 pol A[+] revertant strain was investigated. Most of the activity in this strain apparently is not bound to some large structure. It can be detected only when the enzyme is supplied with an appropriate template-primer-DNA. The freely diffusible state of the DNA polymerase I holds also for in vivo conditions as can be concluded from the work of Hirota et al (7) who showed that anucleated, that is, DNA-less E. coli cells contain high levels of DNA polymerase activity but no DNA dependent RNA polymerase, an enzyme which is thought to be bound efficiently to DNA.

As is shown also in Figure 4, an increased fraction of DNA polymerase I was found associated with E. coli DNA when the cells were irradiated with ultraviolet light in vivo. In the experiment, shown in Figure 4(c) about 25% of the total DNA polymerizing activity was found co-sedimenting with the DNA from UV-irradiated cells, compared to 10% in the untreated control. The fraction of DNA-polymerase I co-sedimenting with the chromosome after UV-irradiation varies from experiment to experiment. No apparent relationship was found between UV dose and amount of enzymatic activity bound. But invariably, the fraction of bound enzyme was higher in extracts from irradiated cells compared to untreated controls. This result points to a possible role of DNA polymerase I in postirradiation repair, as has been suggested by several groups before. The evidence for such a function of DNA polymerase I will now be discussed briefly.

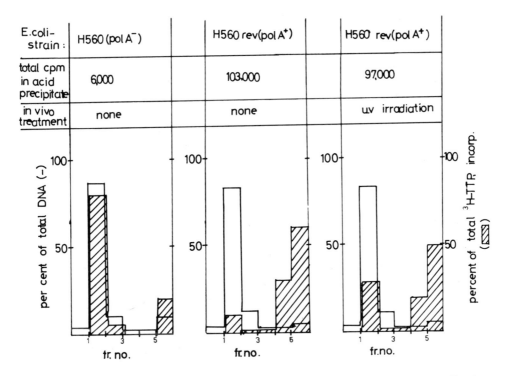

Fig 4. Location of DNA polymerase I. Exponentially growing cells of H 560 pol A1 and H 560 pol A[+] were lysed as described (12). The centrifugation technique and the incorporation assay have been described above.

The dose of ultraviolet light (germicidal lamp at 256 mμ) was 200-400 ergs/mm^2 for a 0.5 ml layer of 1 x 10^9/ml H 560 pol A[+]-cells.

A BIOLOGICAL FUNCTION OF DNA POLYMERASE I

DNA polymerase I contains in a single polypeptide chain, a polymerizing and two exonucleolytic activities; one degrades polydeoxynucleotides from their 3', the other from their 5'-end (14). The latter activity has been shown to excise pyrimidine dimer containing oligonucleotides from ultraviolet-irradiated DNA in vitro (10). Because of this interesting property it became conceivable that DNA polymerase I was a part of a cellular excision-repair system. As discussed extensively elsewhere in this volume, this system is thought 1. to split endonucleolytically a single strand of the DNA duplex in the vicinity of the pyrimidine dimers (endonucleases with a specificity for UV-irradiated DNA were isolated by Yasuda and Sekuguchi (36) and Sadowski and Hurwitz (27)); 2. to remove the damaged section of the DNA by exonucleolytic degradation followed by repair synthesis using the intact complementary strand as template; 3. to rejoin the repaired segment to the continuous parental DNA strand by an polynucleotide ligase-like enzyme. Step 2 of this scheme could be performed by DNA polymerase I as demonstrated by the in vitro experiment of Kelly et al (10). That such a process might also function in vivo was demonstrated first by de Lucia and Cairns (2) and Gross and Gross (5), who found that their pol A1 mutant was about five times more sensitive to ultraviolet light than the wild type parent strain.

However, a typical UVR⁻-strain is 50-100 times more sensitive to UV-irradiation than the corresponding wild type strain (8). Assuming that no active DNA polymerase I is present in pol A⁻-cells, one has to consider whether other enzymes are replacing DNA polymerase I in its function as the polymerizing principle in the excision repair system outlined above or whether pol A1 cells employ another repair system which does not depend on DNA polymerase I.

Such a system has been shown by Rupp and Howard-Flanders (26) to exist in wild type E. coli cells (8,34). These authors presented data suggesting that unexcised pyrimidine dimers in the UV-irradiated DNA are bypassed by the replicating enzymes leaving gaps at the corresponding places in the newly synthesized daughter strands. These gaps are thought to be sealed subsequently in a recombination-like process. This was concluded from experiments which showed that UV-irradiated recombination deficient (rec A⁻)-mutants were killed when they replicated a section of the DNA containing unexcised pyrimidine dimers (25).

This postreplication repair system is probably active in pol A1 cells as shown by Witkin (35) in studies on UV-induced mutagenesis in this strain. This author found the same frequency of induced mutations among the survivors of UV-irradiated wild type cells and those of pol A1 cells. Mutations induced by ultraviolet light are observed only in strains with a functioning postreplication repair system (34). They are not found among the survivors of UV-irradiated recombination deficient (rec A⁻) cells.

That DNA polymerase I is not an indispensable component of the postreplication repair system can also be concluded from the lack of additivity exerted by pol A1- and UVR A-mutations on UV-sensitivity in double mutants. Such an additivity is observed for UVR A⁻ rec A⁻ double mutants (9).

The initiation of the excision-repair process, that is, the excision of pyrimidine dimer containing oligonucleotides, proceeds normally in UV-irradiation pol A1-cells (1). The increased UV-sensitivity of these cells is therefore explained by the lack of the gap-filling activity of DNA polymerase I (35).

DNA POLYMERASE I AND REC-A-GENE PRODUCT(S)

Gross (4) reported unsuccessful attempts to construct rec A⁻ pol A⁻ double mutants. It seems that a combination of these two mutations is lethal for the bacterial cell. Since rec A⁻ single mutants as well as pol A⁻ single mutants are viable it can be concluded that the rec A-gene product(s) and the pol A-gene product can replace each other in a vital cellular process.

The work of Town, Smith and Kaplan (32) suggests that this vital function might be a sealing of single-stranded nicks. These authors found that pol A1-cells and rec A⁻-cells are equally sensitive to X-rays. The major damage induced by X-rays is believed to be single-stranded breaks (8). A sealing of single-stranded nicks seems also to be one of the various biochemical events at the chromosomal growth point during DNA replication as suggested by the work of Okazaki. Okazaki and his colleagues (22) were the first to present evidence that DNA at least partially is replicated in a discontinuous manner. Short fragments seem to be synthesized which are then joined in a subsequent step to form continuous DNA strands.

Since such a joining process is involved in the repair of single-stranded breaks, one might ask whether DNA polymerase I and/or the rec A-gene product are employed in repairing them. Some indication of a role for DNA polymerase I in DNA replication comes from the work of Kuempel and Veomett (1970) and of Moses and Richardson (19) who showed that the DNA fragments produced in a given short time period during DNA replication are of a smaller size in pol A1-cells than in pol A^+-wild type cells as if the joining process were retarded in the mutant strain. It should be mentioned, however, that Geider and Hoffmann-Berling (3) could not detect any difference between pol A^+ and pol A1-strains in the joining of fragments during replication.

Since DNA polymerase I and II perform comparable biochemical reactions in vitro (Fig 2) we and, independently others (4) thought that DNA polymerase II might be the product of the rec A-gene. However, the DNA polymerase II activity in rec A^--cells was found to be normal by Westphal and Knippers (personal communication) and by Kornberg and Gefter (16).

IS DNA POLYMERASE II INVOLVED IN DNA REPLICATION?

As discussed above, and elsewhere (12,30) a DNA synthesizing activity in pol A1-cells cosediments with the bacterial chromosome. The major DNA polymerizing activity which could be solubilized from this fast sedimenting complex is DNA polymerase II. This, of course, does not necessarily mean that this enzyme is the (only) DNA synthesizing activity of the replicating apparatus in bacterial cells. It is quite conceivable that other relevant enzymes can not be detected after biochemical manipulations because 1. we do not know their proper template requirements; 2. they may use precursors different from deoxynucleoside tri- or diphosphates; 3. they may need unknown cofactors; or, 4. they could be extremely fragile.

Indeed, the isolated DNA polymerase II has properties which are difficult to reconcile with the notion that it is the only enzymatic principle operating at the

TABLE I

Optimal Activity of DNA Polymerase II and DNA-Membrane-System
as a Function of pH, KCl and $MgSO_4$ Concentrations

	pH	M KCl	M $MgSO_4$
DNA polymerase II	7.6	0.08	0.008
DNA-membrane-system	7.0	0.05	0.005

chromosomal growth point. First, there are several biochemical differences between the isolated enzyme and the DNA synthesizing activity in situ, that is, at the fast sedimenting structure (Table I). Second, the kinetics and rates of polymerization are different in the DNA membrane system and the isolated DNA polymerase II (Fig 5). Third, the isolated enzyme requires a $3'$-OH-end as a primer site and a single-stranded template strand whose base sequence is copied. In semiconservative replication both strands of the parental DNA, however, are copied (at least approximately) simultaneously with an overall direction of $3' \rightarrow 5'$ in one strand and $5' \rightarrow 3'$ in the other strand.

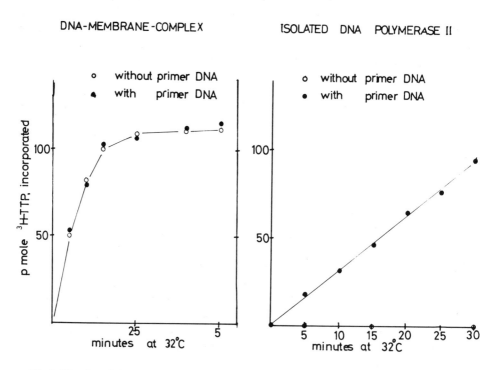

Fig 5. Kinetics of the polymerization reaction. (a) DNA-membrane-complexes were prepared from about 2×10^{10} exponentially growing E. coli H 560-cells (pol A$^-$ endo I$^-$ (33) as described by Strätling and Knippers (30)).

Incorporating activity was assayed as described in the legend of Figure 1. Each point gives the amount of radioactive triphosphates incorporated by a DNA membrane preparation from about 10^9 cells. The chain elongation rate in membrane-DNA-complexes has been reported elsewhere (Strätling and Knippers, (1971)) and amounts to about 2×10^4 nucleotides/minute.

(b) DNA polymerase II was prepared from E. coli H 560 cells by DNA-agarose column chromatography (legend of Figure 1), and further purified by phosphocellulose chromatography and Sephadex gel filtration (details will be published elsewhere).

Phage T7 DNA was treated with exonuclease III (to about 20% acid solubility) and used as primer in a concentration of 4 μg/0.2 ml. Saturating amounts of enzyme completed the partially single-stranded DNA to a DNA duplex under standard assay conditions (Fig 1) in about 40 minutes. From the known molecular weight of T7-DNA (26×10^6; Studier (31)) one can estimate the chain elongation rate as roughly 500 nucleotides/minute (cf the chain elongation rate of DNA polymerase I was estimated to be: 500-1,000 nucleotides/minutes (24)).

Each point gives the amount of radioactive nucleotides incorporated in a 0.2-ml-reaction mixture (plus 4 μg exonuclease III treated T7-DNA) during the time period indicated (legend to Fig 1).

Various models, as reviewed by Goulian (6) and Gross (4), have been proposed to reconcile the unidirectional polymerases with the events supposed to occur at the chromosomal growth point. All these models employ several auxiliary enzymes and factors in addition to a DNA polymerase: endonucleases, ligases, denaturating proteins and so on. These enzymes and factors must work in close spacial arrangement and functional coordination. Therefore, it is not surprising that the overall biochemical characteristics of the DNA-membrane complex are different from those of the isolated DNA polymerase II. More difficult to explain is the much higher rate of polymerization for the replicating apparatus in vivo or in situ.

We do not know yet whether the higher rate in vivo is a consequence of some kind of a pre-arrangement of nucleotides along the parental DNA strand ahead of the replication complex or of a special structure of the parental DNA at the growth point or of the properties of a so-far undiscovered polymerizing enzyme. Among the various temperature sensitive E. coli mutants (4) which are unable to replicate their chromosome at 42°C none has been found so far which contains an altered DNA polymerase II. The strongest point in case for a DNA polymerase as a component of the DNA replicating machinery stems from the work on certain bacteriophages. It is known from genetic analysis and biochemical experimentation that the DNA polymerases of bacteriophages T2, T4 (28) and T7 (Oey, Strätling and Knippers, in press) are essential for phage DNA replication. However, it can not be excluded yet that other so-far undetected polymerizing enzymes are involved also in this process.

From these considerations it becomes quite obvious that we are as ignorant about the biochemical events at the DNA growth point as we have ever been during the past ten years. Does a DNA polymerase catalyze the formation of polydeoxynucleotide chains during replication? Or, is there another enzyme which will appear one day on the scientific scene like a *deus ex machina*, the stage god of the old theater, and which will turn out to be a true replicase performing an authentic semiconservative replication at a rate of several 100,000 nucleotides per minute?

We could show that the DNA polymerizing activity described as peak A in Figure 1 corresponds to the DNA polymerase III of Kornberg and Gefter (1971). DNA polymerase III can be distinguished from DNA polymerase II by their different salt optima (Kornberg and Gefter, 1971; see insert to Figure 1) and by their different sedimentation properties. DNA polymerase II sediments through sucrose gradients with about 4.2 S and DNA polymerase III with about 5.5 S (Ferdinand and Knippers, unpublished report). Gefter, Hirota, Kornberg and Wechsler (1971, in press) discovered a temperature-sensitive DNA polymerase III in an E. coli mutant which is temperature-sensitive in DNA replication.

REFERENCES

1. Boyle, J. M., Patterson, M. C. and Setlow, R. B.: Nature, 226:708, 1970.
2. de Lucia, P. and Cairns, J.: Nature, 224:1164, 1969.
3. Geider, K. and Hoffmann-Berling, H.: Europ. J. Biochem., 21:374, 1971.
4. Gross, J. D.: Current Topics in Microbiology and Immunology, Springer-Verlag, Berlin, Heidelberg, New York, p 57, 1971.

5. Gross, J. D. and Gross, M.: Nature, 224:1166, 1969.
6. Goulian, M.: Ann. Rev. Biochem., 40:855, 1971.
7. Hirota, Y., Jacob, F., Ryter, A., Buttin, G. and Nakai, T.: J. Molec. Biol., 35:175, 1968.
8. Howard-Flanders, P.: Ann. Rev. Biochem., 37:175, 1968.
9. Howard-Flanders, P. and Boyce, R. P.: Radiat. Res., Suppl. 6, 156, 1966.
10. Kelly, R. B., Atkinson, M. R., Huberman, J. A. and Kornberg, A.: Nature, 224:495, 1969.
11. Knippers, R.: Nature, 228:1050, 1970.
12. Knippers, R. and Strätling, W.: Nature, 226:713, 1970.
13. Knippers, R., Razin, A., Davis R. and Sinsheimer, R. L.: J. Molec. Biol., 45:237, 1969.
14. Kornberg, A.: Science, 163:1410, 1969.
15. Kornberg, T. and Gefter, M. L.: Biochem. Biophys. Res. Commun., 40:1348, 1970.
16. Kornberg, T. and Gefter, M. L.: Proc. Nat. Acad. Sci. USA, 68:761, 1971.
17. Kuempel, P. L. and Veomett, G. E.: Biochem. Biophys. Res. Commun., 41:973, 1970.
18. Mitra, S., Reichard, P., Inman, R. B., Bertsch, L. L. and Kornberg, A.: J. Molec. Biol., 24:429, 1967.
19. Moses, R. E. and Richardson, C. C.: Proc. Nat. Acad. Sci. USA, 67:674, 1970,a.
20. Moses, R. E. and Richardson, C. C.: Biochem. Biophys. Res. Commun., 41:1557, 1970,b.
21. Okazaki, T. and Kornberg, A.: J. Biol. Chem., 239:259, 1964.
22. Okazaki, R., Okazaki, T., Sakabe, K., Sugimoto, K. and Sugino, A.: Proc. Nat. Acad. Sci. USA, 59:598, 1968.
23. Okazaki, R., Sugimoto, K., Okazaki, K., Imae, Y. and Sugino, A.: Nature, 228:223, 1970.
24. Richardson, C. C., Schildkraut, C. L., Aposhian, H. V. and Kornberg, A.: J. Biol. Chem., 239:222, 1964.
25. Rupert, C. S. and Harm, W.: Adv. Radiat. Biol., 2:1, 1966.
26. Rupp, W. D. and Howard-Flanders, P.: J. Molec. Biol., 31:291, 1968.
27. Sadowski, P. D. and Hurwitz, J.: J. Biol. Chem., 224:6192, 1969.
28. Smith, D. W., Schaller, H. and Bonhoeffer, F.: Nature, 226:711, 1970.
29. Speyer, J. F. and Rosenberg, D.: Cold Spring Harbor Symp. Quant. Biol., 33:345, 1968.
30. Strätling, W. and Knippers, R.: J. Molec. Biol., 61:471, 1971 and Europ. J. Biochem., 20:330, 1971.
31. Studier, F. W.: Virology, 39:562, 1969.
32. Town, C. D., Smith, K. C. and Kaplan, H. S.: Science, 172:851, 1971.
33. Vossberg, H. P. and Hoffmann-Berling, H.: J. Molec. Biol., 58:739, 1971.
34. Witkin, E. M.: Ann. Rev. Genet., 3:525, 1969.
35. Witkin, E. M.: Nature, 229:81, 1971.
36. Yasuda, S. and Sekiguchi, M.: Proc. Nat. Acad. Sci. USA, 67:1839, 1970.

THE DIFFERENCE BETWEEN DNA REPLICATION AND REPAIR

Rudolf Werner[1]

Department of Biochemistry
University of Miami School of Medicine
Miami, Florida

It has been known for several years that two different types of DNA synthesis exist in the living cell, the duplication of the chromosome, also called replication, and repair synthesis (1). Although it is generally assumed that these two reactions are closely related, there is no indication that their mechanisms are very similar. DNA polymerase I, the enzyme isolated from Escherichia coli by Kornberg (2), is now generally believed to be involved in repair synthesis. This does not preclude its possible participation in the replication process, however. In fact, there is evidence that replication is always accompanied by some kind of repair synthesis: Although a bacterium can live without polymerase I, it is not viable if the product of the rec A gene is missing as well (3). The rec A mutation alone is not lethal, however. It seems, therefore, that polymerase I and the rec A gene product participate in two distinct repair systems at least one of which has to be functional. In phage T4, a mutation in gene 43, the structural gene for the DNA polymerase of the polymerase I-type, is lethal, probably because there is no rec A repair system that could take over as in E. coli.

EXPERIMENTAL DATA

Recent experiments in my laboratory on the synthesis and function of "Okazaki pieces," small single-stranded DNA pieces that have been considered intermediates in the synthesis of long DNA, have led to two new conclusions about the mechanism of DNA replication (4).

First, Okazaki pieces are not engaged in extensive strand elongation, as the model of discontinuous DNA replication had predicted (5), but are created in an event that follows, rather than accompanies, replication. This was concluded from the observation that very short pulses of tritiated thymine given to Escherichia coli under steady-state conditions were incorporated preferentially into large DNA and only later appeared in Okazaki pieces. In contrast, short pulses of tritiated thymidine were incorporated predominantly into Okazaki pieces. These results led to a new model for the relationship between Okazaki pieces and DNA replication. It sees the creation of Okazaki pieces as a consequence of the action of a specific nuclease upon one of the two new daughter strands. This nuclease presumably recognizes specific base sequences located at intervals of about 3,000 nucleotides in one of the two new DNA strands. It seems possible that these strand interruptions

[1] This work was supported by research grants from the National Science Foundation and the American Cancer Society, and was done during the tenure of an Established Investigatorship of the American Heart Association.

function as swivel points for the rotation of the daughter helices during the replication of the circular chromosome. Similar strand interruptions, therefore, may occur in the parental strand of the other daughter duplex. This is suggested by the finding that some thymidine is incorporated into parental DNA. The interruptions in the parental strand even may be created ahead of the fork, thus providing the necessary swivel point for the unwinding of the parental double helix, and persist through the replication region into one daughter helix where they are eventually sealed. Recent electron micrographs, by Salzman (6), of the structure of replicating polyoma DNA support the idea that all swivel points are located near the replicating fork. Salzman observed that unreplicated regions of the polyoma chromosomes were often supercoiled. It seems unlikely that the torque created by the unwinding process could be transmitted through the supercoiled section to some swivel point at the origin of replication. Of course, the single-strand interruptions near the replication fork may have additional functions, for example, in transcription (4,7) or in the repair of replication mistakes.

The predominant incorporation of tritiated thymidine into Okazaki pieces seems to suggest that thymidine is preferentially used for a repair-type of DNA synthesis that precedes the sealing of the Okazaki pieces to long DNA. This would also explain the observation that the total incorporation of thymidine accounts only for a small fraction of the total DNA synthesis in a bacterium. The apparent ability of the cell to distinguish between thymine and thymidine and to use them separately for two different reactions, DNA replication and repair synthesis, led to the second conclusion, namely, that the two reactions draw their precursors from two distinct pools. Although these results do not prove that the precursors for the two types of DNA synthesis are chemically different, the idea that DNA replication uses precursors different from deoxyribonucleoside triphosphates seems rather attractive. Comparing the two reactions, replication and repair, we know that DNA replication has to be controlled precisely in relation to cell division and may not occur at all times during the cell cycle. Repair synthesis, on the other hand, must be available at all times. The use of different precursors would facilitate such different regulation and could prevent interference between the two types of DNA synthesis.

The only known fact about the nature of the in vivo precursor for DNA replication is that it must be some $5'$-nucleotide or derivative thereof (8). To find out more about the nature of the DNA replication precursor, I have studied the flow of thymine through the various nucleotide pools into DNA (9). Under steady-state conditions, where all intracellular pool sizes remain constant, the immediate precursor of DNA is expected to reach its maximal specific activity at the same time or slightly before the rate of incorporation of radioactive label into DNA becomes maximal. Both TDP and TTP pools show this kind of kinetics, except that the rate of incorporation of label into DNA consistently becomes maximal slightly before the TTP pool reached its final specific activity.

In the presence of unlabelled thymidine or any other deoxyribose donor, however, the incorporation of tritiated thymine into DNA reaches its maximal rate much sooner than under steady-state conditions, while the specific activity of the TTP pool increases only slowly. It seems, therefore, that under these conditions of accelerated thymine uptake, thymine bypasses most of the TTP pool on its way to DNA. The very rapid establishment of full incorporation rate suggests that the real DNA precursor pool must be very small, possibly as small as one tenth of the normal deoxyribonucleoside triphosphate pool. Of course, I cannot rule out the possibility that there exists a small separate TTP pool that is not mixed with the larger TTP pool which is used for repair synthesis. However, the previously mentioned results obtained with thymidine, which seems to be used preferentially for a repair-type of DNA synthesis, make a compartmentation of the deoxyribonucleoside triphosphate pool somewhat unlikely.

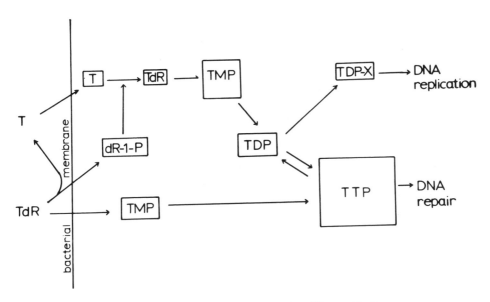

Fig 1. Tentative scheme of thymine and thymidine metabolism.

DISCUSSION

Figure 1 shows a tentative scheme of the intermediary metabolism of thymidine nucleotides. Let me explain how the cell might be able to use thymine or thymidine for two seemingly similar reactions, DNA replication and repair synthesis: Under steady-state conditions, thymine is converted intracellularly sequentially to thymidine, TMP, TDP and finally TTP. The postulated precursor for DNA replication, TDP-X, is derived from TDP which is in complete equilibrium with TTP, the precursor for repair synthesis, thus leading to the observed labelling pattern of both TDP and TTP pools. Normally, a wild-type bacterium contains no intracellular deoxyribose pool. It is unable, therefore, to incorporate thymine. A thymine-requiring bacterium, however, which was used for all of these studies, has a small intracellular pool of deoxyribose-1-phosphate. In the presence of a deoxyribose donor in the medium, like thymidine or deoxyadenosine, the intracellular pool of deoxyribose-1-phosphate increases dramatically, thus causing a large expansion of the TMP pool (10). This in turn leads to an expansion of the TDP as well as the TTP pool and, at least temporarily, blocks the back-reaction from TTP to TDP. Therefore, the TTP pool is no longer equilibrated with the TDP pool, and thymine can enter DNA via TDP without being mixed with the TTP pool. Although presumably most of the thymidine is broken down by thymidine phosphorylase to thymine and deoxyribose-1-phosphate (11), some of the thymidine escapes this breakdown, at least as long as the activity of the thymidine phosphorylase is low, and is converted directly to TTP via a separate, possibly membrane-bound, TMP pool. TTP can only participate in DNA replication via TDP; this pathway, however, is blocked because of the simultaneous increase in the thymine-derived TMP and TDP pools, caused by the simultaneously-occurring breakdown of thymidine to deoxyribose-1-phosphate. Consequently, during a short pulse, tritiated thymidine will be used only for repair synthesis while thymine goes preferentially into replication. Of course, during longer pulses, this exclusive handling of thymidine will disappear.

The scheme in Figure 1 also offers an explanation of the phenomenon that hydroxyurea blocks DNA replication but has little effect on repair synthesis (12). It has been shown that hydroxyurea inhibits the enzyme ribonucleoside diphosphate reductase which catalyses the main entrance route into the deoxyribonucleotide pool (13). If the precursors for DNA replication and repair synthesis were the same, it would be difficult to explain how a block in the precursor synthesis could inhibit only one of the two reactions, while the other one goes on. With different precursors, however, the phenomenon can be explained easily: It is known that the inhibition of DNA replication has little, if any, effect on the viability of the cell. If, however, the ability of the cell to repair damaged regions in the DNA were abolished for only a short time, this might well be lethal. The cell, therefore, may have a mechanism that, as soon as it senses a decline in the deoxyribonucleoside triphosphate pool, interrupts the conversion of deoxyribonucleoside triphosphates into the replication precursor via the diphosphates. This would ensure the cell of enough precursors for repair synthesis for a long time to come. The inhibitory effect of carbon monoxide or cyanide upon DNA replication but not repair could be explained similarly (14).

As to the nature of the real DNA replication precursor, it seems most likely that it is derived from the deoxyribonucleoside diphosphate. The very small size of the DNA precursor pool may provide some clue as to its nature. The pool of all four deoxyribonucleoside triphosphate in E. coli amounts to only about 1.2×10^5 molecules per cell which is about 1% of its total DNA content (15). Considering the relative concentrations of both ribo- and deoxyribonucleotides as well as the rates of RNA and DNA synthesis, Maniloff (16) recently has calculated that the average lifetime of a deoxyribonucleoside triphosphate molecule at the active site of the DNA polymerase is almost two orders of magnitude shorter than that of a ribonucleoside triphosphate molecule on the RNA polymerase. Assuming that the time required for proper recognition of the monomer by the polymerase is approximately the same for RNA and DNA synthesis one wonders whether the intracellular concentration of deoxyribonucleoside triphosphates is sufficient to support the observed rate of DNA replication by means of a random diffusion and collision process. With the discovery that the DNA precursor pool is even smaller, possibly by as much as an order of magnitude, we are compelled to consider processes of monomer selection other than random collision between precursors and polymerase.

The problem of a rate-limiting recognition time may be circumvented by allowing the DNA precursor to align on the parental DNA template ahead of the fork so that the DNA polymerase would only have to connect these nucleotides and itself may have no function in recognizing and selecting the proper nucleotides (Fig 2). As the alignment process would occur simultaneously over an extended region, the collision lifetime of an individual nucleotide with the template no longer would be limiting to the rate of DNA

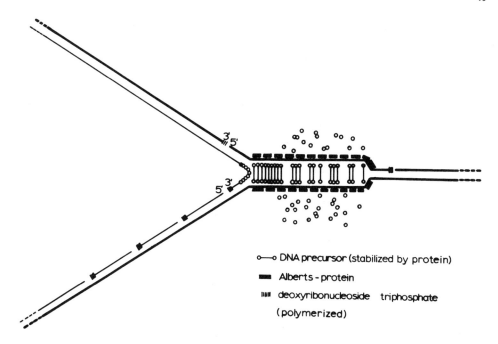

Fig 2. Model of DNA replication. The two daughter strands are thought to be covalently connected and elongation occurs by insertion of nucleotides at the apex.

replication. Since nucleotide DNA complexes are rather unstable, one would have to postulate that the precursor is stabilized on the DNA template with the help of some protein. In phage T4, the gene 32 protein is believed to facilitate the unwinding of the parental helix (17). No doubt proteins analogous to the gene 32 product will be found in E. coli and other organisms. With the recent finding by Gisela Mosig (personal communication) that certain temperature-sensitive T4 mutants in gene 32 are mutagenic, it seems possible that the gene 32 protein has an additional function, namely, that of stabilizing the precursor on the DNA template. Of course, there may be other proteins that provide this function.

From an evolutionary point of view, it seems likely that DNA replication originally occurred by a nonenzymatic crystallization process using the inherent ability of the DNA strand to bind complementary nucleotides (18). The replication process, as it occurs today, still may employ the same principle albeit with the help of an enzyme. In contrast, repair synthesis presumably has evolved much later, perhaps after the transcription process came to life. Since transcription and repair have much in common, it is conceivable that the repair reaction has evolved from transcription rather than replication.

In summary, it appears possible that DNA replication uses precursors different from deoxyribonucleoside triphosphates, the known precursors for repair synthesis. It may prove futile, therefore, to search for other DNA synthesizing activities in extracts prepared from polymerase I-less mutants applying the same assaying procedures developed by Kornberg for polymerase I. Although this method may lead to the detection of still other repair enzymes, its usefulness for discovering the real replication enzyme is questionable. Before we set out to find the real replication enzyme, we should at least know the substrate requirements of this enzyme.

REFERENCES

1. Pettijohn, D. E., and Hanawalt, P. C.: Biochim. Biophys. Acta, 72:127, 1963.
2. Kornberg, A.: Science, 131:1503, 1960.
3. Gross, J. D., Grunstein, J. and Witkin, E. M.: J. Molec. Biol., 58:631, 1971.
4. Werner, R.: Nature, 230:570, 1971.
5. Okazaki, R., Okazaki, K., Sakaba, K., Sugimoto, K., Kainuma, R., Sugino, A. and Iwatsuki, N.: Cold Spring Harbor Sympos. Quant. Biol., 33:129, 1968.
6. Sebring, E., Kelly, T. J. Jr., Thoren, M. and Salzman, N.P.: Fed. Proc., 30:1177, 1971.
7. Riva, S., Cascino, A. and Geiduschek, E. P.: J. Molec. Biol., 54:103, 1970.
8. Price, T. D., Darmstadt, R. A., Hinds, H. A. and Zamenhof, S.: J. Biol. Chem., 242:140, 1967.
9. Werner, R.: Nature, 233:99, 1971.
10. Munch-Petersen, A.: Biochim. Biophys. Acta, 161:279, 1968.
11. Razzell, W. E. and Casshyap, P.: J. Biol. Chem., 239:1789, 1964.
12. Cleaver, J. E.: Radiat. Res., 37:334, 1969.
13. Krakoff, I. H., Brown, N. C. and Reichard, P.: Cancer Res., 26:638, 1968.
14. Cairns, J. and Denhardt, D. T.: J. Molec. Biol., 36:335, 1968.
15. Neuhard, J.: Biochim. Biophys. Acta, 129:104, 1966.
16. Maniloff, J.: J. Theor. Biol., 25:339, 1969.
17. Alberts, B. and Frey, L.: Nature, 227:1313, 1970.
18. Watson, J. D. and Crick, F. H. C.: Nature, 171:964, 1953.

Part II

PHOTOENZYMATIC REPAIR

PHOTOENZYMATIC REPAIR OF DNA

I. INVESTIGATION OF THE REACTION BY FLASH ILLUMINATION[1]

Walter Harm, Claud S. Rupert and Helga Harm

Division of Biology, University of Texas at Dallas
Dallas, Texas

INTRODUCTION

It has long been known that ultraviolet (UV) irradiation of microorganisms with wavelengths below 300 nm leads to inactivation. The fraction of inactivated individuals increases with the UV exposure and there is ample evidence that this is a consequence of an increasing number of UV photoproducts formed in the genetic material, which is usually DNA (13). Several kinds of DNA photoproducts are known; the most prominent ones, as far as frequency of occurrence and significance for biological effects is concerned, are cyclobutyl type pyrimidine dimers. Their formation involves two neighboring pyrimidine bases of the same DNA strand, whose 5,6-double bonds are converted into a cyclobutane ring.

To escape the lethal effects of UV or other damaging agents, organisms have developed various repair mechanisms. They operate in two principal ways: 1. Either the UV lesion is *reversed,* that is, the photochemically altered base is restored to its original condition or to something functionally equivalent; or, 2. a DNA segment containing a lesion is *replaced.* It is interesting to notice that these two principles found in nature are the same as those used by men for the maintenance of technical equipment.

While the replacement principle is variably employed by different dark repair systems, the only case known so far to use the reversion principle is photoenzymatic repair. Its mechanism is simpler than that of any known type of dark repair since it involves the action of only a single enzyme: the photoreactivating enzyme (PRE). This enzyme monomerizes UV-induced pyrimidine dimers in situ, that is, it reverses the potentially lethal lesion while leaving the DNA structure fully intact. The action of PRE has an absolute requirement for an outside factor, *light,* which makes experimental control of the reaction rather easy. Therefore, it is not surprising that photoenzymatic repair has been investigated in more detail than any other kind of repair.

The wavelengths effective in promoting photoenzymatic repair range from about 310 to 480 nm and for this reason yellow light is used for all manipulations except for the controlled illumination with photoreactivating light. Different action spectra have been found for photorepair of different organisms (6); for E. coli and the yeast Saccharomyces cerevisiae we found a broad maximum of effectiveness in the wavelength region 355 to 385 mm.

[1] Supported by Research Grants GM 12813, GM 13234, GM 16547, and Research Career Development Award (to W.H.) GM 34963 from the National Institute of General Medical Sciences.

The most detailed information about the mechanism of photoenzymatic repair has been obtained by using an in vitro system. It employs UV-irradiated transforming DNA of Hemophilus influenzae and extracts of yeast cells (Saccharomyces cerevisiae) containing the photoreactivating enzyme (7). The biological activity of the DNA, expressed by the number of transformed cells, permits quantitative determination of the amounts of UV photoproducts formed and repaired. Study of this biological effect on dependence of various experimental parameters has established the following reaction scheme (8,9):

$$E + S \; \underset{k_2}{\overset{k_1}{\rightleftharpoons}} \; ES \; \overset{\text{light}}{\underset{k_3}{\longrightarrow}} \; E + P$$

According to this scheme a molecule of the photoreactivating enzyme (E) binds in a reversible, light-independent reaction to a substrate molecule (S) (a pyrimidine dimer in DNA) to form a complex (ES). Upon absorption of photoreactivating light the complex is photolysed, thereby liberating the enzyme molecule and converting the substrate to the repair product (P) (the monomerized dimer).

Experimental work of various investigators over the past ten years has confirmed this scheme not only for the in vitro reaction, but also for photorepair within cellular systems. In recent years we have applied a new technique for such studies, that is, the use of single intense light flashes instead of continuous illumination. This technique permits a closer look at the repair process in terms of the physical-chemical events and their biological implications. The results obtained with the in vitro system as well as with E. coli cells and bacteriophages will be summarized briefly here and in the subsequent paper (10). For experimental details the reader is referred to the original publications (1, 3-5).

THE USE OF LIGHT FLASHES IN OUR STUDIES

Initial Considerations:

A detailed analysis of the photoenzymatic repair requires separate investigation of the first step of the reaction, "complex formation," and the second, "photolysis of complexes." This is difficult to achieve with the conventional technique of continuous illumination, since PRE molecules liberated by photolysis of existing complexes can enter the light-independent reaction again and lead to more repair. In contrast, a high intensity light flash of millisecond duration photolyses (and thus repairs) only those enzyme-substrate complexes ("ES complexes") which are present at the moment of the flash. For this reason, the flash technique permits separate quantitative study of the two reaction steps, provided the following requirements are met:

1. A single flash must cause a measurable repair effect in the biological system used.

2. One must be able to relate the magnitude of the observed effect with the number of physical-chemical events (that is, dimers monomerized) by which it is caused.

3. One must know what fraction of the ES complexes present are repaired by a single flash.

We will see that all of these requirements have been satisfied in our experimental work which was carried out with a rather simple device described elsewhere (1,5). It consists of four or six electronic flash units designed for photographic use, mounted symmetrically around a center where the sample is located. The flash units are discharged either simultaneously or successively, the light being filtered through blue glass.

Conditions for Observing a Biological Effect:

It is implicit from the reaction scheme that a single flash can cause a measurable biological effect only under conditions where an appreciable fraction of the UV lesions

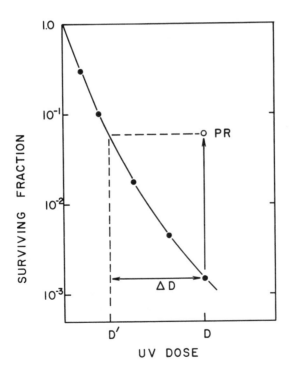

Fig 1. Quantitative characterization of photoenzymatic repair by the dose decrement.

exists in complexed form. With the in vitro system this requirement is easily met by choosing suitable concentrations of PRE and UV-irradiated DNA for the reaction mixture. To find appropriate conditions for studying the in vivo reaction is more difficult, since E. coli cells contain only a rather small number of PRE molecules, a point to be discussed later. An appreciable survival increase by a single flash therefore can be expected only in very UV-sensitive systems, where the survival is markedly affected by a difference of a few UV photoproducts. For this reason we used mainly cells of the dark-repair-defective strain B_{s-1}.

Relation Between Photoreactivation Effect and Number of Dimers Repaired:

The example in Figure 1 illustrates our considerations for relating quantitatively the observed biological effects with the molecular events occurring at the sites of the UV photoproducts. A UV dose D leads to a certain survival in the dark. As a result of photoenzymatic repair by a flash (or by any kind of illumination) the survival increases to the level marked "PR," which is identical with the dark survival obtained with a (smaller) UV dose D'. We call the difference $D-D'$ (or ΔD) the *dose decrement*. It is the portion of the UV dose whose inactivating effect is annulled by the photoreactivating treatment.

We can assume reasonably that the number of dimers repaired, as expressed by the dose decrement ΔD, closely resembles the number of dimers produced by an equal dose increment ΔD. The latter is known for 254 nm radiation[2] and for the DNA's used in our experiments (11,14). A dose decrement of 1 erg mm^{-2} corresponds to repair of about 6.5 dimers in the E. coli chromosome (4), and about 2.2×10^9 dimers per μg of Hemophilus DNA (1). All our calculated numbers or concentrations of dimers produced, dimers repaired and complexes present, are based on these figures.

Fraction of ES Complexes Repaired by a Single Flash:

The following results show that a single light flash as used in our experiments photolyses virtually all of the ES complexes present at that time. The evidence is two-fold: (a) Figure 2 shows that the level of photoreactivation of phage T1 or of transforming DNA obtained with a 4-unit flash is the same as with a 3-, 2- or 1-unit flash; only at a still lower flash intensity would the effect begin to drop. We conclude from this result that the extent of the photorepair cannot be limited by the amount of light, even in the case of a 1-unit flash, but must be limited by the number of ES complexes present. (b) We will see later that under certain conditions, one single flash is sufficient to produce the same maximal level of photoreactivation that is obtainable with continuous illumination. This is only feasible if the probability for photolysis by one flash is very close to unity.

[2]All our UV-irradiations were carried out with a low-pressure mercury-vapor lamp which emits in the far UV almost monochromatic 254 nm radiation.

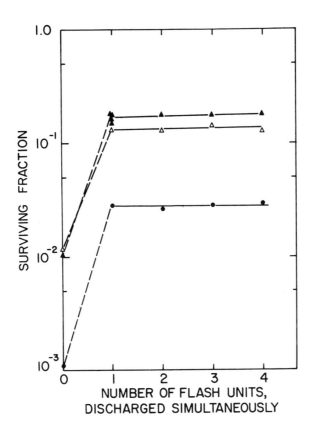

Fig 2. Survival increase resulting from a single flash of varying strength. •, Phage T1 (280 erg mm^{-2} UV) in B$_{s-1}$ cells, ▲, △, Hemophilus transforming DNA (2000 erg mm^{-2} UV); two experiments with different PRE/substrate ratios.

KINETICS OF COMPLEX FORMATION IN THE DARK

To illustrate the potentiality of the flash method for studying photoenzymatic repair, we will show first its use for establishing the kinetics of ES complex formation. In a typical experiment, a single flash is applied to a sample at various times after PRE and substrate begin to react. For the in vitro system time zero is when PRE is added to the irradiated DNA; for the cellular system it is the time at which the substrate is created by irradiation. The results of such experiments are shown in Figures 3 and 4.

We see in Figure 3 that it takes about five minutes at room temperature for the B$_{s-1}$ cells to reach the dark equilibrium of complex formation. The ordinate, $\Delta D/\Delta D_{max}$, expresses the fraction of complexed lesions among the total photorepairable lesions. If

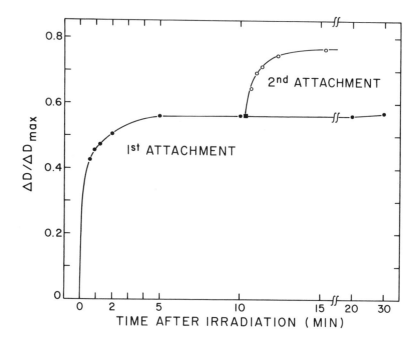

Fig 3. Kinetics of ES complex formation in the dark for E. coli B_{s-1} cells irradiated with 4.8 erg mm^{-2}.

the first flash is given after the equilibrium is reached, and a second flash is applied at fixed intervals thereafter, a new "round of complex formation" is observed due to liberation of PRE molecules by the first photolysis. In E. coli the kinetics of the second round is similar to the first.

For the same kind of experiment done with the in vitro system, the first and second rounds of complex formation can differ appreciably, as seen in Figure 4. Under the conditions of this particular experiment the concentrated mixture requires at least two to four minutes for reaching the equilibrium in the first round, while a 5-fold diluted mixture requires 30 minutes. In the second round the concentrated mixture requires only a few seconds and the diluted mixture not more than four minutes for reaching the new equilibrium. Theoretical considerations suggest that this difference is due to clustering of the substrate: each DNA molecule contains more than a hundred dimers, but even in the higher concentrated reaction mixture individual DNA molecules are well separated from each other. Thus, the average distance which an enzyme molecule has to travel for the first attachment is considerably greater than for the second attachment, where it is already close to the remaining substrate. Such a difference is not expected in E. coli cells containing only a single DNA molecule which is highly coiled.

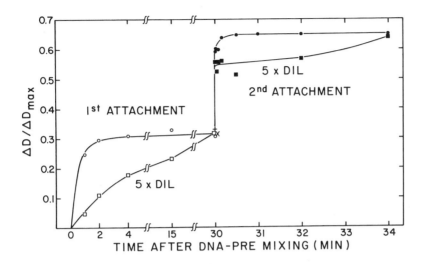

Fig 4. Kinetics of ES complex formation in the dark for Hemophilus transforming DNA in vitro. ●, ○, Reaction mixture containing 0.17 μg/ml DNA, UV-irradiated with 2400 erg mm^{-2} and 1.33 mg/ml PRE-containing extract (5 to 10-fold purified over crude extract). ■, □ Reaction mixture containing 1/5 the above concentrations.

The relative slow kinetics of complex formation in our experiments is mainly due to the low concentrations of *both* enzyme and substrate. It is not the result of a low reaction rate constant k_1, as will be seen in the following paper (10). Since calculating this rate constant requires knowledge of the absolute number of PRE molecules involved, we will describe first how this number is determined.

Determination of the Number of PRE Molecules:

In essence, our quantitative analysis of the data involves the following logical steps: 1. we observe a biological effect resulting from a single flash; 2. we calculate from it the number of dimers repaired; 3. we equate this number with the number of ES complexes photolysed; and, 4. we equate this with the number of ES complexes present at the time of the flash.

By the same reasoning we are also able to determine the number of photoreactivating enzyme molecules in the in vitro reaction mixture or in a cell. All that is required is to have the substrate in excess, sufficient to bind virtually all of the enzyme. Under these conditions the number of ES complexes, of course, equals the number of PRE molecules. It is understood that for these types of experiments the time allowed before flashing must be sufficient to guarantee maximum complex formation.

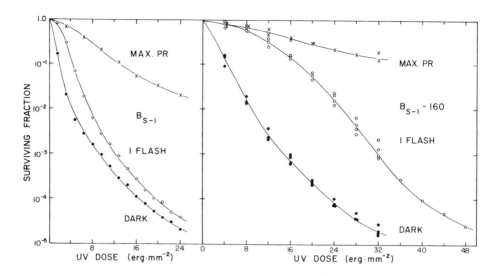

Fig 5. Survival of irradiated stationary phase E. coli cells. •, without photorepair; ○, with photo-repair by a single flash; x, with maximum photorepair by continuous white light illumination. Left panel: strain B_{s-1}. Right panel: strain B_{s-1}-160.

E. coli B_{s-1}: If UV-irradiation of cells creates enough substrate to bind all PRE molecules, the number of ES complexes (and thus the dose decrement) should have its maximum value and should not increase upon further UV irradiation. The left panel of Figure 5 shows results obtained with stationary phase B_{s-1} cells, where the dose decrement by a single flash was studied as a function of the UV dose.

At all exposures between 6.4 erg mm^{-2} and 24 erg mm^{-2} the dose decrement by a single flash stays constant at about 3 erg mm^{-2} (Fig 6), corresponding to repair of about 20 pyrimidine dimers per cell. Consequently, not more than about 20 (active) PRE molecules seem to be present in such a cell.

Other E. coli strains: With the same method we obtained even lower estimates of 12 to 15 molecules per cell for UV-sensitive derivatives of E. coli K12. To test whether in UV-resistant strains the PRE content might be higher, we infected comparatively B_{s-1} and B/r cells (the latter representing the wild-type resistance) with UV-irradiated T-even phages (T4v^-x^-) and studied their photorepair after a single flash. Both UV inactivation and photorepair of the phage were virtually the same in the two host strains, suggesting that the low PRE content is characteristic of E. coli in general.

B_{s-1} mutants: In view of the low PRE content we considered the possible occurrence of mutants producing more PRE as a result of some regulatory defect. Using as a criterion the expected greater survival increase by a single flash, we screened for such mutants after mutagenic treatment with N-methyl-N′-nitro-N-nitrosoguanidine, and indeed found several. Strain B_{s-1}-160, which has the highest PRE content, gives the flash effects shown on the right panel of Figure 5. We see that at sufficiently low UV doses a single flash leads to maximal photoreactivation of this strain.

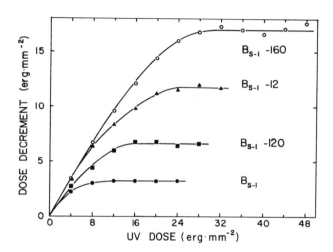

Fig 6. Dose decrements resulting from a single flash exposure in E. coli B_{s-1} and three mutant strains, as a function of UV dose. The plateau level permits calculation of the number of PRE molecules per cell in the different strains.

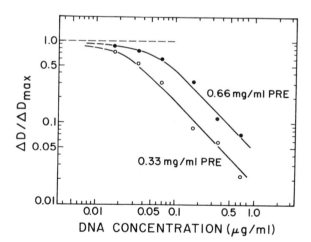

Fig 7. Determination of the number of PRE molecules in vitro. The dose decrement obtained with a single flash, relative to the maximally possible dose decrement, is plotted as a function of the concentration of irradiated DNA (1920 erg mm^{-2}) for two concentrations of the PRE-containing extract. With the information given in the text, one calculates a content of approximately 7×10^{10} and 1.4×10^{11} PRE molecules per ml for the two extract concentrations.

The dose decrements obtained at various UV doses with the original B_{s-1} strain and with our mutants are summarized in Figure 6. From the plateau levels of ΔD we calculate numbers of 20, 43, 75 and 110 PRE molecules, respectively.

In vitro reaction mixtures: The flash technique has been used in the analogous manner to determine the number of PRE molecules contained in yeast cell extracts used for studies of the reaction in vitro. Again, at a sufficient excess of substrate all PRE should be complexed and ΔD should become constant. Therefore, $\Delta D/\Delta D_{max}$ (that is, the fraction of lesions repaired by a single flash among the total repairable lesions) is expected to decrease proportionally with increasing substrate concentration.

The approximately $45°$ slope in the log-log plot of Figure 7 indicates that this is the case. Theoretical considerations show that straight extrapolation of the curves to a $\Delta D/\Delta D_{max}$ value of 1 gives on the abscissa the DNA concentration at which the number of substrate molecules equals the number of PRE molecules. The latter can thus be calculated by taking into account the particular UV dose applied in this experiment. Assuming that the molecular weight of PRE does not exceed 10^5 daltons (12) we can estimate that the PRE constitutes less than 10^{-5} of the total protein in yeast cells. This is the same order of magnitude which one calculates for E. coli B_{s-1}.

CONCLUSIONS

I wish to finish my paper with a few thoughts concerning the very low number of PRE molecules found in E. coli cells. Natural UV-radiation in the form of sunlight is always accompanied by high intensity photoreactivating light. Sunlight exposure of PRE-containing cells and, comparatively, of mutant cells lacking PRE activity has indicated that PRE is of considerable advantage for the cell survival (2). The small amount of PRE under most circumstances is sufficient to guarantee rapid removal of the lesions; therefore, any greater enzyme content would be wasteful for the cell.

On the other hand, the low number of PRE molecules may make it understood why this enzyme is found in many bacteria which are only occasionally exposed to UV. A regulatory system which would produce PRE only when it is needed would probably be more "costly" for the cell in terms of metabolism than the production of the small amount of PRE at all time. Similar considerations might apply for higher organisms, where the enzyme has been found in tissues in which it does not have any obvious function. One could simply assume that the enzyme is there because the organism profits from its photorepair function in other cells (perhaps during early developmental stages) and that its production cannot be shut off in cells where it is not needed.

In this paper we have discussed the potential value of the flash photolysis method for studying photoenzymatic repair and the basic considerations which enable us to use this method for a quantitative analysis. We have shown a few applications of the method, that is, establishing the net reaction kinetics of complex formation and determining the number of PRE molecules. This information serves as a background for the following paper by Rupert et al, dealing mainly with the physical-chemical characterization of the individual reaction steps.

REFERENCES

1. Harm, H. and Rupert, C. S.: Mutat. Res., 6:355, 1968.
2. Harm, W.: In: Symposium on the Mutation process. The Physiology of Gene and Mutation Expression. Edited by M. Kohoutova and J. Hubacek. Academia, Prague, pp 51-59, 1965.
3. Harm, W.: Mutat. Res., 8:411, 1969.
4. Harm, W., Harm, H. and Rupert, C. S.: Mutat. Res., 6:371, 1968.
5. Harm, W., Rupert, C. S. and Harm, H.: In: Photophysiology. Edited by A. C. Giese, Vol 6, pp 279-324, 1971. Academic Press, N.Y.
6. Jagger, J., Takebe, H. and Snow, J. M.: Photochem. Photobiol., 12:185, 1970.
7. Rupert, C. S.: J. Gen. Physiol., 43:573, 1960.
8. Rupert, C. S.: J. Gen. Physiol., 45:703, 1962a.
9. Rupert, C. S.: J. Gen. Physiol., 45:725, 1962b.
10. Rupert, C. S., Harm, W. and Harm, H.: This Symposium, p 64, 1971.
11. Rupp, W. D. and Howard-Flanders, P.: J. Molec. Biol., 31:291, 1968.
12. Saito, N. and Werbin, H.: Biochemistry, 9:2610, 1970.
13. Setlow, R. B.: Science, 153:379, 1966.
14. Setlow, R. B. and Carrier, W. L.: J. Molec. Biol., 17:237, 1966.

PHOTOENZYMATIC REPAIR OF DNA

II. PHYSICAL/CHEMICAL CHARACTERIZATION OF THE PROCESS[1]

Claud S. Rupert, Walter Harm and Helga Harm

Division of Biology, University of Texas at Dallas
Dallas, Texas

INTRODUCTION

The photoenzymatic repair of ultraviolet damage to DNA, as an explicitly recognized mechanism which could be carried out in vitro, has its fifteenth birthday this month, born here at The Johns Hopkins Medical Institutions in the laboratory of Professor Roger Herriott (6,25). The large magnitude of the phenomenon, and its precise controllability by light, firmly established the reality of DNA repair and the importance of this restoration in cellular recovery from radiation injury (27). Thus it may have served as a stimulus toward recognition of other DNA repair processes (3,11,12,31).

Besides being the first such repair process to be discovered, it is also the simplest: a single enzyme acting on a single class of pyrimidine photoproducts to reconvert them to the original bases. Therefore, it is probably the most primitive in an evolutionary sense. Since it removes harmful photoproducts produced in DNA by the shortest wavelengths of normal sunlight, utilizing the energy of longer wavelengths which arrive at the same time (26,30), we can imagine it playing a role in the first successful incursions of life into the open daylight, a possibility consistent with its presence in all orders of living things today.

Yet, although this mechanism still confers a survival advantage on cells exposed to sunlight (13) and would presumably continue to be selected for under these circumstances, it is far less versatile in the range of damage it can handle than the excision-resynthesis and recombination repairs covered by other speakers in this Symposium. Indeed, apparently it has become superfluous in cells of the higher mammals, since it cannot be detected there at all (4). Consequently one might ask why, aside from idle curiosity, it should be worth the trouble to characterize its detailed steps.

An answer lies in the unique experimental control afforded by its dependence on light, which opens the way for information not readily obtainable with other DNA enzymes. Like the incising endonuclease which performs the initial step of excision-resynthesis repair, and like DNA-dependent RNA polymerase, the photoreactivating enzyme (PRE) must recognize and attach to appropriate sites on the nucleic acid. The forces leading to such recognition and attachment have a general interest beyond the particular enzyme system in which they are studied. Only to the extent that we ultimately

[1] Supported by Research Grants GM 16547, GM 13234, GM 12813 and Research Career Development Award (to W.H.) GM 34963 from the National Institute of General Medical Sciences.

understand them can one hope to design agents with deliberately intended effects on DNA metabolism (for example, drugs inhibiting repair to increase the radiation sensitivity of target cells during radiotherapy) rather than simply to proceed by trial and error. The photorepair process, occurring within the enzyme-substrate complex after attachment, involves excited states of nucleic acid components which are related to those involved in creation of the original damage, and hence have their own interest. It seems appropriate, therefore, to utilize any opportunities for understanding the elementary steps of this easily manipulated repair reaction, both in vivo and in vitro.

The work summarized here represents a beginning in this direction. Most of the practical experimental details are outlined in other recent publications (7-9,14-16).

THE MEASUREMENT OF REACTION RATE CONSTANTS

Two things limit the clarity with which we can analyze the fundamental events in this system. The first, described by Harm et al (17) (referred to subsequently as Paper I) is the confinement of the substrate sites to large pieces of DNA which are relatively isolated from each other in solution. Within each of the resulting substrate clusters the "local" substrate concentration, c_L, is larger than the average concentration, c_A, over the bulk solution in vitro. Because the chemical potential of the substrate depends on both these concentrations, the attachment kinetics simply cannot be described in full using only one of them, along with the concentration of the enzyme and a single rate constant. From the average fragment size in the DNA preparation ($\approx 20 \times 10^6$ daltons) the known dimensions of DNA in solution (22) and the number of dimers per unit of DNA (estimated as in Paper I) it is clear c_L/c_A may be at least 10 or more at the DNA concentrations of many reaction mixtures. As a first approximation, however, we ignore this problem and deal only with the average concentrations.

The second limitation lies in the heterogeneity of the substrate. The three different types of pyrimidine dimers, $\widehat{TT}$, $\widehat{CC}$ and $\widehat{CT}$, formed by UV-irradiation of DNA are known to disappear at different rates during photoreactivation (32) showing that they behave differently in at least one part of the reaction. Even ignoring the difference between $\widehat{CT}$ and $\widehat{TC}$, and any influence of nearest neighbors, we therefore are dealing with a mixture of substrates, and for the most part obtain only weighted averages of their measured properties. The relative contribution of different substrate types to these averages will generally not be the same for the different rate constants measured.

Within the uncertainties imposed by these factors we can determine the three rate constants appearing in the reaction scheme (outlined in Paper I): k_1, the second order rate constant for enzyme-substrate complex formation; k_2, the first order constant for dark dissociation of complexes; and k_3, the first order rate constant for their photolysis, a constant which depends on light intensity.

The constant k_1 is most readily measured when the reverse reaction (dark dissociation) is negligible, which will be true whenever there is sufficient illumination intensity to give $k_3 \gg k_2$. A practical equivalent to this condition is provided by frequent flash illumination (about one per second), each flash converting nearly all of the existing ES to E + P. The sufficiency of the flash rate is assured if changing it moderately still gives the same results. Under these conditions the concentration [ES] fluctuates in a range of very small values, and the enzyme concentration remains almost constant at the initial value $[E]_o$, while the substrate, initially at concentration $[S]_o$, disappears in a pseudo-first-order manner: $-d[S]/dt \approx k_1 [E]_o [S]$, or, $\ln [S]_t/[S]_o = -k_1 [E]_o t$. Measuring the fraction of the initial substrate remaining at various times t after mixing enzyme and irradiated DNA under these circumstances gives $k_1 [E]_o$. When $[E]_o$ is determined (as described in Paper I) k_1 can be found. The effects of substrate clustering in vitro will tend to make this k_1 value higher than would be the case if the substrate were randomly distributed, although the ratios of total enzyme and substrate are chosen to minimize this.

Panel A of Figure 1 shows the result of such a measurement in an in vitro reaction mixture of yeast photoreactivating enzyme and irradiated Hemophilus influenzae transforming DNA. The fraction of the substrate remaining is measured by the corresponding dose decrement (described in Paper I): $[S]_t/[S]_o = 1 - (\Delta D/\Delta D_{max})$. The

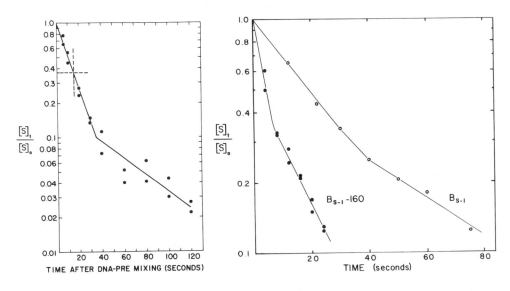

Fig 1. Measurement of the reaction rate constant k_1. The fraction of photorepairable damage remaining unrepaired is shown as a function of time after PRE is mixed with substrate under frequent flash illumination.
A. For a mixture of yeast PRE and transforming DNA in vitro. The reciprocal of the time at which 37% remains is taken as $k_1 [E]_o$.
B. For E. coli B_{s-1} and B_{s-1}-160 cells, the entire UV dose being given within one second at t = 0. (From H. Harm and Rupert (9) and W. Harm (14))

expected heterogeneity is evident, but from the initial slope a weighted average k_1 of about 2.6×10^7 liter mole^{-1} sec^{-1} can be obtained. Varying both the DNA and enzyme concentrations leads to the same measured k_1, but the value varies with temperature, pH, ionic strength and to some degree with the exact ionic make-up of the reaction mixture. As will be seen below, employing an entirely different method for estimating $[S]_t/[S]_o$ leads to similar k_1 values.

Panel B of Figure 1 shows the result of applying this technique to two strains of E. coli cells, the measured time under flash illumination beginning with a one-second-long UV-irradiation which creates the substrate. Strain B_{s-1}-160, containing about five times as many PRE molecules as B_{s-1}, shows a $k_1 [E]_o$ between four and five times as large. Assuming cell volumes of about 10^{-15} liters this corresponds to $k_1 \approx 1 \times 10^6$ liter mole^{-1}.

These different values for k_1 in vitro and in vivo actually are fairly consistent. It can be shown, by adding glycerol or sucrose to reaction mixtures in vitro, that k_1 is inversely proportional to the viscosity, and it is known that the intracellular viscosity is of the order of 25 times that of water (23).

The constant k_2 can be determined in several ways, none entirely free of objection, which, however, are in rough agreement. The first depends simply on the attainment of dark equilibrium between enzyme and substrate. Under these conditions

$$\frac{[ES]_{eq}}{([E]_o - [ES]_{eq})([S]_o - [ES]_{eq})} = \frac{k_1}{k_2}$$

The fraction of the total substrate complexed, $[ES]_{eq}/[S]_o$, is measured by the fraction which can be abolished by a single flash. In a properly designed reaction mixture all the other quantities can be determined with sufficient accuracy to calculate k_1/k_2, and if k_1 is measured under the same conditions, k_2 can be found.

Two other methods both start with an equilibrium in which a high proportion of substrate is complexed. A change then is introduced abruptly into the reaction mixture which interferes with re-formation of any dissociating complexes. If no complexes whatever could re-form (that is, if $k_1 = 0$) we would observe decay of the existing complexes: $d[ES]/dt = -k_2[ES]$, or $\ln [ES]_t/[ES]_{t=o} = -k_2 t$. Single flash illumination applied to samples of the reaction mixture at successively later times, then would show the relative number of complexes remaining (since ΔD is proportional to $[ES]$), and permit a measure of k_2. In practice some re-formation of complex occurs, and the system only shifts toward a new equilibrium with much lower complexing. However, k_2 can be estimated from the first order rate of approach to this new equilibrium.

One method for hindering re-formation of complexes is to add a large excess of biologically distinguishable, heavily irradiated DNA (for example, calf thymus) which can compete with the substrate for newly-liberated enzyme. Another way is to add a relatively high concentration of caffeine, which complexes with the substrate and tends to block attachment of the enzyme. The first procedure detects only those dissociations where the enzyme diffuses far enough from the DNA on which it was originally bound to reach a competing substrate cluster, and may therefore underestimate k_2. The caffeine on the other hand actually might facilitate the dissociation of otherwise stable complexes and correspondingly overestimate the constant.

With the in vitro system the equilibrium and competing substrate methods give similar k_2 values of the order of 2×10^{-3} sec^{-1} at 23°C (depending also, however, on pH and ionic strength). Results with the caffeine method are about 4-fold higher but somewhat less reproducible.

In vivo the competing substrate method can be applied to irradiated T1 phage infecting E. coli cells, using chloramphenicol to arrest phage development during the measurement manipulations. After equilibration of the cell's enzyme with the substrate in phage DNA, the competing substrate is created by irradiating briefly the infected cell. This may be done by using a dose which produces little additional phage inactivation, but adds a great excess of competing substrate, because of the large ratio of bacterial to phage DNA. The result gives a k_2 value similar to that obtained in vitro, around 2×10^{-3} sec^{-1}. On the other hand, the equilibrium method applied to B_{s-1}-160 cells gives about 5×10^{-3} sec^{-1}, while the caffeine method gives a still higher value of about 1.3×10^{-2} sec^{-1}.

Heterogeneity of the substrate with respect to k_2 values is evident with both the competing substrate and caffeine methods, in vivo and in vitro.

The constant k_3, depends on the light intensity, I, and is zero in the dark. It is consequently convenient for purposes of analysis to define a photolytic constant k_p by setting $k_3 = k_p I$. Under the simplest conditions, k_p is independent of I (that is, k_3 is directly proportional to the light intensity). Otherwise it is simply a coefficient describing the intensity dependence of k_3.

If all substrate is complexed with enzyme, $[ES] = [S]_o$ and we have for continuous illumination $-d[S]/dt = k_p I [S]$. If k_p is independent of $[S]$ this integrates to $\ln [S]_t/[S]_o = -k_p L$, where $L = It$ is the incident light dose measured in erg mm^{-2}, or equivalent units. The condition $[ES] = [S]$ is met if single-flash illumination applied to a sample gives the same dose reduction as long-applied continuous light.

Under these circumstances the decrease in $[S]_t/[S]_o$ as a function of light dose can be determined by the dose decrement (described in Paper I). Again the reaction shows a heterogeniety of the reacting material. The weighted average k_p, indicated by the initial rate, is of the order of 10^{-3} mm^2 erg^{-1} for the most effective wavelengths in vivo and in vitro.

Despite the uncertainties mentioned, these methods enable us to measure approximately the individual rate constants and not merely some combination of them as in the case in many other enzyme systems. The exact values of the constants are of less interest than their general magnitude and the manner in which they are affected by environmental parameters, since it is these details which relate to mechanisms of the individual steps in the reaction.

THERMODYNAMICS OF COMPLEX FORMATION

The thermodynamic quantities governing dark formation of the enzyme-substrate complex are each determined by several factors of varying interest in questions of mechanism. The enthalpy of complex formation, ΔH, depends not only on all changes in bonding during this process, but also on $\int_o^T \Delta C_p dT$, where ΔC_p is the increase in specific heat at constant pressure in complexing. For macromolecular interactions the latter term could be rather large (2). The entropy of complex formation, ΔS, depends on the increase in disorder of the entire system (enzyme, substrate and solvent), including that entailed in the free diffusion of the components through the solution. For two reactants forming one product, the latter contribution depends on concentration, and ΔS therefore is usually expressed as the "standard" entropy change, ΔS^o, occurring when reactants and product are all at 1 M. However, because this choice is arbitrary the change also sometimes is given as the "unitary" entropy change, ΔS_u; that is, the entropy change *excluding* the part due to the translational diffusion of all components. It can be shown that in very dilute aqueous solution $\Delta S_u \approx \Delta S^o + 8$ kcal mole^{-1} (19).

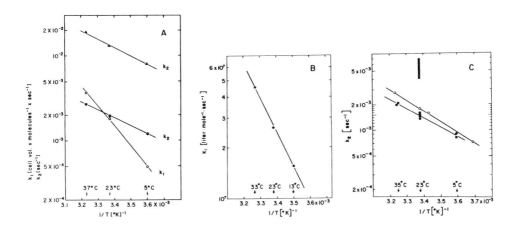

Fig 2. Temperature dependence of rate constants k_1 for complex formation and k_2 for dissociation presented as Arrhenius plots.
A. Values of constants in cells of E. coli B$_{s-1}$, showing for k_2 the different results given by the caffeine method (▲) and the competing substrate method (●). (The numerical values for k_1, given in cell volumes molecule^{-1} sec^{-1} can be converted approximately to liter mole^{-1} sec^{-1} by multiplying by 6 x 10^8).
B. Values for k_1 in vitro.
C. Values for k_2 in vitro, showing the different results by the competing substrate method (●) and the equilibrium method (o). The shaded vertical bar at 23°C shows the range of values obtained by the caffeine method at this single temperature. (From W. Harm (14) and H. Harm and Rupert (9))

The same things can be said of the enthalpies and entropies of activation, $\Delta H\ddagger$ and $\Delta S\ddagger$, associated with each rate constant, which express the changes in these thermodynamic quantities on passing to the "activated" state from which the forward or reverse reaction occurs.

All these quantities may be estimated from the variations of rate constants k_1 and k_2 with temperature. The results of such measurements in vivo and in vitro are shown in Figure 2 and Table I. Both rate constants are well described by Arrhenius expressions with similar activation energies and frequency factors for the same constants in vivo and in vitro. Because the frequency factors, in effect, are measured by long extrapolations of the experimental curves to $1/T = 0$ they are only roughly determined. The

TABLE I

Arrhenius Expressions for k_1 and k_2

The value of each rate constant in Figure 2 can be expressed as a function of temperature by $k = A \exp(-E_A/RT)$, using the frequency factors A and the activation energies tabulated below.

System	Rate Constant	A	E_A
E. coli PRE in vivo	k_1	$1.5 \times 10^{14} M^{-1} sec^{-1}$	11 kcal mole^{-1}
	k_2 (Compet. Substr. Method)	4.3 sec^{-1}	4.5 kcal mole^{-1}
	k_2 (Caffeine Method)	29 sec^{-1}	4.5 kcal mole^{-1}
Yeast PRE in vitro	k_1	$1.6 \times 10^{14} M^{-1} sec^{-1}$	9.3 kcal mole^{-1}
	k_2 (Compet. Substr. Method)	7 sec^{-1}	5.1 kcal mole^{-1}
	k_2 (Equilib. Method)	30 sec^{-1}	5.7 kcal mole^{-1}

uncertainty is more obvious for k_2 because of the additional differing results of different measurement methods, but it exists also for k_1. Hence, although the general similarity in magnitude of these factors in vivo and in vitro is significant, close agreements may be only accidental.

The equilibrium constant $K = k_1/k_2$ at each temperature can be determined from the data of Figure 2. (In the case of the open circles in Panel C of Figure 2, K was the quantity actually determined, from which the plotted k_2 was calculated.) From this we obtain the standard free energy of the complex-forming reaction as a function of temperature: $\Delta F° = -RT \ln K$, and therefore can resolve $\Delta F°$ into its enthalpy and entropy terms: $\Delta F° = \Delta H - T\Delta S°$.

For the yeast enzyme in vitro this gives for the various determinations $\Delta H = 3.6$ to 4.2 kcal $\cdot$ mole^{-1}, and $\Delta S° = 58$ to 61 cal $\cdot$ mole$^{-1} \cdot$ deg^{-1}. For the E. coli enzyme in vivo we find $\Delta H = 6.5$ kcal $\cdot$ mole^{-1} and $\Delta S° = 58$ to 62 cal $\cdot$ mole$^{-1} \cdot$ deg^{-1}. The striking fact both in vitro and in vivo is that complex formation is *endothermic* ($\Delta H > 0$). The only reason for stability of the complex, and the large equilibrium constant, which is able to maintain the enzyme and substrate in highly complexed form at concentrations around $10^{-9} M$, is the large entropy increase during coupling.

A number of other examples of entropy-driven reactions involving macro-molecules are known. The binding of isoleucyl-tRNA synthetase to isoleucine-tRNA falls in this class (34), as does the binding of DNA-dependent RNA polymerase to DNA (P. Witonsky, personal communication). Further cases arising in protein reactions have been tabulated by Kauzmann (19) who lists arguments that such behavior is consistent both with salt linkages (that is, ionic bonds between oppositely charged groups) and with hydrophobic bonds (that is, the tendency of nonpolar structures to be squeezed out of aqueous surroundings into association with other nonpolar groups).

In terms of absolute reaction rate theory (for example, Glasstone et al (5)), any rate constant can be expressed as $k = (kT/h)e^{\Delta S^{\ddagger}/R} e^{-\Delta H^{\ddagger}/RT}$, where k and h are Boltzmann's and Planck's constants, respectively. By comparison with the Arrhenius expressions (Table I) $\Delta H^{\ddagger} = E_A - RT$, which, within the errors of measurement, is the same as E_A. These enthalpies of activation are in a range typical of many enzymes (21).

$\Delta S^{\ddagger}$ can be calculated from the measured frequency factors by the above relation: $\Delta S_1^{\ddagger}$ (associated with k_1) is about 4 cal mole^{-1} deg^{-1}, and $\Delta S_2^{\ddagger}$ (associated with k_2) about -54 to -58 cal mole^{-1} deg^{-1}. Before attempting to compare these it should be noted that, although $\Delta S_1^{\ddagger} - \Delta S_2^{\ddagger} = \Delta S^{\circ}$, both $\Delta S_1^{\ddagger}$ and ΔS° include the same arbitrary additive contribution stemming from the choice of a 1 M standard state, while $\Delta S_2^{\ddagger}$ does not (since no rendezvous of two molecules is involved in the activation ES $\rightarrow$ ES‡). One can compare better the unitary entropies with $\Delta S_2^{\ddagger}$: $\Delta S_{1u}^{\ddagger} \approx \Delta S_1^{\ddagger} + 8 = 12$ cal mole^{-1} deg^{-1} and $\Delta S_u \approx 66$ to 70 cal mole^{-1} deg^{-1}.

For complex formation (k_1) the entropy of activation is positive; that is, the activated state is statistically favored, although in the temperature range where the enzyme is stable (for instance, below 320 °K) it compensates less than half of $\Delta H^{\ddagger}$, and leaves the free energy of activation positive. In the case of k_2, however, the activation entropy is large and negative, amounting to a major part of the total entropy decrease during dissociation. Thus, a relatively high degree of order must be introduced into the complex and/or surroundings before dissociation even can begin. This, rather than the formation of very strong bonds, is the reason for the low probability of dissociation.

ELECTROSTATIC EFFECTS IN COMPLEX FORMATION

The existence of electrostatic forces in macromolecular interactions can be shown by the effects of electrolyte concentration. In the present case such forces might affect the structure of the enzyme, the structure of the substrate (which lies at a locally denatured region when it occurs in a double-stranded DNA), or their interactions.

Measurements of k_1 and k_2 in reaction mixtures of different ionic make-up show that both constants are extremely sensitive to the ionic strength μ. In the case of k_1, a three-fold change in μ above or below the optimum decreases the constant by an order of magnitude. While it is difficult to measure k_2 when k_1 is small (on account of the difficulty in obtaining sufficient complex formation initially), k_2 changes at least as rapidly as k_1 in the low μ region.

A well-authenticated theory by Brønsted predicts that if two small ions of algebraic charge Z_A and Z_B react in water at 25°C, the forward rate constant at very low ionic strength can be expressed by $\log_{10}k = \log_{10}k^\circ + 1.02\, Z_A Z_B \sqrt{\mu}$, k° corresponding to the zero-ionic-strength rate (for example, Glasstone et al (5)). Thus a logarithmic plot of k vs $\sqrt{\mu}$ will have a slope essentially equal in sign and magnitude to $Z_A Z_B$. With macromolecules the situation is more complex, but a linearity of log k with $\sqrt{\mu}$ may nevertheless hold in some cases (20).

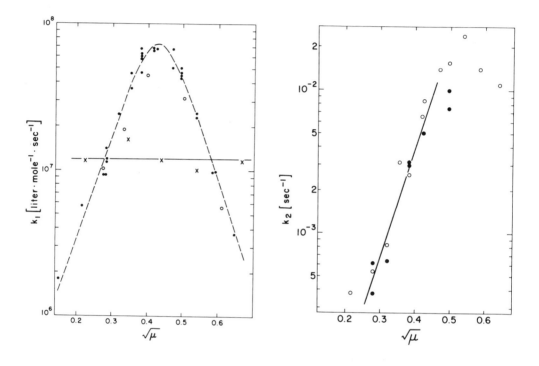

Fig 3. Dependence of rate constants k_1 and k_2 on ionic strength μ.
A. Data for k_1. Measurements with irradiated H. influenzae DNA using either dose decrement (•) or competitive inhibition (o) fit the empirical expression given in the text (dashed curve). Measurements with irradiated dA:dT (x) show no variation with μ.
B. Data for k_2 determined by either the equilibrium method (o) or the competing substrate method (•). (In part from H. Harm and Rupert (9))

Such a plot is shown in Panel A of Figure 3 (solid data points) for k_1 in our reaction. The result is linear over the low μ range up to about 0.14, with a slope of approximately + 7. At higher ionic strength it deviates from this, as is not surprising, since the simple theory should not be expected to hold this high. What is remarkable is the rapid shift to another linear relation having a slope of the same magnitude but opposite sign. The dashed empirical curve in the figure is $1/k_1 = 1/k_{1a} + 1/k_{1b}$, with $k_{1a} = 1.1 \times 10^5$ exp $(16.4 \sqrt{\mu})$, and $k_{1b} = 1.7 \times 10^{11}$ exp $(-16.4 \sqrt{\mu})$ liter mole^{-1}sec^{-1}. Evidently the smaller of the two quantities k_{1a} and k_{1b} determines k_1.

Over the restricted range where k_2 can be measured, an analogous plot in Panel B of Figure 3 can be represented as $k_2 = 3.5 \times 10^{-6} \exp (16.4 \sqrt{\mu}) \sec^{-1}$. The two rate constant expressions are clearly related.

It is possible in the k_1 measurement to employ other means than the biological dose reduction for determining the values of $[S]_t/[S]_o$ plotted in Figure 1. If irradiated nontransforming DNA is added to a reaction mixture of irradiated transforming DNA and PRE the rate of photorecovery is competitively inhibited (28). As shown schematically in the upper panel of Figure 4, the time required for repair is increased by the same factor at all levels of recovery, so that on a logarithmic time plot the recovery curve (lower panel

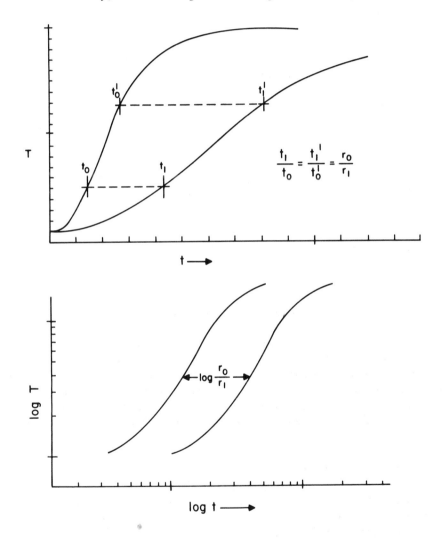

Fig 4. Schematic representation of competitive inhibition of transforming DNA repair by irradiated extraneous DNA. The inhibition multiplies the time required to reach any level of recovery by the same factor. T represents the number of bacterial transformants produced under standard conditions by a mixture of transforming DNA and PRE illuminated for time t, with and without inhibition.

of Figure 4) is simply displaced along the time axis. If we call the rate of the uninhibited reaction r_o and the rate with inhibition r, this curve displacement gives r_o/r directly. The inhibition, defined as (r_o/r)-1, is found proportional to the concentration of competing DNA when a fixed dose has been administered, or to the dose given this DNA when it is present at a fixed concentration; that is, it is proportional to the concentration of competing damage. Consequently if we mix samples of irradiated nontransforming DNA with PRE and immediately apply repeated light flashes for various times before deproteinizing and dialyzing them, we can use their competitive inhibitory power, as revealed in a subsequent test, to determine $[S]_t/[S]_o$, and thus construct an analog of Figure 1. This procedure does not depend on any assumed relation of biological activity to the fraction of pyrimidine dimers removed.

The results of such a procedure applied to genetic-marker-free H. influenzae DNA are shown by the open circles in Panel A of Figure 3. Although these determinations were carried out nearly a year after the biological dose-reduction determinations, and used a different, more highly purified enzyme preparation, they clearly indicate similar ionic strength dependence. This not only confirms the ionic strength effect, but also supports the dose-reduction method of analysis.

The competitive inhibition method permits the measurement of rate constants in biologically inactive DNA, such as the synthetic dA:dT, which consists of paired homopolymer strands. The only photoreactivable UV damage produced in this polymer is thymine dimer. We have repeated the k_1 measurements at different ionic strengths with the results shown by the crosses in Panel A of Figure 3. Surprisingly, there is no clear dependence on μ over the entire range tested! Thus the ionic strength effect seems influenced strongly by the detailed structure of the *substrate,* and may reflect that feature more than details of the enzyme or enzyme-substrate interaction.

THE LIGHT-DEPENDENT REACTION

Cyclobutane-type pyrimidine dimers can be split into their constituent bases by ultraviolet wavelengths short enough for them to absorb directly, although this splitting is only partial in polynucleotides because these same wavelengths also form dimers. Low-efficiency sensitized dimer splitting has been obtained at wavelengths too long for direct absorption with derivatives of tryptophane (18) and anthraquinone (1). The photoenzymatic monomerization of dimers may be considered a highly effective form of sensitized splitting.

The initial photolysis rate in the enzyme-substrate complex is proportional to light intensity and, above $0°C$, is only marginally affected by temperature. Such behavior is consistent with photolysis of the complex by absorption of a single photon. For such a reaction it can be shown that k_p is related to the product of ϵ the molar extinction coefficient of the complexes and ϕ the quantum yield for photolysis (29):

$$\epsilon\phi \text{ [liter mole}^{-1} \text{ cm}^{-1}] = k_p \text{ [mm}^2 \text{ erg}^{-1}] \frac{5.2 \times 10^9}{\lambda \text{ [nm]}}$$

This relation applied to k_p for a series of monochromatic wavelengths with the yeast enzyme in vitro gives the *absolute* action spectrum shown in Figure 5 (the open triangles representing light intensities 10 times as high as the solid triangles).

We have recently obtained a mutant of a UV-sensitive strain of yeast, somewhat analogous to the B_{s-1}-160 strain of E. coli, which contains 4 to 5 times as many PRE molecules per cell as the parent strain. In cells of this strain it is possible to secure complexing of about 90% of the inactivating UV lesions in the cell at low doses, which is sufficient for approximate determination of the absolute action spectrum in vivo. The result is essentially the same as in Figure 5, except at 313 nm where the apparent $\epsilon\phi$ is lower due to some inactivation of the cells.

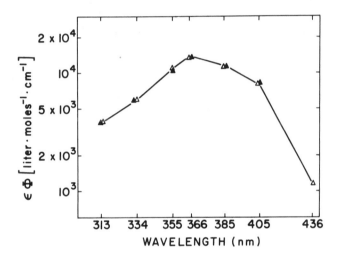

Fig 5. Absolute action spectrum for yeast PRE in vitro corresponding to the initial repair. (From H. Harm and Rupert (10))

With B_{s-1}-160, where essentially complete complexing of the substrate in vivo can be obtained, $\epsilon\phi$ for the most effective wavelengths is clearly higher than in the yeast system: about 2.4×10^4 liter mole^{-1} cm^{-1} at 385 nm compared with 1.4×10^4 at 366 nm in yeast.

These measured values set limits on ϵ and ϕ. Since $\phi \leq 1$, ϵ is not less than the measured value of $\epsilon\phi$ at each wavelength. Since it is unlikely that $\epsilon > 10^5$ liter mole^{-1} cm^{-1} for usual organic structures, ϕ is probably greater than 0.1 to 0.2, and may even approximate 1.

The apparent simplicity of the light reaction for the initial stages of repair disappears after about half the dimers have been removed. Below this value k_p decreases and becomes dependent on the intensity and continuity of illumination, as well as on the previous history of illumination of the enzyme.

A dependence on intensity implies that more than one photon must act within a limited period of time under these circumstances. Figure 6 illustrates the importance of the time interval over which the light is applied when $[S]_t/[S]_o$ is below 0.5. Here the effect of polychromic ("white") light delivered continuously for varying times is compared with different intensities of single-flash illumination, the dose scales being adjusted to agree in the initial repair range. Clearly complexes involving between 50% and 60% of the substrate, which show a k_p 5-fold smaller than the most rapidly repaired group under moderate continuous light intensity, can be photolyzed with the high initial k_p if they receive all their illumination within a millisecond.

The virtual independence of k_p and temperature found above $0^{\circ}C$ changes to a decrease with decreasing temperature below this range. A similar effect occurs both for E. coli PRE in cells and yeast enzyme in vitro (employing 20% glycerol in both cases to

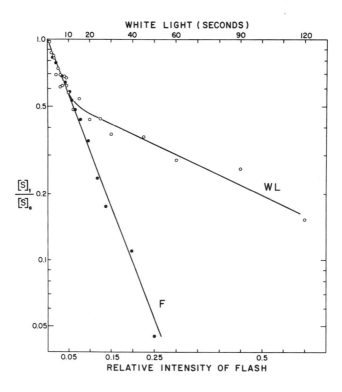

Fig 6. Fraction of fully-complexed substrate still unreacted as a function of relative light energy delivered either as a single flash (F), or as continuous "white" light (WL). (From H. Harm (7))

prevent ice crystal formation). As measured by flash illumination, k_p diminishes to about 5% of its room temperature value at $-120^\circ C$. Over this temperature range DNA undergoes a conformational change which changes the nature and amounts of the major thymine photoproducts (24) and it would seem likely that this fact is related to the observed change in $\epsilon\phi$ of the enzyme-substrate complexes.

CONCLUSION

The information which can be obtained about this enzymatic repair is clearly of a kind which concerns the elementary processes of individual reaction steps. Just as clearly it does not yet delineate any of them. It is not expected that the basic processes will be simple, for this or any other enzyme, since nature designed enzymes to perform needed functions, not merely to be easy to understand. It is entirely possible that a mix of mechanisms, including electrostatic and hydrophobic interactions, conformational changes and solvent effects, occurs in all parts of the reaction. Sorting out these possibilities and determining even the major influences acting at each stage will take more information than outlined here. However, more should be readily available.

The pH, for example, affects all steps, including the light-dependent one, but this has not been thoroughly explored. The effects of dielectric constant of the medium, as well as the interactions of pH and the ionic strength effect also remain to be worked out. For these purposes the availability of different forms of substrate, using the competitive inhibition assay for irradiated synthetic polydeoxynucleotides, or the newly-developed synthetic substrate $(pT)_4 p\widehat{TpT}(pT)_4$ (33) (which can be assayed by purely chemical means) will be indispensible. The great difference between DNA and dA:dT with respect to ionic strength shows that we cannot treat all substrates as equivalent.

The photoenzymatic repair process, in spite of its apparently secondary importance in cellular survival today, remains curiously close to the leading edge of our knowledge about repair processes, which is where it stood 15 years ago. By analogy and example it still seems capable of illustrating things about nucleic acid enzymes, including repair enzymes, which are hard to study in other systems. Thus, we may expect to see this adolescent subject continue to grow a while longer.

REFERENCES

1. Ben-Hur, E. and Rosenthal, I.: Photochem. Photobiol., 11:163, 1970.
2. Benzinger, T. H.: Nature, 229:100, 1971.
3. Boyce, R. P. and Howard-Flanders, P.: Proc. Nat. Acad. Sci. USA, 51:293, 1964.
4. Cook, J. S. and McGrath, J. R.: Proc. Nat. Acad. Sci. USA, 58:1359, 1967.
5. Glasstone, S., Laidler, K. J. and Eyring, H.: The Theory of Rate Processes. McGraw-Hill Book Co., Inc., New York. Chapter 8. 1941.
6. Goodgal, S. H., Rupert, C. S. and Herriott, R. M.: In: The Chemical Basis of Heredity. Edited by W. D. McElroy and B. Glass. Johns Hopkins Press, Baltimore. pp 341-343, 1957.
7. Harm, H.: Mutat. Res., 7:261, 1969.
8. Harm, H. and Rupert, C. S.: Mutat. Res., 6:355, 1968.
9. Harm, H. and Rupert, C. S.: Mutat. Res., 10:291, 1970.

10. Harm, H. and Rupert, C. S.: Mutat. Res., 10:307, 1970.
11. Harm, W.: Z. Vererbungsl., 90:428, 1959.
12. Harm, W.: J. Cell. Comp. Physiol., 58:Suppl. 1, 69, 1961.
13. Harm, W.: In: Symposium on the Mutation Process. The Physiology of Gene and Mutation Expression. Edited by M. Kohoutova and J. Hubacek. Academia, Prague, pp 51-59, 1965.
14. Harm, W.: Mutat. Res., 10:277, 1970.
15. Harm, W., Harm, H. and Rupert, C. S.: Mutat. Res., 6:371, 1968.
16. Harm, W., Rupert, C. S. and Harm, H.: In: Photophysiology. Edited by A. C. Giese, Academic Press, N.Y., Vol 6, pp 279-324, 1971.
17. Harm, W., Rupert, C. S. and Harm, H.: This Symposium, p 53, 1971.
18. Helene, C. and Charlier, M.: Biochem. Biophys. Res. Commun., 43:252, 1971.
19. Kauzmann, W.: Advances Protein Chem., 14:1, 1959.
20. Kistiakowsky, G. B., Manglesdorf, P. C., Rosenberg, A. J. and Shaw, W. H. R.: J. Amer. Chem. Soc., 74:5015, 1952.
21. Laidler, K.: The Chemical Kinetics of Enzyme Action. Clarendon Press, Oxford. Chapter 7, 1958.
22. Lang, D., Bujard, H., Wolff, B. and Russell, D.: J. Molec. Biol., 23:163, 1967.
23. Lehman, R. C. and Pollard, E. C.: Biophys. J., 5:109, 1965.
24. Rahn, R. O., Setlow, J. K. and Hosszu, J. L. Biophys. J., 9:510, 1969.
25. Rupert, C. S., Goodgal, S. H. and Herriott, R. M.: J. Gen. Physiol., 41:451, 1958.
26. Rupert, C. S.: In: The Comparative Effects of Radiations. Edited by M. Burton, J. S. Kirby-Smith and J. L. Magee. John Wiley & Sons, Inc., N.Y., pp 49-71, 1960.
27. Rupert, C. S.: J. Cell. Comp. Physiol., 58:Suppl. 1, 57, 1961.
28. Rupert, C. S.: J. Gen. Physiol., 45:703, 1962.
29. Rupert, C. S.: J. Gen. Physiol., 45:725, 1962.
30. Rupert, C. S.: In: Photophysiology. Edited by A. C. Giese, Academic Press, N.Y., Vol 2, pp 283-327, 1964.
31. Setlow, R. B. and Carrier, W. L.: Proc. Nat. Acad. Sci. USA, 51:226, 1964.
32. Setlow, R. B. and Carrier, W. L.: J. Molec. Biol., 17:237, 1966.
33. Williams, D. L., Hayes, F. N., Varghese, A. J. and Rupert, C. S.: Biophysical Society Abstracts 15th Annual Meeting, 191a, 1971.
34. Yarus, M. and Berg, P.: Anal. Biochem., 35:450, 1970.

PHOTOENZYMATIC REPAIR IN ANIMAL CELLS[1]

John S. Cook

Biology Division, Oak Ridge National Laboratory
Oak Ridge, Tennessee

Enzymatic photoreactivation—an enzyme-mediated, light-dependent reversal of ultraviolet radiation damage to DNA—has been demonstrated in a variety of plant and microbial cells and is almost ubiquitously distributed throughout the animal kingdom, as seen in Table I (3,27). Moreover, in any animal species in which photoreactivating enzyme (PRE) activity is found, it is found in virtually *all* the tissues. A major exception to these generalizations is seen in the placental mammals, where neither biological photoreactivation nor PRE activity have been unequivocally demonstrated (1-3,29). Although PRE activity can be demonstrated readily in the dedifferentiated fibroblasts of fish, amphibia, reptiles, birds and marsupials, it is not found in the fibroblasts of man, hamster or mouse. Although skin is the tissue most vulnerable to ultraviolet radiation (UV) and potentially

TABLE I

Photoreactivating Enzyme Activity in Metazoa

Mollusca	
Fresh-water snail	+
Echinodermata	
Sea urchin	+
Sand dollar	+
Arthropoda	
Flower moth	+
Land crab	+
Lobster	+
Brine shrimp	+
Vertebrata*	
Fish (3)	+
Amphibia (3)	+
Reptiles (3)	+
Birds (1)	+
Mammals	
Marsupialia (3)	+
Placentalia (5)	All negative

*Number of species tested in parentheses.

[1] Supported jointly by the National Cancer Institute and the U.S. Atomic Energy Commission under contract with Union Carbide Corporation.

the most susceptible to photoreactivation, PRE activity could not be demonstrated in mammalian skin from a variety of sources (13). Finally, although eggs and zygotes of many animals are exposed to the environment and are susceptible to inactivation and concurrent photoreactivation by solar radiation, the embryos of rats and cattle show no PRE activity even in very early stages of embryogenesis. To this extent, at least, their ontogeny fails to recapitulate phylogeny.

Despite the absence of PRE activity in placental mammals, I wish to reemphasize that such activity is probably present in nearly all the cells of all other animals. In fact, in some of the work to be described in this paper, we performed experiments with tissues from animals which we had not previously screened for PRE activity; we were confident that these tissues would show the desired activity, and in no case were we disappointed.

Photoreactivation in the cells of metazoa, just as in microbial cells, may be observed by a number of criteria: the survival of UV-irradiated cells may be enhanced in the light; the inhibited growth rate of irradiated cells may be partially restored in the light, as may the rates of DNA synthesis. Cyclobutyl pyrmidine dimers, which are the principal photoproducts in the DNA of UV-irradiated cells, are the only known substrate for PRE,

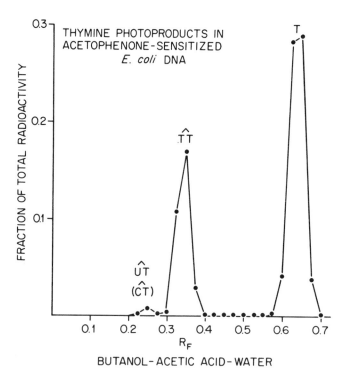

Fig 1. Radiochromatogram of a formic acid-hydrolysate of E. coli DNA which had been labeled with ^{3}H-thymine, then irradiated with light of wavelength greater than 310 nm in the presence of the photosensitizer acetophenone. Chromatography in butanol-acetic acid-water (80:12:30). The peak at R_F .63 is thymine, at R_F .35 it is thymine-thymine dimer, and at R_F .35 it is uracil-thymine dimer arising from cytosine-thymine dimer by deamination during hydrolysis.

and their disappearance (reversal to pyrimidine monomers) may be observed in vivo as a consequence of exposure to photoreactivating light. In vitro, the enzymatic activity from cell extracts can be shown with the sensitive Hemophilus assay first described by Goodgal et al (10). In all of our experience with metazoan cells, we have never found a case in which one of these assays was positive while another was negative. Photoreactivation in metazoa appears to operate by a mechanism identical to that first described for microbial systems and summarized in Cook (2).

For our work with metazoan tissues, we have found it convenient to work with yet another assay. I shall first describe that assay together with some of the data we obtained during its development, since in that work we were using the yeast enzyme, and some of the results are pertinent to other papers in this Symposium (12,26). I shall then

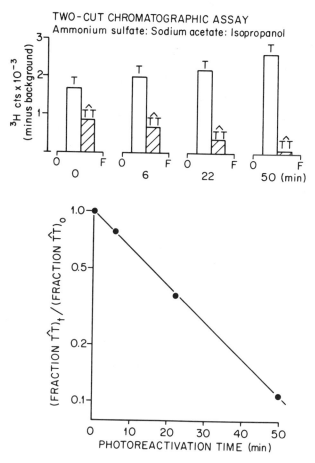

Fig 2. Two-cut chromatographic assay for pyrimidine dimers. The upper four bar graphs represent paper-strip chromatograms developed in saturated ammonium sulfate, 1 M sodium acetate, and isopropanol (40:9:1, v/v/v) of hydrolysates of DNA treated with yeast PRE in the presence of light for the times indicated (0, origin; F, front). Thymine is located on the strips by optical marker. The entire chromatogram runs about 16 cm and the length of the cuts corresponds to the width of the bar graphs as indicated. The fraction of initial dimers remaining as determined from these four chromatograms is plotted as a function of time in the lower graph.

discuss some of the more recent data we have obtained on the physiology of photoreactivating enzyme in several animal systems.

ASSAY FOR PRE ACTIVITY

It has been shown in a number of laboratories that when DNA is irradiated with
light of 310 nm and longer in the presence of acetophenone, there is a very substantial
photoproduction of thymine dimers to the exclusion of nearly all other photoproducts
(14,15). Figure 1 shows a chromatogram of radioactivity from DNA labeled with ^{3}H-
thymine and irradiated in the presence of acetophenone, hydrolyzed and chromatographed
in a solvent system that separates thymine-thymine dimers from thymine-cytosine dimers.
This DNA contains about one third of its thymine as $\widehat{TT}$ dimer but only about one percent of its thymine as $\widehat{CT}$ dimer. Ninety-six percent of the nonthymine radioactivity in
this DNA may be converted back to thymine by treatment with PRE in the presence of
light. Such a DNA is a useful substrate for assaying for PRE activity, because the assay
may be performed with nanogram quantities of DNA, yielding a sensitivity comparable
to the Hemophilus bioassay, and because it measures directly the conversion of the chemical substrate of the enzyme. The principal virtue of using a DNA containing such a high
concentration of dimers is not that there are so many dimers but that there is, relatively,
so little of the radioactive thymine which ordinarily makes difficult and laborious the
quantitation of dimers in DNA that has been UV-irradiated without photosensitizers.

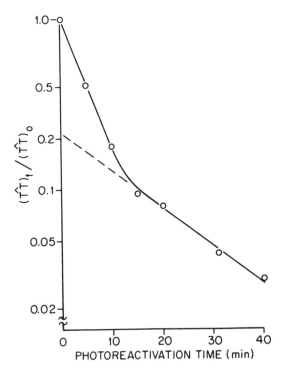

Fig 3. Time course of photoreactivation of thymine-thymine dimers in acetophenone-sensitized
E. coli DNA in the presence of yeast PRE and saturating light conditions.

In practice we illuminate this substrate in the presence of the enzyme preparation to be assayed, precipitate with TCA, hydrolyze and chromatograph in a solvent system in which the dimers move rapidly than the thymine (Fig 2). Two cuts from the paper chromatogram are all that are needed to determine the fraction of dimers which have been repaired. As may be seen in the upper part of the figure, the decrease in radioactivity in the "dimer cut" is accompanied by an increase in the "thymine cut." Under conditions of saturating light, the reaction is first-order until it is at least 90% complete.

As an aside, if the reaction with the yeast enzyme is followed beyond the first 90% of repair, we observe (Fig 3) that the curve breaks sharply and the slope of the second portion of the curve is decreased by a factor of 2 or more. If we extrapolate this slope to the ordinate, it appears that over 20% of the dimers are being repaired at the slower rate. This finding corresponds to a similar observation by H. Harm and Rupert (11), but in the present case cannot be ascribed to photoreactivation at different rates of different homo- and hetero-dimers, since the substrate here is almost solely the *cis-syn* thymine-thymine homodimer. For reasons we shall describe elsewhere we believe this change in rate represents a change in configuration of substrate and consequently the enzyme's affinity for it.

For our assay, we use only the first (and major) portion of the repair curve, where the slope is proportional to the enzyme concentration of the extract we assay (Fig 4). Using this system, we have investigated a number of the properties of yeast PRE activity, two of which I will describe here.

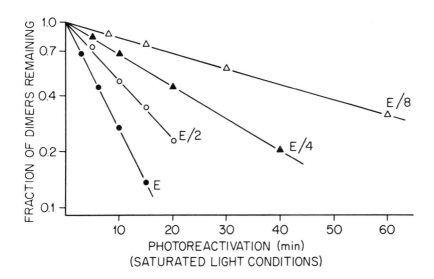

Fig 4. Time course of photoreactivation of thymine-thymine dimers in acetophenone-sensitized E. coli DNA in the presence of various dilutions of yeast PRE and saturating light conditions. Concentration of crude extract "E" was 170 μgm protein per ml; dilutions as indicated.

STUDIES WITH YEAST PRE

      We have estimated the molecular weight of the enzyme by gel filtration through
Sephadex G-150 and by sucrose gradient analysis with appropriate markers. In our first
experiments with the gel columns, we found that the PRE activity came through in the
void volume; this may have been due either to aggregation or to nonspecific binding of
the enzyme to nucleic acids still present in the crude preparations. In later experiments
we used more highly purified preparations containing no detectable nucleic acid, but
even with the cruder material the problem with aggregation could be avoided by carrying
out the separations in 1 $\underline{M}$ KCl (Fig 5 and 6). Under these conditions, the molecular
weights in five determinations varied from 61,000 to 73,000, with a mean of 63,000.

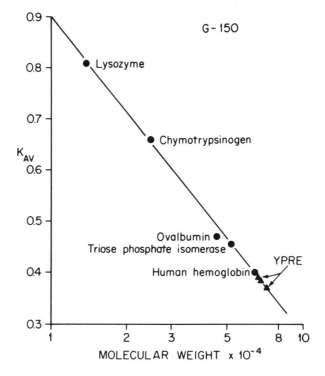

Fig 5. Sephadex chromatography (G-150) of yeast PRE. Column calibrated with maker proteins as
indicated. Markers were located by optical density of purified materials, yeast PRE by activity in crude
extracts (35-55% ammonium sulfate cut from autolysed cells). All columns were run in 1 $\underline{M}$ KCl buffered with .01 $\underline{M}$ sodium phosphate, pH 7.0.

This is more than twice the value given a few years ago by Muhammed (19) who used
optical analytical-ultracentrifuge methods with a protein solution which, it is now known,
was less than 1% photoreactivating enzyme. Apart from the nonspecific aggregates, we
have not seen any activity in any smaller or larger fraction than the 63,000 molecular
weight; from activity criteria we have no evidence for subunits, but definite answers to
this and similar questions must await purification of the enzyme. That work is being
done elsewhere (17).

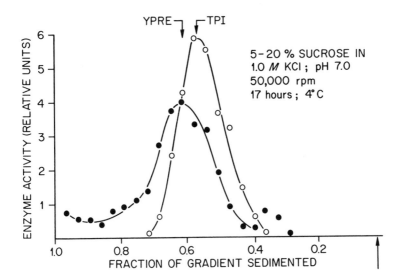

Fig 6. Sucrose-gradient sedimentation of yeast PRE (closed circles) together with rabbit-muscle triose phosphate isomerase (open circles) as marker. The molecular weight of TPI has been taken as 54,000 (21).

A second property of the yeast enzyme, which we explored further in relation to the PRE activity in animal cells (and discussed later in this paper), is the response of

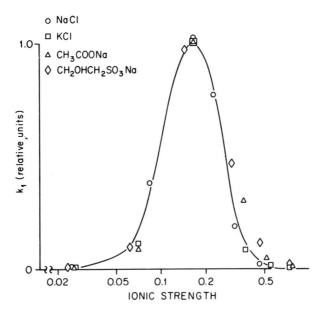

Fig 7. Relative ionic-strength dependence of yeast PRE's forward rate constant, k_1, assayed under saturating light conditions. Salts used as indicated.

the yeast enzyme to media of various ionic strengths. This work follows directly from that of H. Harm and Rupert (11). Using our dimer assay and their flash-photolysis technique for determining enzyme concentration, we have repeated their observations that the forward rate constant (k_1) for the reaction with yeast enzyme shows a maximum activity at an ionic strength 0.17, falling off sharply and symmetrically on both sides of this value (Fig 7), and that the peak value is almost exactly 1×10^8 liters mole^{-1} sec^{-1} at 36°C. Moreover, this curve is quite insensitive to the ionic species used. The reference curve in Figure 7 is that for NaCl, and the data for the other salts are normalized to it at the peak point; hence the units of the ordinate are a relative scale. Nevertheless, the peak activity at an ionic strength of 0.17 was the same, within 20%, for all the salts used. We tested the several other uni-univalent salts for very definite reasons: KCl in comparison to NaCl because K is the principal intracellular (although not necessarily intranuclear) cation in most cells, sodium acetate because many cells are low in chloride and maintain electroneutrality with organic anions; and sodium isethionate because in at least one large group of animals, marine cephalopods, this anion is the principal nondiffusing anion in certain excitable cells and is found in concentrations as high as 450 milliequivalents per liter of cell water. The yeast enzyme is affected by all of these ionic species in the same way, with a peak activity near 0.17 regardless of the salt used.

EFFECTS OF IONIC STRENGTH ON PRE ACTIVITY
IN EXTRACTS OF ANIMAL CELLS

As with the yeast enzyme, photoreactivating activity in many animals living in environments representing extremes of ionic composition shows similar sensitivity to ionic strength (Fig 8). The curve drawn in this figure is the same as that for the yeast enzyme in Figure 7. The points are relative values, again normalized to the peak activity of the yeast curve, for PRE activity from cell extracts of the animals listed in the legend to the figure. Specifically, the tissues are: snail muscle, unfertilized sea urchin eggs, lobster ovary, whole brine shrimp nauplii and Xenopus fibroblasts grown in culture. Either NaCl or KCl was used to regulate the ionic strength; all experiments were done at pH 7.1 and at 33-35°C. Clearly, the PRE activity from all these divergent sources shows very nearly the same response to ionic strength: in all cases the enzyme peaks at 0.17 but is inactive below 0.03 or above 0.5. It is instructive to compare this activity range with the ionic compositions of the animals and their environments. As shown in the top of Figure 8, these animals originate in aqueous environments ranging from fresh water of near-zero ionic strength to the NaCl-saturated Great Salt Lake. Even the marine animals live in an environment in which the salt concentration is too high for the photoreactivating enzyme to function. As is well known, however, the cells of most of these animals are not in direct contact with their environment, but with their blood plasma or hemolymph, which is frequently maintained at salt compositions quite different from the environment. Even so, the salt concentrations in the plasma of marine crustacea, or of fresh water molluscs, to say nothing of the sea water environment of the free-living echinoderm eggs, are still outside the limits of the activity of the enzyme. However, the cells themselves represent a further step in ionic regulation, and here we find the intracellular milieu quite different in some cases even from the hemolymph. Now we see that PRE activity spans the entire range of intracellular ionic composition. I do not mean to imply that animals regulate their ions so as to maintain their PRE activity. This particular enzyme is not at all unique

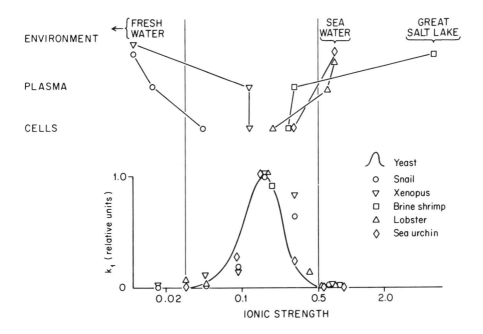

Fig 8. Lower: Dependence on ionic strength of the forward rate constant, k_1, for the formation of enzyme-substrate complex of PRE activity from a variety of sources, assayed under saturing light conditions. The curve drawn for yeast enzyme was taken from Figure 7. Sources of animal enzymes as indicated on the right of the figure, with specific tissues given in text. Upper: Ionic strengths (same abscissa as for lower curve) of various milieus for animals whose tissues were assayed in the lower curve, with the same symbols for each animal. Values are the best available estimates for most closely related species where literature values for the exact species were not available. Sources for these values were: amphibian plasma and muscle water, marine crustacean plasma and muscle water from Prosser and Brown (23); unfertilized sea urchin eggs from Rothschild and Barnes (25); brine shrimp from Croghan (5); fresh water mollusc plasma and muscle from Potts (22).

in these respects. It is known, for example, that a KCl solution of the same ionic strength as sea water is a very satisfactory solvent for dissolving muscle myosin or the mitotic apparatus even of marine animals. It is interesting to note, however, that the optimum ionic strength (and temperature, for that matter) for PRE activity from all sources is characteristic for that one order of animals in which it is not found—placental mammals.

PHOTOREACTIVATION OF MITOCHONDRIAL DNA IN XENOPUS

We know, then, that PR enzyme is of very wide distribution among animals, and that its properties, insofar as they have been studied, are very similar from one animal to another and very similar to the yeast enzyme. What we know much less about is the physiological functioning of this enzyme in vivo. Our most recent approach to this problem starts with the recognition that in cells of higher organisms the DNA is not all of a unique sequence on a single chromosome, but is organized much more complexly. We have elected to look at which classes of DNA are subject to repair, and under what conditions. As a first step in the classification of repair on this basis, we have examined the photoreactivation of mitochondrial DNA in Xenopus laevis (4).

Several years ago, we (24) demonstrated photoreactivation in cell line A8W2 derived from Xenopus by K. A. Rafferty and cloned by J. D. Regan. In that line we observed that UV inhibition of growth and of DNA synthesis could be photoreactivated, and that PRE activity could be detected in crude cell lysates when assayed in the Hemophilus system. Although in this line we find a small amount of repair replication in the dark (unpublished results) the excision of pyrimidine dimers in the dark from acid-insoluble material is negligibly small (Fig 9) and probably not real. Twenty-four hours after irradiation, virtually all of the dimers are still there (there has been little or no cell division after this UV dose) but in the light, these persistent dimers may be readily reversed by photoreactivation. All these observations were made in the analysis of whole cells and the results pertain almost entirely to nuclear DNA.

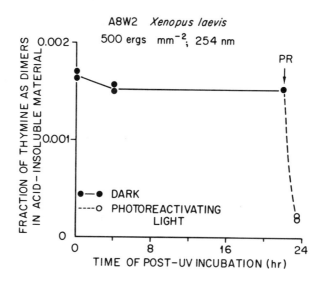

Fig 9. Acid-insoluble pyrimidine dimers in Xenopus cells following UV-irradiation. Cells were maintained at 25°C throughout the experiment. Photoreactivating light intensity was supramaximal.

Earlier (3), we had also looked for PRE activity in fractions from the liver of another amphibian, Rana pipiens, and had concluded that the enzyme was concentrated in nuclei, where more than 80% of the total cellular activity could be located. The remainder was recovered in the soluble fraction of the homogenates, but there was reason to believe that most of this soluble activity had been leached out of nuclei. A subcellular fraction rich in mitochondria but free of nuclei contained no detectable PRE activity, but the assay conditions we had used in this work were not sufficiently sensitive to resolve less than about 5% of the total cellular activity.

The A8W2 cells in culture offered a number of advantages for re-examining the question of mitochondrial photorepair; these were advantages already known for the study of repair phenomena in cultured cells (ease of labeling, ease of obtaining mono-layers of cells for UV-irradiation, to mention a few) plus the known presence of a func-tional PR enzyme and the lack of a vigorous excision-repair system. In addition, the properties of the mitochondrial DNA of this species had been investigated extensively by Dawid and his coworkers (6-9).

Our first step in dealing with this problem was to find a simple procedure for separating mitochondrial DNA (Mt-DNA) from nuclear DNA (Nu-DNA) so that numerous samples of each could be obtained easily for analysis in the course of each experiment. After separation of mitochondria from nuclei and DNase treatment of the mitochondria by standard methods (20), the organelles were lysed and the DNA's released. As previous-ly reported (9) these DNA's have very similar buoyant densities in CsCl, reflecting their nearly identical overall base compositions. They may be separated in CsCl gradients con-taining ethidium bromide, but this technique is preparatively laborious even if analytically useful. A simpler separation technique became available by the recognition of the

THERMAL DISSOCIATION OF *XENOPUS* DNA

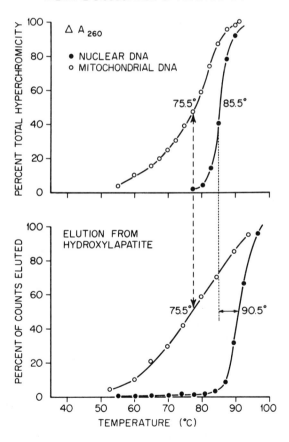

Fig 10. Thermal dissociation of Xenopus DNA's determined either by hyperchromicity (total hy-perchromicity greater than 30% for both DNA's) in the upper curve or by elution of radioactive DNA from hydroxylapatite in the lower curve. Solvent in both cases was 0.12 M sodium phosphate, pH 6.8.

disparate melting properties of the two DNA's. Xenopus nuclear DNA is exceptional in having a very steep melting curve (Fig 10). The Mt-DNA has a much shallower melting curve, presumably reflecting a greater degree of heterogeneity of base sequences despite the similarity of overall base composition to Nu-DNA. The disparities between the two DNA types are even greater when the analysis is made, not by absorbance methods, but by elution of ^{3}H-thymidine-labeled DNA from hydroxylapatite columns (18) where the greater size of the Nu-DNA is an additional factor in retarding its elution (lower curves in Figure 10). We treat the lysed mitochondrial and nuclear suspensions with isoamyl alcohol:chloroform overnight to deproteinize them (16) and the next day apply the aqueous phase to hydroxylapatite columns in 0.12 $\underline{M}$ sodium phosphate buffer. The material eluting at 80°C from the mitochondrial fractions we take as Mt-DNA, and that eluting in high salt from the nuclear fractions we take as Nu-DNA (Fig 11).

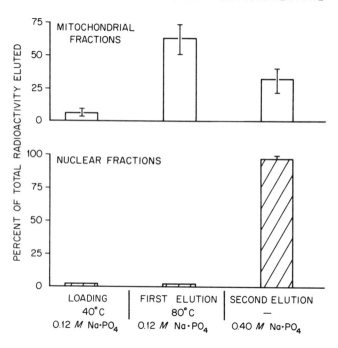

TWO-STEP ELUTION OF *XENOPUS* DNA FROM HYDROXYLAPATITE

Fig 11. Typical elution patterns (average of six points from a single experiment) of mitochondrial and nuclear DNA's from hydroxylapatite. The material eluting at 80°C from the mitochondrial fractions was taken as Mt-DNA for further analysis of pyrimidine dimers, and that eluting in 0.4 $\underline{M}$ sodium phosphate from nuclear fraction was taken as Nu-DNA for similar analyses.

With this technical background, we used cells labeled with ^{3}H-thymidine to look first at the rate of dimer production in the two types of DNA as a function of UV dose; the dimers were measured by standard methods (28). The results are shown in Figure 12. Paired points from a single cell sample are enclosed within the dotted circles. The experiments were extended to very high UV doses to enhance the accuracy of the measurements. For both kinds of DNA, 0.3% of the DNA thymine is converted to pyrimidine dimer by

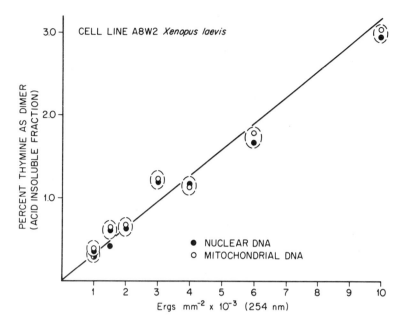

Fig 12. Rate of thymine-containing dimer production in Xenopus DNA's.

each 1000 ergs mm^{-2} (254 nm). The similarity of the results for the two DNA types again reflects the similarity of their base composition as determined by CsCl ultracentrifugation (9). Starting with lower UV doses, we have irradiated Xenopus cells and subsequently photoreactivated them in vivo, with the results shown in Figure 13. After two hours,

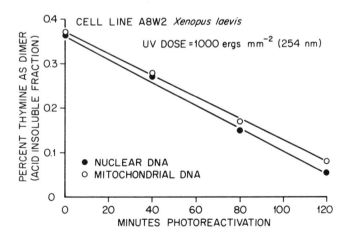

Fig 13. Photoreactivation in vivo of the thymine-containing dimers from Xenopus DNA's. Photoreactivation was carried out at 25°C starting immediately after the UV-irradiation, and approximately 3×10^8 cells per sample were removed at the times indicated for fractionation and analysis.

nearly 90% of the dimers are gone, presumably reverted to monomeric thymine. More-over, the rate constants for in vivo photorepair are about the same for both Mt-DNA and Nu-DNA. The significance of this latter observation is not certain, but the most obvious interpretation is that the number of PRE molecules per unit length of DNA is the same in both the mitochondria and nuclei. Although the experiment shown here was done at quite high UV dose from the biological standpoint, similar results may be obtained at lower doses, but with necessarily less precision in the data.

As noted above, our earlier attempts (3) to find PRE activity in amphibian mito-chondria were not successful. The fact that Mt-DNA was photoreactivable persuaded us to try again. In our previous work, we had noted that the enzyme was easily, and irre-versibly, leached out of nuclei by too high an ionic strength in the homogenizing medium. Since the enzyme appeared to be bound so loosely to the organelles, we attempted to in-crease the binding by a simple trick well known to those who do affinity chromatography. We irradiated cells with high (2000 ergs mm^{-2}) doses of UV and isolated mitochondria and nuclei in the dark. Since, for the yeast enzyme at least, the dissociation constant of the enzyme-substrate complex is of the order of 10^{-11} $\underline{M}$ (11) we anticipated that this

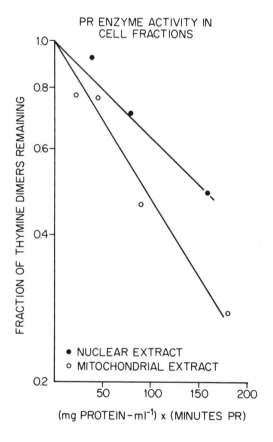

Fig 14. Activity of the PRE enzyme in cell fractions from Xenopus. Fractions were isolated by dif-ferential centrifugation of cell-free homogenates (20) and assayed under saturating light conditions with the acetophenone-dimer assay shown in Figures 2 and 4.

introduction of substrate dimers into DNA would trap PRE molecules in mitochondria as well as nuclei during dark-isolation procedures. After isolation, we exposed the organelles to strong illumination to rid them of endogenous substrate, lysed them by several freeze-thaw cycles in phosphate buffer and assayed them for PRE activity using the aceto-phenone-dimer method described above. The results are shown in Figure 14, where it may be seen that the specific activity of PRE in mitochondrial protein in fact is somewhat greater than in nuclear protein.

We still cannot be certain of where these PRE molecules originate. It is possible that in unirradiated cells they are present only in the nuclei, and migrate to mitochondria after irradiation. We believe it more likely that they are present in mitochondria all along. This interpretation is not only simpler, but also accounts for the fact that there is no apparent lag in the onset of photoreactivation of Mt-DNA (Fig 13) and that a full complement of PRE activity is to be found in mitochondria of irradiated cells which have been homogenized immediately after irradiation.

These results strengthen our conviction that the photoreactivating enzyme is nearly ubiquitously distributed wherever DNA is found in metazoa, always excepting placental mammals. How it functions in relation to other nucleic acid enzymes and chromosomal proteins, of course, still is quite unknown.

ACKNOWLEDGMENTS

I wish to thank T. E. Worthy for expert assistance. Some of the biological materials and advice regarding their use were generously provided by J. D. Regan, F. C. Hartman, D. M. Skinner, L. E. Roberson and W. L. Carrier, all of the Biology Division at Oak Ridge.

REFERENCES

1. Cleaver, J. E.: Biochem. Biophys. Res. Commun., 24:569, 1966.
2. Cook, J. S.: In: Photophysiology. Edited by A. C. Giese, Vol 5, p 191, Academic Press, Inc., New York, 1970.
3. Cook, J. S. and McGrath, J. R.: Proc. Nat. Acad. Sci. USA, 58:1359, 1967.
4. Cook, J. S. and Worthy, T. E.: 15th Annual Biophysical Society Abstracts, 191a, 1971.
5. Croghan, P. C.: J. Exp. Biol., 35:219, 1958.
6. Dawid, I. B.: J. Molec. Biol., 12:581, 1965.
7. Dawid, I. B.: Proc. Nat. Acad. Sci. USA, 56:269, 1966.
8. Dawid, I. B. and Wolstenholme, D. R.: Biophys. J., 8:65, 1968.
9. Dawid, I. B. and Wolstenholme, D. R.: In: Biochemical Aspects of the Biogenesis of Mitochondria. Edited by E. C. Slater, J. M. Tager, S. Papa and E. Quagliariello, p 283. Adriatica Editrice, Bari, Italy.
10. Goodgal, S. H., Rupert, C. S. and Herriott, R. M.: In: The Chemical Basis of Heredity. Edited by W. D. McElroy and B. Glass, p 341, Johns Hopkins Press, Baltimore, Md., 1957.
11. Harm, H. and Rupert, C. S.: Mutat. Res., 10:291, 1970.
12. Harm, W., Rupert, C. S. and Harm, H.: This Symposium, p 53, 1971.
13. Johnson, B. E., Daniels, F. Jr. and Magnus, I. A.: In: Photophysiology. Edited by A. C. Giese, Vol 4, p 139, Academic Press, Inc., New York, 1968.

14. Lamola, A. A.: Photochem. Photobiol., 9:291, 1969.
15. Lamola, A. A. and Yamane, T.: Proc. Nat. Acad. Sci. USA, 58:443, 1967.
16. Marmur, J.: J. Molec. Biol., 3:208, 1961.
17. Minato, S. and Werbin, H.: 15th Annual Biophysical Society Abstracts, 190a, 1971.
18. Miyazawa, Y. and Thomas, C. A., Jr.: J. Molec. Biol., 11:223, 1965.
19. Muhammed, A.: J. Biol. Chem., 241:516, 1966.
20. Nass, M. M. K.: J. Molec. Biol., 42:529, 1966.
21. Norton, I. L., Pfuderer, P., Stringer, C. D. and Hartman, F. C.: Biochemistry, 9:4952, 1970.
22. Potts, W. T. W.: J. Exp. Biol., 35:749, 1958.
23. Prosser, C. L. and Brown, F. A., Jr.: Comparative Animal Physiology, 2nd edition. W. B. Saunders Co., Philadelphia, 1961.
24. Regan, J. D., Cook, J. S. and Lee, W. H.: J. Cell. Physiol., 71:173, 1968.
25. Rothschild, Lord, and Barnes, H.: J. Exp. Biol., 30:534, 1953.
26. Rupert, C. S., Harm, W. and Harm, H.: This Symposium, p 64, 1971.
27. Setlow, J. K.: In: Research Progress in Organic-Biological and Medicinal Chemistry. Edited by U. Gallo and L. Santamaria. Vol 3, 1972 in press. North Holland Publishing Co., Amsterdam.
28. Setlow, R. B. and Carrier, W. L.: J. Molec. Biol., 17:237, 1966.
29. Trosko, J. E., Chu, E. H. Y., Carrier, W. L.: Radiat. Res., 24:667, 1965.

DISCUSSION

Dr. Roger M. Herriott (Baltimore) You have heard three very interesting papers on the photo-reactivating system. I think it may be worth noting that in photo-reactivation the change induced by the ultraviolet radiation is presumably reversed. This is different from the dark or excision-repair reactions in which the damaged region is removed and new bases correctly introduced for the latter involves at least three enzymes.

I shall now ask for questions and discussion from panel members.

Dr. John S. Cook (Oak Ridge) I would like to ask Dr. Harm if he has any thoughts on the localization in E. coli of the PRE molecules.

Dr. Walter Harm (Dallas) Well, actually I have none.

Dr. Cook You haven't tried anything like the gentle lysis with Brij or things of this kind, to see if it is associated with the membrane fraction?

Dr. Harm No, we haven't done this kind of experiment.

Dr. C. S. Rupert (Dallas) Dr. John Cook, you may have done more localization experiments than you told us about here. Didn't you find some localization in the eukaryotes?

Dr. Cook We found 80% of the total activity localized in the nuclei, and I think it was more than that, in fact.

Dr. Rupert Well then, how is it that so much of it seems to be in the mitochondria?

Dr. Cook In the graph I showed the abscissa was milligrams-protein times time; that is a specific activity graph.

Dr. Rupert Ah, that's not cellular content?

Dr. Cook It's not cellular content, it is not total protein. There is very much less in the mitochondrial fraction in terms of total enzyme.

Dr. Rupert Is there a qualitative difference between the mitochondrial and the nuclear enzyme as you finally get it out of the cell?

Dr. Cook No, it just seems to be that in the mitochondrial protein PRE is more concentrated than it is in nuclear protein. But the amount of mitochondrial protein we get is a very small fraction of the total protein.

Dr. Harm   You showed one graph according to which the removal of dimers by the photoreactivating enzyme of marsupital cells is very slow. Does this refer to the absolute number of dimers removed or is it on a relative scale? Could it just be a matter of the ratio of photoreactivating enzyme molecules to pyrimidine dimers, or does one have to conclude that the enzyme actually works slower in that case?

Dr. Cook   I think that from our measurements it seems that the enzyme is really inhibited in some way from acting at its maximal rate. We get about the same amount of enzyme out of marsupial cells as we get out of Xenopus cells and there's more DNA in Xenopus cells in fact. And yet the rate for photoreactivation in Xenopus is much faster; and it's even faster in echinoderms.

Dr. Rupert   You mean the in vitro assay?

Dr. Cook   The in vitro assay, yes. The in vitro assay is about the same. The in vivo is much lower. I think that the DNA is well coated with something in marsupials. The enzyme can't get at it.

Dr. Rupert   That sharp melting curve of Xenopus DNA is unusual, isn't it?

Dr. Cook   I think it's the sharpest melting curve I know of. You'd expect it the other way around, that the mitochondrial DNA would be more uniform and the nuclear DNA spread out over a big range.

Dr. Herriott   Have any of you tried to dissociate the enzyme from the substrate without the use of light, that is, using high salt and then see if there is any modification of the DNA or whether the dimers are still present? The presently accepted picture is that light is needed to repair the damage but it may be that the light merely releases the enzyme after repair takes place.

Dr. Rupert   I'm not sure, because we never deliberately did it. Therefore, I don't quite know whether these indirect indications can mean anything or not. We have put the transforming DNA with enzyme under conditions where raising the salt concentration prevents the photoreactivation from occurring. However, if one doesn't design experiments specifically to test something, I don't quite believe what it says. The dimers can be split by short wave lengths (240 mm) that they can absorb. In a polynucleotide, of course, this just leads to a steady state, because the short wave lengths also make dimers. With longer wave lengths and anthraquinone derivatives or tryptophan derivatives one can also get a sensitized splitting and my prejudice is that the enzyme is simply a very efficient and highly specific form of sensitized splitting and it takes light to do it, but that's only my prejudice.

Dr. Rupert	The fact that UV'd transforming DNA can be put on and dissociated without high salts and without repair suggests that light is needed for repair. When you first complex the enzyme and UV'd transforming DNA and then throw in a big excess of other UV'd DNA you find very little repair of transforming DNA, but, of course, that isn't answering quite the question you were asking either. The complex has formed and the DNA has come back off but nothing has apparently happened.
Dr. Rolf Knippers (Tübingen)	Has anybody tried to purify the enzyme, and if so, is there a chromophore?
Dr. Rupert	The purest stuff that is available now on a regular basis is, I think, being produced by Harold Werbin in Dallas, who gets it up toward 10^5-fold purification. Remember that Dr. Harm has told us it is present in only about one part in 10^5 of the cell protein, so that purification is a big problem. With the small amounts of enzyme he gets, he finds a flourescence that goes with the enzyme, in purification, but which can be dissociated from it by inactivating treatments. He has the activation and fluorescent spectra, but whether or not this is really the chromophore is still an open question. We should know the answer to that question before too many months or years.
Dr. Knippers	Could one use some affinity chromatography like the DNA complex, for example, just using irradiated DNA?
Dr. Rupert	That's what Werbin does in one of his later purification steps.
Dr. Cook	Jane Setlow and Muhammed also used that method and they found that it was a very fastidious, a very finicky enzyme.
Dr. Rupert	Of course part of the problem is that whenever you have very little enzyme present you end up with such dilute solutions after high purification that it's prone to loss, namely sticks to the glass. We hope that the yeast mutant we have, which produces about five times as much enzyme as the wild cell, maybe can be a help. If one can get an order of magnitude headstart on purification for Harold Werbin, he's got an order of magnitude smaller job to do for the same end result.
Dr. Harm	I think there is always a problem with the stability. I have heard from Jane Setlow that the photoreactivating enzyme became less and less stable the more she purified it.
Dr. Cook	She autolysed a half a ton of yeast.
Dr. Herriott	I can vouch for the difficulties, because we've been working on the purification for a very long time, and it has a number of difficulties

that have been suggested. It can be stabilized, but unfortunately, two different lots of yeast from the same manufacturer behaved so differently that I have had to shift methods after perfecting one.

Dr. Rupert   That is a problem we found too.

Dr. Knippers   You could, of course, use the mutant of Dr. Harm.

Dr. Herriott   Then you have the problem of growing and harvesting the yeast. When you can buy freshly prepared commercial yeast for a few cents a pound, I doubt if you save much by setting up a laboratory unit to grow a strain that contains only ten times as much enzyme.

Dr. Harm   Did you mean the yeast mutant or the E. coli mutant? E. coli presents other problems because they have more nucleases, which I think was the reason why Stan Rupert used yeast enzyme rather than E. coli enzyme for most of his in vitro studies.

Dr. Rupert   It might be possible. Dr. Sutherland working with Dr. Chamberlain in Berkeley has had some success purifying the enzyme out of E. coli. The first steps of purification in E. coli were discouraging to us because of the nuclease problems and in the early days we simply abandoned that source.

Dr. Herriott   The other thing was that the assay depended upon doing the transformation, which required a 24-hour period or longer to get the assay in.

Dr. Robert   Dr. Cook, I believed you described an in vitro measure of PR
Stoller   enzyme activity using a sea urchin egg extract. I would imagine that the
(Rockville)   DNase activity which might be present in the extract would degrade the transforming DNA. Did you use any DNase inhibitors?

Dr. Cook   We use a lot of calf thymus DNA along with that, yes. As a matter of fact, in the dark controls you see the activity is falling off quite a lot in some of them because of the nucleases. If you use enough calf thymus DNA, that also will compete very strongly with the enzyme.

Dr. Rupert   Even unirradiated, you begin to get some kind of interaction.

Dr. Cook   Unirradiated double-stranded calf thymus DNA is competivie.

Dr. Rupert   I've probably never used as much in it as you had. Usually a double-stranded DNA doesn't compete significantly, but a single-stranded one or one with single-stranded regions in it, does compete in some general sort of way showing a weak binding with the enzyme.

Dr. Cook   That's true, the single-stranded is about ten times more effective.

Dr. Rupert   Unirradiated?

Dr. Cook   Unirradiated, yes.

Dr. Harm   Perhaps this is the reason why the enzyme, as Jane Setlow claims, has some affinity for unirradiated double-stranded DNA. One could assume that double-stranded DNA always contains some short denatured regions to which the enzyme would bind.

Dr. Rupert   It might be of practical use to keep the enzyme in the right region of the cell where it is available for use rapidly, rather than wandering around loose.

Dr. Cook   As a matter of fact, there are some data on that which I think are of interest to this question of localization. Two of the graduate students at Oak Ridge, Malcolm Paterson and Ken Roozen have been working with the mini-cell system, (E. coli cells that split off about one tenth of the total cell volume with no DNA in them). These cells are thought to contain no PRE. They have this system now operating with R-DNA which contains ribosomal markers; the R-DNA is about 60 million molecular weight. It is UV-inactivable and photoreactivable with about the same rate constants as in the whole cell. So apparently, some photoreactivating enzyme is going with this relatively small plasmid into the mini-cell.

Dr. R. W.
Tuveson
(Urbana)   A couple of years ago Hanawalt suggested that the photoreactivating enzyme might have a function in the dark which was localization of or recognizing damage for a dark repair system. Is there any evidence from purification that there are other activities that purify along with the photoreactivating activity?

Dr. Rupert   Any accompanying nuclease activities would be evident from the change in the activity of transforming DNA on incubation in the dark, and these clearly do not stay with the enzyme during purification. I don't know how many other different enzyme activities have been looked for in purified preparations. We ourselves have done nothing on that.

Dr. Tuveson   Do you have any estimate of the possible size?

Dr. Rupert   Yes. The enzyme size is a little murky yet, but between 50 and 100 thousand Daltons, depending upon who does it.

Dr. Harm   If the photoreactivating enzyme would have dark activity of any kind, this should not be a vital function, since mutant strains producing no photoreactivating enzyme (at least no active photoreactivating enzyme) nevertheless, live perfectly well, and you can't see any disadvantage, other than when exposed to ultraviolet light.

Dr. Rupert   Of course, what these cells lack, Walter, is photoreactivating enzyme activity. You don't know that the entire protein is missing in these particular mutants but only that it is altered. Until one knows what is being looked for, I don't know quite how to answer this question. The only fact is, I think, nobody has any evidence as yet that the PR enzyme has any other activity.

Dr. Alan   It seems to me in this system you've got at least two enzymes,
Bruce   a dark repair enzyme and a photoreactivating enzyme, both of which
(Buffalo)   are competing for the same substrate. What I'd like to ask is, how much interference in the results may there be from these two systems? How much does PR affect dark repair, and how much do dark repair enzymes affect PR? We had an answer from Dr. Cook that some of this has been done in cells not having dark repair; however, the absence of dark repair doesn't mean the first enzyme in the system may not be there complexed with the substrate. At low doses it seems to me there would be a real problem in coming up with definite answers on the system.

Dr. Rupert   In most cases, (Dr. Walter Harm has done most of this), the UVR-cell, which includes B_{s-1}, is believed to lack the first step in the repair, and so the work that Dr. Harm has reported here is presumably minus the major excision dark repair needs. There are plenty of interactions between dark and light repair, in wild type cells, which he studied rather extensively, both in phage and bacteria.

Dr. Harm   In fact, under conditions of most extensive dark repair we don't find photorepair, although we find it with the same strains under usual dark repair conditions. In principle, dark repair can do everything that photorepair does. The reason why one observes photorepair in these strains at all is that dark repair usually does not operate with maximum effectiveness; therefore, a decrease of the leftover damage is what one sees as photorepair.

Dr. Herriott   Are you suggesting that there is a single enzyme that will dark repair?

Dr. Harm   The dark repair uses a multienzyme system; but, what he was referring to, I think, is the first step in the repair.

Dr. F. Hutchinson   It was pointed out in the presentations, that one of the reasons
(New Haven)   for working with this enzyme was its ability to recognize altered bases in a DNA sequence, and that this might be a valuable model to follow up in finding out how other enzyme systems identify the errors in the DNA. What's known about this? You have a good system, what do you know about it? Does it work on dinucleotides in solution?

Dr. Rupert   No, it does not work on dinucleotides. As far as is known, it will work only on the cis-syn isomers of cyclobutyl pyrimidine dimers and only when those are located in sufficiently long sequences. For a thymine sequence shorter than nine, we can detect no interaction. That comes out of work that Jane Setlow did with Fred Bollum a few years ago, combined with our earlier findings that shorter ones didn't work at all.

Irradiated PT-9 mer will competitively inhibit in vitro PR of transforming DNA very weakly, while PT-8 does not work at all, no matter how much it is irradiated; that is, the enzyme just isn't bound at all by it.

Recently, in collaboration with Lloyd Williams and Newt Hayes at Los Alamos Scientific Laboratory, we have constructed a synthetic substrate of exactly known structure, where we put the dimer of thymine exactly in the middle of a ten-nucleotide long sequence: four nucleotides on each side, and the radioactive dimer in the middle. With this, you do a purely chemical assay of the repair process, detecting the change by hydrolysis and chromatography. All the radioactivity begins in the dimer fraction of hydrolysates and shifts over into the monomer fraction as you carry out the light dependent enzymatic reaction with it.

Dr. Harm
Maybe the enzyme doesn't see the dimer as such but sees the distorted region.

Dr. Rupert
The synthetic substrate molecules that we're talking about are single-stranded, which is a little abnormal. Ordinarily, it is only the dimer region of a double-stranded DNA plus the next neighboring bases that are not hydrogen-bonded, since model building shows that beyond these nearest neighbor bases, everything else can form a Watson-Crick helix. However it is clear that an irradiated single-stranded polynucleotide will work with PR enzyme if it is long enough, nine being the absolute minimum for polythymidilic acid. (We don't know what it would be for polycytidylic acid.) There must also be adjacent pyrimidines in the chain in order to form the cis-syn isomer of the pyrimidine dimer during irradiation. I guess you might conceivably form it in other ways, but that's the only one we've seen.

Dr. Cook
As a matter of fact, Ronald Rohn has depurinated alternating poly-d(A-T)n, irradiated it and gotten photoreactivable dimers. It's obviously a somewhat different structure.

Dr. Rupert
When the purines are out of the way, then the things can get together.

Dr. Cook
With the purines out of the way, you can then dimerize the pyrimidines.

Dr. K. Lemone
Yielding
(Birmingham)
I'd like to ask whether any other specific modifications of the DNA will produce materials which will compete for the irradiated DNA as a substrate. I'm thinking specifically, for example, of the use of

fradulent bases which interrupt the normal stacking interactions of DNA, or otherwise interrupt the normal hydrogen bonding. It seems to me that it is a question of whether it is a primary recognition of the thymine dimer, or whether in fact, it is a distortion of the strands.

Dr. Rupert   The only thing that anybody has ever shown to act as substrate for this enzyme is pyrimidine dimers. If you merely alkylate the DNA and leave it unirradiated, it doesn't work. The same is true if you make it single-stranded, create breaks in it with nucleases, or treat with nitrous acid. I don't know what other things one can think of right off hand. Putting bromouracil in it in place of thymine also doesn't do anything, if it's unirradiated, but of course that doesn't interrupt the hydrogen bonding the way you were suggesting.

Dr. Yielding   Also, is it possible that some of the UV reactivation we see of infecting particles might be based on providing a substrate which could find a photoreactivating enzyme, and therefore permit access of the excision enzymes to the base of host DNA? That might possibly be one role in which a competitive relationship could be demonstrated between photoreactivation and excision.

Dr. Rupert   It might be. There are only about 20 molecules of enzyme in E. coli to get in the way, but there could be conceivably 20 critical regions that might be interfered with, a little bit.

Dr. John Boyle (Manchester)   Mike Patrick and his colleagues recently presented data in Photochemistry and Photobiology concerning the photoreactivation of $\widehat{TT}$ dimers and $\widehat{CT}$ dimers at 313 and 405 nanometers. The ratio of monomerization of $\widehat{TT}$ dimers compared to $\widehat{CT}$ was, I think, greater at 405 nanometers than 313. Have you any thoughts about the reason for this differential photolysis at different wave lengths?

Dr. Rupert   On the face of it, it sounds like the action spectrum may be a little bit different for the different dimers. However, when you're doing this, unless you have all the substrates completely complexed, the relative affinity of the enzymes for the different dimer types at the relative rates at which it is going on and coming off, each is also involved, and I really wouldn't be sure of any interpretation without setting up, or seeing somebody set up, an experiment designed to test whatever hypothesis you had.

Dr. James Jackson (Narragansett)   I have two simple questions. One is, does X-ray or other part ionizing radiation cause any dimer formation? And the other is, do green plants that are always exposed to both ultraviolet and visible light have the photoreactivating system?

Dr. Cook   To answer the question about green plants, yes, they do. As a matter of fact, they have two kinds, probably, and E. coli also might have two kinds. The second kind being one that repairs dimers in RNA, under certain special conditions. Milton Gordon's been working on this question with RNA from tobacco mosaic virus, and its photoreactivation. That's a question of RNA repair. Dr. Jackson's first question had to do with dimers from X-rays and the answer is no.

Dr. Telino (Columbus)   Has anyone done, even though the enzyme has not been purified to that great an extent, any work on the type of moiety that absorbs the photon energy for the activation process? What type of structural moiety quantity is it?

Dr. Rupert   All I can say is, I think Werbin has this fluorescent material that's associated with the enzyme he purified 10^5-fold. That's the only indication of a chromophoric substance I know about, and until he gets enough of this out, for somebody to characterize a little more, there's not much more to say about it.

Dr. Hutchison   Did Dr. Cook mean to imply that the dimers in ribose polymers are not broken by the ordinary yeast enzyme?

Dr. Cook   That's right.

Dr. Rupert   The ordinary yeast photoreactivating enzyme does not act on RNA photoproducts. Only on DNA.

Dr. Herriott   I want to point out that there is another short paper which will be presented at this time. I think we should suspend the discussion at this moment.

THE REPAIR OF FREEZING INJURY IN MAMMALIAN CELLS RECOVERED FROM LIQUID NITROGEN[1]

David M. Robinson

The American National Red Cross
Blood Research Laboratory
Bethesda, Maryland

Exposure to many kinds of environmental stress may produce potentially lethal injury. The ability of cells to repair such damage and so avoid death has been amply demonstrated in the case of certain radiation- and chemically-induced lesions. This report will indicate the presence of a repair mechanism in mammalian cells grown in culture, probably associated with the cell surface, by means of which the cells are able to remain alive following exposure to very low temperature.

The cell line (CHA) used in these experiments is "Clone A" originally isolated by T. T. Puck from ovary of Chinese hamster and which has been grown continuously in serial culture for about twelve years. The rates of cooling and warming used produce damage as a result of exposure to increasingly concentrating solute molecules as water crystallizes as ice in the external medium around the cells. There is very little likelihood of the production of intracellular ice in CHA cells at these rates of change in temperature (1). All values of survival quoted here have been measured by an assay of colony-forming ability, whereby the number of cells, each capable of producing a macroscopic colony of descendants after ten days of incubation, is expressed as a percentage of the original population.

It has already been reported (2,3,4) that CHA cells in isotonic solutions, containing neither serum nor cryoprotective agents, may be cooled slowly (1 to 5°C/minute) to -196°C and warmed quickly (about 200°C/minute) yet still retain viability provided they are placed into "conditioned medium" immediately on return to 37°C. Conditioned medium (CM) is that taken from old cultures of CHA cells which have remained as confluent monolayers for several days. Such cells placed in fresh complete growth medium (FM) immediately after thawing, all die.

The first series of observations was made on cells recently removed from monolayers and frozen and thawed in suspension in medium without serum. Cells placed in CM for a recovery period of 20 hours prior to incubation in FM produced 80% survival, whereas cells placed directly into FM all died. It should be noted that these cells are still suffering the insult of trypsinization, which is known to have effects on radiation response (5) and on the uptake of precursors of DNA and RNA synthesis (4). In the last mentioned case it is known that CM goes someway towards ameliorating the effects of trypsin, in that recently trypsinized cells placed in FM will not take up ^{3}H-uridine at one hour after

---

[1]Contribution No. 232 from the Blood Research Laboratory, American National Red Cross, Bethesda, Maryland 20014.

plating, yet cells placed in CM all take up the nucleoside at that time. If the effects of freezing and thawing per se are to be investigated, clearly it is necessary to exclude the effects of trypsinization from the experimental system.

Accordingly, a second series of observations was made on cells which had been allowed to attach to cover slips for several hours after trypsinization and which, therefore, had recovered from its damaging effects. Cells in this state behaved in the same way as cells frozen and thawed in suspension, in that when they were placed into FM immediately on return to 37°C they all died. However, cells attached to cover slips and placed into CM for 20 hours immediately after freezing and thawing produced 100% survival.

In an attempt to determine the nature of this reparable injury, cells were frozen and thawed in a perfusion chamber under a phase contrast microscope. Upon thawing, the cells were perfused either with FM or with CM. Cells left to recover in CM showed no visible signs of injury. However, cells allowed to recover in FM developed membranous vesicles at the external surface after about 30 minutes; these vesicles eventually broke away and the cells finally disintegrated. The assumption was made that the primary damage due to freezing and thawing could not be visualized in the light microscope and that, if left unrepaired, a subsequent progression of events would lead to the production of surface vesicles.

It has already been proposed that the most likely cause of damage in this type of freezing is a result of exposure to the high concentration of solutes produced as water is removed as ice. Following this assumption cells were placed in a solution of 10 times isotonic sodium chloride and kept at 37°C. After one hour, surface vesicles appeared; these had essentially the same appearance as those produced by freezing. Large numbers of vesicles were prepared in this way, isolated from the cells by gentle shaking and concentrated by ultracentrifugation. A chemical analysis of this preparation of vesicles was made, with the finding that vesicles differ most strikingly from normal plasma membrane preparations in their very low content of phospholipid and their complete lack of sialic acid.

If surface vesicles do arise from sites of primary injury, the normal cell surface constituents that are reduced or missing in vesicles may be involved in the initial damage. Indeed the role played by CM in the repair process may be to replace such compounds, since CM prevents vesicle formation. Phospholipid would seem to be a good candidate in this context, since it is turned over quickly and secreted into the medium by mammalian cells in culture (6). To investigate this further, cells were grown in ^{3}H-choline and ^{3}H-myo-inositol, precursors of two of the main membrane phosphatides in hamster cells. The cells were washed and exposed to concentrated sodium chloride solution in order to produce vesicles. The cells with vesicles were fixed by osmium tetroxide and autoradiographs prepared. Cells grown in ^{3}H-choline showed the same intensity of labeling over the vesicles as over the unaffected portions of the plasma membrane, but cells grown in ^{3}H-myo-inositol produced vesicles with a grain count approximately one half that of normal plasma membrane. Phosphatidyl-inositol, therefore, appears to be removed from the cell surface prior to the formation of vesicles. However, the addition of phosphatidyl-inositol (Fraction 1) or inositol to FM during the recovery period after freezing and thawing did not result in any increase in cell survival.

The finding that the vesicles had no sialic acid prompted a further study of surface carbohydrates. CHA cells grown on cover slips were fixed with osmium tetroxide and stained with ruthenium red, a dye which produces intense red coloration by binding to charged polysaccharides. Normal cells, neither frozen nor thawed, but maintained at 37°C, showed intense staining. However, cells which had been frozen to -196°C then thawed and fixed immediately afterwards, showed very little uptake of ruthenium red. This was taken to indicate that the freezing and thawing process had resulted in a loss of some cell surface carbohydrate.

If, indeed, carbohydrate molecules, particularly sialic acid, are involved in reparable freezing injury, then a qualitative comparison of the carbohydrate content of FM and CM might be expected to show some differences. A preliminary analysis of FM and of CM, using SDS gels, gave no detectable differences. Specific analysis of sialic acid content after acid hydrolysis similarly gave no differences. However 50% of the sialic acid in CM exists as the free monosaccharide and is detectable prior to acid hydrolysis. In FM, all the sialic acid is bound. These limited analyses indicate the removal of carbohydrate from the cell surface on freezing and thawing and the presence of free monosaccharide in conditioned medium.

It would not be surprising to find that cells in prolonged serial culture, such as those investigated here, exposed to trypsinization at frequent intervals over long periods of time, were characterized by very efficient surface repair mechanisms. That CM accelerates recovery from trypsin-induced injury (4) and that trypsinization removes surface glycoproteins (7), make it tempting to postulate that the repair of freezing injury which takes place in CM might involve a multi-glycosyl transferase system capable of repairing damaged surface oligosaccharide chains. The existence of such enzymes at cell surfaces is known in other animal systems (8) and although there is no evidence to suggest their presence here, it is obvious that cell surface carbohydrates are at least involved in freezing injury and presumably in its repair.

REFERENCES

1. Mazur, P.: Science, 168:939, 1970.
2. Robinson, D. M.: Cryobiology, 6:573, 1970.
3. Robinson, D. M. and Meryman, H. T.: Biophys. J., 11:94a, 1971.
4. Robinson, D. M. and Harris, L. W.: Nature, in press.
5. Berry, R. J., Evans, H. J. and Robinson, D. M.: Exp. Cell Res., 42:512, 1966.
6. Pasternak, C. A. and Bergeron, J. J. M.: Biochem. J., 119:473, 1970.
7. Harris, E. D. and Johnson, C. A.: Biochemistry, 8:512, 1969.
8. Roth, S., McGuire, E. J. and Roseman, S.: J. Cell Biol., 51:536, 1971.

DISCUSSION

Dr. Herriott   I think we might throw this paper open for discussion for a few moments. Yes, Dr. Cook.

Dr. Cook   I was curious whether you have done any electron micrographs on this, and whether you see any association of Golgi with the vesicle formation and repair.

Dr. Robinson   We've just managed to get enough money to do some electron microscopy with that in view.

Dr. B. Strauss (Chicago)   Just a practical question. Do you get this effect if you freeze glycerol medium or with dimethylsulfoxide?

Dr. Robinson   Yes, one imagines that glycerol and dimethylsulfoxide are acting in a purely colligative fashion in reducing the amount of ice that develops at any particular temperature, and so reducing the concentration of solutes, and perhaps reducing the damaging effects that occur. So you get protection in this way, but of course you can't get 100% recovery following freezing with this kind of protective agents, if you put the cells into conditioned medium, whereas you might not get 100% recovery, if they were put directly into fresh medium.

Part III

CELLULAR REPAIR PROCESSES I

DNA SYNTHESIS, REPAIR AND CHROMOSOME BREAKS IN EUCARYOTIC CELLS[1]

Bernard Strauss, M. Coyle,[2] M. McMahon, K. Kato and M. Dolyniuk

Department of Microbiology, The University of Chicago
Chicago, Illinois

Both metabolic inhibitors and alkylating agents cause chromosome breaks (13) and it is our belief that this is due to their effect on DNA synthesis. The monofunctional alkylating agents induce single-strand breaks in isolated DNA molecules. On the other hand, the inhibitors of DNA synthesis such as hydroxyurea and fluorodeoxyuridine do not act directly on DNA. Their chromosome-breaking activity, therefore, must be due to their effect on the metabolic systems of the cell. In this paper we will discuss some of the experiments which have led to the conclusion that both types of compounds act by virtue of their effect on a common system.

The eucaryotic cells used in these experiments were a strain of HEp.2 (8) obtained from Microbiological Associates, at frequent intervals, and cultivated as previously described (6). We used the monofunctional alkylating agent, methyl methanesulfonate (MMS) as a chromosome-breaking compound. Breaks in pre-existing DNA molecules invariably follow treatment with this compound of either organisms or of DNA in vitro. Although the action of MMS is complex (20), it is no more so than that of ultraviolet light which, aside from inducing the formation of different pyrimidine dimers, also, at physiological doses, induces unidentified covalent crosslinks between DNA and protein molecules (19). The chromosome-breaking inhibitors of DNA synthesis were fluorodeoxyuridine (FUdR) (22) and hydroxyurea (HU) (3,23). Our attention was drawn to these compounds because of their wide use in the analysis of the phenomena of DNA replication and repair. In the course of their use for such analysis, we became interested in their action per se.

EXPERIMENTAL RESULTS

We analyzed the fragmentation of DNA by the same technique as that used in the rapid preparation of polyoma DNA (10). This technique, referred to in this paper as the "Hirt technique," is based on the insolubility in 1M NaCl and detergent of endogenous DNA molecules of size greater than about 20S. Both large molecular size and attachment of DNA to some cellular constituent are required for precipitability since large DNA molecules added to a cell suspension before lysis do not precipitate as completely as endogenous DNA (6). Molecules of DNA found in the soluble or

[1] Supported in part by grants from the National Science Foundation (GB 8514), the National Institutes of Health (GM 07816) and the Atomic Energy Commission (AT(11-1) 2040).
[2] Dr. Coyle's present address is Temple University, Health Sciences Center, School of Medicine, Philadelphia, Pa. 19140.

111

supernatant fraction after the Hirt fractionation are double-stranded as evidenced by their density in CsCl and, when isolated from cells treated with inhibitors or alkylating agents, have a sedimentation value of about 20S (Fig 1). Only small amounts of material from normal, untreated cells are found in the Hirt supernatant and these generally sediment more rapidly. We interpret this difference to mean that the material in the supernatant from untreated cells has a different origin.

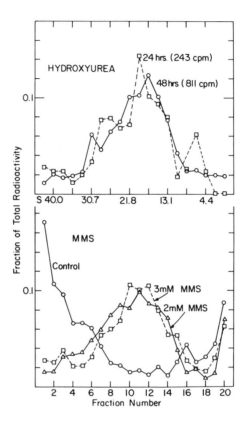

Fig 1. Sedimentation of material from the Hirt supernatant through a neutral sucrose gradient. The supernatant was dialyzed and layered on a 5-20% neutral sucrose gradient 1M with respect to NaCl. Top: supernatant from hydroxyurea-treated cultures (24 hrs --- ; 48 hrs ——). Bottom: control and MMS-treated. S values are calculated as described by McEwen (14). Sedimentation was for 4 hrs at 35,000 rpm at 20° in a Beckman L2 centrifuge using a SW50.1 rotor.

When cells are treated with MMS and then incubated with tritiated thymidine for one hour, or are allowed to incorporate thymidine in the presence of FUdR or HU and are then incubated for an additional period with these inhibitors, the isotope incorporated initially precipitates in the Hirt pellet after fractionation. However, within about 24 hours of incubation, the DNA isolated from inhibited or alkylated cultures is fragmented (Table I). This is not the degradation to be expected in dying cells since our methodology requires that cells remain attached to the surface of culture dishes and "dead" cells rapidly detach from such plates. We wish to emphasize both findings:

TABLE I

Degradation of DNA as Determined by the Hirt Procedure

Set	Inhibitor	Time Incubated (hours)	Ratio of Acid Precipitable Radioactivity: Supernatant / Pellet
1.	Control	4	0.08
	MMS - 2 mM	4	0.06
	Control	24	0.09
	MMS - 2 mM	24	0.38
2.	Control	10	0.14
	HU - 2.5 mM	10	0.16
	Control	24	0.09
	HU - 2.5 mM	24	0.17
	Control	48	0.21
	HU - 2.5 mM	48	0.72
3.	Control	24	0.08
	FUdR - 0.1 mM	24	0.46
	Control	48	0.16
	FUdR - 0.1 mM	48	1.52

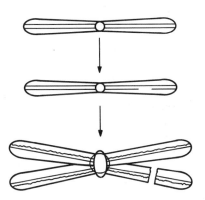

Fig 2. Interpretation of the relationship between the formation of chromatid breaks and the replication of broken DNA molecules.

(a) newly synthesized DNA, formed by alkylated cells, initially precipitates with the bulk of the cellular DNA, and (b) DNA from such cultures separates from the bulk of the cell DNA and is found in fragments of about 20S (Fig 1) within approximately one cell generation after its synthesis. Both facts require explanation. We need to know how the DNA is formed initially and also how the cells are altered so that this newly-formed DNA either is released or degraded after a cell generation.

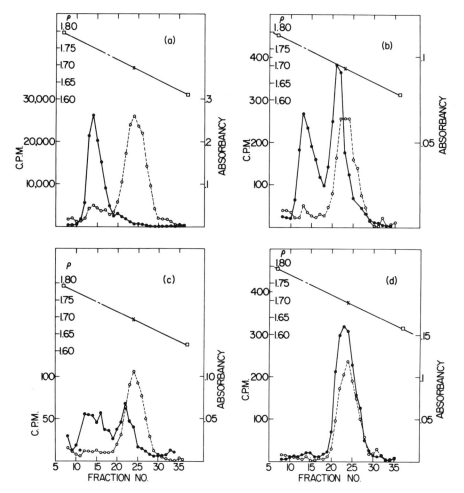

Fig 3. Effect of hydroxyurea on ^{3}HBUdR incorporation. HEp.2 cells were pre-incubated for 2 hours in medium with 5 μg/ml BUdR in the presence of 10^{-6}M FUdR. They then were treated for 60 min with 2.5 x 10^{-3} M MMS in BUdR containing medium plus 10^{-6}M FUdR and 5 x 10^{-3}M hydroxyurea where indicated. The MMS was removed and the cells were incubated for 60 min in medium containing ^{3}H BUdR (0.95 Ci/mM; 5 μg/ml) plus FUdR or for 120 min in medium containing ^{3}HBUdR plus FUdR and hydroxyurea. Chlortetracycline (10 μg/ml) was added at the start of incubation with BUdR and was present throughout the experiment, but the cells were grown in the absence of other antibiotic. a) Control, no MMS; b) MMS-treated; c) Control plus hydroxyurea; d) MMS-treated plus hydroxyurea.

Symbols: filled circles, radioactivity; open circles, absorbancy at 260 mμ; squares, density as calculated from refractive index.

Chromatid breaks are generally assumed to be the result of DNA synthesis using molecules with single-strand breaks as template (Fig 2). Whole chromosome breaks can occur by double-strand scission and, it is assumed, need not involve DNA synthesis. If changes in chromosome structure can be interpreted in terms of changes in DNA molecules, that is, if it is possible to translate molecular into biological structure, our experiments imply that chromatid breaks result from DNA replication before the operation of some repair mechanism, very likely an excision-repair mechanism. Alternatively, the results of our experiments indicate that repair must occur before semiconservative synthesis starts, if the newly synthesized DNA is to behave normally in subsequent replication.

These experiments were performed as follows: HEp.2 cells were grown attached to the surface of plastic dishes. Alkylation was performed by addition of medium containing freshly dissolved MMS. The MMS solution was siphoned off after one hour's incubation, the cells then were rinsed with medium, and fresh medium (Eagles' MEM with 10% calf serum) was added. Washing and the replacement of medium could be done quickly since the cells remain attached to the culture dish. This ease of replacement permitted protocols in which isotope was added for limited periods of time. We observed no effect of fresh as opposed to conditioned medium.

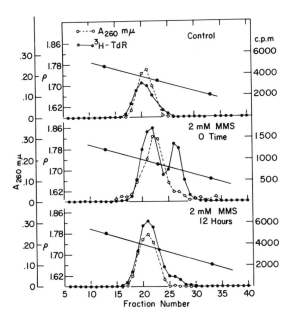

Fig 4. Replication of the DNA synthesized by HEp.2 cells after alkylation. Cells were treated with 2mM MMS for one hour and then incubated with [3]HTdR (5 μCi/ml, 3 Ci mM) for one hour either immediately (center) or twelve hours after treatment. After an additional incubation for 21 hours in unlabelled medium following incubation with [3]HTdR they were incubated in medium with unlabelled BUdR (5 μg/ml) for 48 hours. DNA was isolated and subjected to centrifugation through a CsCl gradient as described in the text.

Symbols: dotted line, absorbancy at 260 mμ; solid line, radioactivity in cpm. The superimposed line indicates density as determined from refractive index.

Both semiconservative and nonsemiconservative synthesis occur immediately after treatment of HEp.2 cells with 2 mM MMS, a dose permitting about 50% survival (Fig 3). Nonsemiconservative, or "repair" synthesis, was demonstrated by incubation of MMS-treated cells with ^{3}H-BUdR (tritiated bromodeoxyuridine) in the presence of hydroxyurea. It is an experimental observation that hydroxyurea inhibits semiconservative synthesis but does not inhibit UV- or alkylation-induced nonsemiconservative synthesis in mammalian cells (1,4) although the reason for this selectivity of inhibition is not understood.

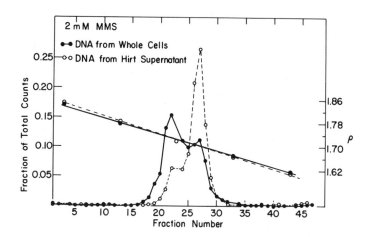

Fig 5. Density distribution of DNA from whole cells and from the Hirt supernatant after incubation in BUdR. HEp.2 cells were treated with 2mM MMS for one hour, labelled with ^{3}HTdR (5 μCi/ml; 3 Ci/mM) for an additional hour, incubated in unlabelled medium for 22 hours and then in BUdR (5 μg/ml) for 48 hours. The DNA was purified and centrifuged to equilibrium through a CsCl gradient. Symbols: closed circles and solid curves, DNA preparation from whole cells; open circles and broken line, DNA from Hirt supernatant. Slanted lines (ρ) density calculated from refractive index.

A portion of the DNA made by semiconservative synthesis in the first hour after alkylation does not replicate and is degraded. This conclusion is demonstrated as follows:

1. The cell cycle for HEp.2 cells is about 24 hours. We determined whether DNA made after alkylation could replicate by an experiment involving three incubation periods. Cells alkylated with MMS were (a) incubated with ^{3}HTdR for one hour, (b) in unlabeled medium for the next 21 hours, and then (c) incubated with BUdR (5μg/ml) for 48 hours. Only cells which replicated the DNA synthesized after alkylation should produce hybrid, labeled DNA. We found that all of the DNA synthesized by control cells was hybrid after such a protocol. In contrast, a portion of the DNA initially synthesized by MMS-treated cells did not replicate (Fig 4). This portion was dose-dependent, being higher in cultures treated with larger MMS doses.

2. Nonreplicated, newly-formed DNA was preferentially degraded. Cells were treated as described above and the cell suspension was divided into two portions. In the first

portion, DNA was extracted from whole cells. A Hirt supernatant was prepared from the second portion of cells and the DNA in this supernatant was purified and analyzed in a CsCl gradient (Fig 5). Comparison of gradients from the whole cell and from the supernatant preparations shows that DNA that had not replicated after the initial thymidine incorporation concentrated in the Hirt supernatant.

3. The newly synthesized, degraded DNA in the Hirt supernatant includes DNA produced by semiconservative synthesis. Cells were alkylated, treated with ^{3}H-BUdR and then incubated in unlabeled medium before harvest. It was found that the DNA in the Hirt supernatant distributed itself in an equilibrium CsCl gradient as though it were a mixture of material synthesized by semiconservative and nonsemiconservative synthesis (Fig 6). This indicates that much of this DNA was synthesized by a "normal" mechanism.

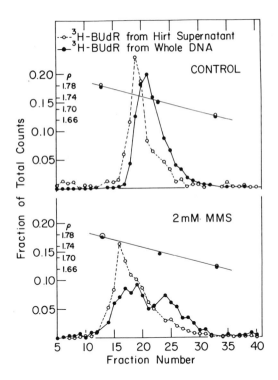

Fig 6. Distribution of density of [3]HBUdR labelled material in the Hirt supernatant as compared to cellular DNA. HEp.2 cells were pretreated with BUdR (5 μg/ml) for 2 hrs, treated with 2mM MMS in the presence of BUdR, labelled with [3]HBUdR (5 μg/ml; 0.95 Ci/mM) for one hour and chased with unlabelled BUdR (5 μg/ml) for an additional three hours. The cells were incubated 21 hours in unlabelled medium, collected and a cellular DNA and Hirt supernatant DNA were prepared and centrifuged to equilibrium in a CsCl gradient.

Symbols: solid circles, radioactivity from whole DNA; open circles, radioactivity from supernatant DNA; slanted lines, density as calculated from refractive index. The total radioactivity was normalized for the comparison.

We also found that if a period of incubation intervened between alkylation and [3]HTdR incorporation, the incorporated [3]HTdR replicated normally. If a period of 12, or even 5 hours, elapsed between alkylation and isotope addition, the incorporated thymidine was replicated (Fig 7). We therefore conclude that DNA repair occurs in the interval and that the ^{3}H-containing DNA replicated because it was synthesized from a repaired template. The DNA made in the first hour neither was normal nor was it subsequently repaired because it was not transferred to hybrid density. Furthermore, our data can not be

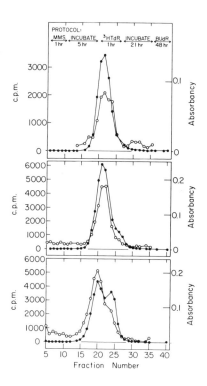

Fig 7. Replication of the DNA synthesized by HEp.2 cells five hours after treatment with MMS. Cells were treated as indicated in the protocol (top). Concentrations and conditions were as in the legend to Figure 4. a) Top, control; b) middle, treatment with 2mM MMS; c) bottom, treatment with 3mM MMS.

Symbols: closed circles, radioactivity; open circles, absorbancy at 260 mμ.

explained by supposing that there is some selective inactivation process which prevents cells unable to produce DNA capable of replicating from incorporating any thymidine at all, since HEp.2 cells treated with 3 mM MMS did take up thymidine at both 5 and 12 hours after MMS treatment even though a large portion of this thymidine was not transferred subsequently to a hybrid density (Fig 8). The same result argues against a selective degradation process which removes newly synthesized DNA molecules unable to replicate. We, therefore, conclude that DNA synthesized from a damaged template is unable to replicate but that, as proposed by Painter, Umber and Young (16) repaired-DNA replicates normally. Although our experiments do not describe fully the nature of the repair process,

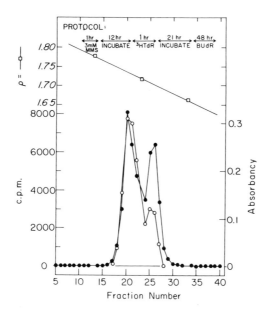

Fig 8. Failure of DNA synthesized 12 hrs after treatment with 3mM MMS to replicate further. Protocol as described in the legend for Figure 4 except that treatment was with 3mM MMS for one hour. Symbols: closed circles, radioactivity; open circles, absorbancy at 260 mμ.

we have demonstrated nonsemiconservative replication within the required 5 hour time period. The result of MMS-treatment is an increase in hydroxyurea-insensitive [3]HTdR incorporation by HEp.2 cells (Table II) and nonsemiconservative incorporation of ^{3}H-BUdR can be detected after MMS treatment in hydroxyurea inhibited cultures (Fig 3). Most of the repair is completed in less than 4 hours after MMS treatment (Table II).

Table II

DNA Synthesis in the Presence of 5 mM Hydroxyurea

MMS Concentration (x 10[3] M)	Time of [3]HTdR Pulse after MMS (hr)	Acid Precipitable (c.p.m.)	Fraction of Uninhibited Incorporation
0	0-1	158	0.024
2		416	0.23
3		568	0.56
0	2.5-3.5	187	0.26
2		209	0.062
3		317	0.15
0	5-6	237	0.024
2		245	0.058
3		294	0.13

Since the structure and replication of eucaryotic chromosomes are so little understood, any attempt at explanation requires a consistent point of view of the available facts and hypotheses (5,9,11,17,21). We, therefore, assume: (a) that the DNA of the eucaryotic chromosome exists as a single Watson-Crick molecule without interruption throughout its entire length; (b) that in each chromosome there are a number of fixed initiation sites for replication; (c) that the initiation sites do not reproduce simultaneously but have a specific order of replication during the S phase; that individual replicons have a fixed size and that replication stops once that size has been reached; (d) that replication starts at a point at which DNA is associated with the nuclear membrane and that it involves the introduction of single-strand breaks in the DNA (the equivalent of the "swivel" in bacterial DNA replication); (e) that once started, synthesis of a replicon continues until completion (in the presence of an inhibitor, new replicons are not initiated); and (f) that nucleases are present which can attack DNA at growing points.

We assume that semiconservative DNA synthesis converts single-strand breaks into scissions, irreparable by simple excision-repair, since replication removes the complementary strand required to serve as a template (Fig 2). Any repair after DNA replication should require additional steps in order to provide an undamaged complementary strand as a model, that is, as in the scheme for recombinational repair suggested by Rupp and Howard-Flanders (18). Failing such alternative mechanisms, newly synthesized DNA must have double-strand breaks which separate the chromosome into centric and acentric fragments. One would expect to find chromatid breaks and acentric fragments at lower doses and fragmentation and DNA pieces at higher doses of alkylating agent because the higher the dose of alkylating agent, the greater will be the interruptions in the continuity of the single DNA molecule which we assume makes up a chromosome. Aberrations of this type are, of course, observed (13).

This interpretation of the course of formation of chromatid breaks assumes that DNA synthesis takes place regardless of breaks in the template, and that the synthetic mechanism is able to bridge the alkylation-induced gap. The analysis ignores the possibility that some cells may sense damage by an unknown mechanism and may delay replication until that damage has been repaired. Semiconservative synthesis by HEp.2 cells during the first hour after treatment shows that DNA synthesis does occur. The fact that the fragments of DNA formed by MMS-treated cells gradually become larger (Fig 9B) implies that pieces of DNA smaller than "normal" can be formed. "Bridging a gap" might occur if either single-strand breaks serve as sites of initiation for DNA synthesis (2) or if the synthetic mechanism ignores a loss of continuity in one of the template strands.

Why might DNA with single-strand breaks replicate in contradistinction to DNA with double-strand (that is, chromotid) breaks? Several explanations are possible. Alkylated cells might start but not finish the first S period after treatment. The experiments of Myers and Strauss (15) which illustrate the normal timing of the first S period and of the first cell division following alkylation, rule out this explanation. On the other hand, a portion of cells containing DNA fragments might not start a second S period. Critical DNA segments lacking a centromere might be lost at mitosis, cells with less than a complete chromosomal complement might not produce the enzymes necessary for replication, or

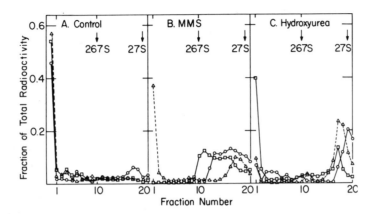

Fig 9. Sedimentation of incorporated ³H-thymidine through an alkaline sucrose gradient.

A. Control. Cells incubated an initial 30 min with ³HTdR were incubated an additional 30 min (0); 2 hrs (□) or 24 hrs (△) before lysis.

B. MMS-treated. Cells treated with 2 mM MMS were incubated with ³HTdR and then an additional 30 min (0); 2 hrs (□) or 24 hrs (△) before lysis.

C. HU-treated. Cells were allowed to incorporate thymidine in the presence of HU (5mM) and then were incubated an additional 30 min (0) or 24 hrs (△) before lysis. One set of cells was removed from HU after 2 hrs and incubated an additional 2 hrs in HU-free medium (□).

Sedimentation was for 60 min at 20,000 rpm and 20°C in the SW50.1 rotor of the Spinco L-2 centrifuge. The gradient was 5-20% sucrose in 0.9 M NaCl + 0.1 M NaOH.

the DNA fragments produced by alkylated cells may not contain the necessary sequences for attachment at the "initiation sites" on the cell membrane.

RESULTS OF STUDIES WITH HYDROXYUREA

Our experiments with one of the inhibitors of DNA synthesis, hydroxyurea (HU), can be summarized as follows (7):

1. Cells incubated in the presence of HU continue to incorporate a small amount of thymidine.

2. Thymidine incorporated by control cells sedimented as an aggregate when lysates of more than 10^4 cells were placed on an alkaline sucrose gradient (Fig 9A). A one-hour pulse of thymidine incorporated by cells incubated with HU prior to, during and after the incorporation did not sediment with the aggregate but rather as much smaller acid precipitable material (Fig 9C). Removal of inhibitor after 20-24 hours incubation produces a change in the cells so that after a short additional incubation without inhibitor, thymidine-containing material sediments with the aggregate. After 24 hours the effect of inhibitor is no longer reversible.

3. Very little of the thymidine incorporated in the presence of HU is found in the Hirt supernatant for 20-24 hours. After 24 hours incubation in the presence of inhibitor

newly synthesized DNA appears in quantity in the Hirt supernatant along with DNA
synthesized before addition of the inhibitor (Table I).

DISCUSSION

Treatment with alkylating agents or with inhibitors of DNA synthesis leads to
breakdown of newly synthesized DNA. Is there some fundamental relationship between
these two phenomena? We assume (Fig 10) as suggested by Hearst and Botchan (9) that
the initiation of DNA synthesis occurs only at particular sites attached to the nuclear
membrane. Single-strand breaks acting as initiation sites at any other point in the chromosome lead to the synthesis of DNA with double-strand breaks as previously discussed.
When the chromosome is released from the nuclear membrane at the onset of mitosis,
such double-strand breaks appear visually as chromatid breaks (Fig 2). Alkali denaturation
of newly replicated pieces leads to their immediate release from the bulk of the DNA
(Figs 10, 11).

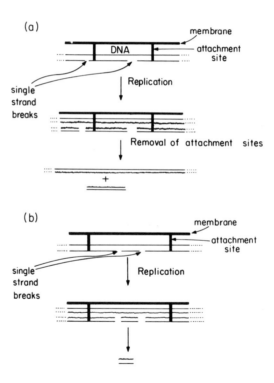

Fig 10. An interpretation of the origin of DNA fragments as a result of replication at: (a) low
doses: (b) high doses of alkylating agent.

The following variation of this hypothesis accounts for the induction of breaks
as a result of prolonged incubation in the presence of inhibitors (Fig 11): If synthesis of
an already active replicon continues and new replicons are not initiated as the amounts of
precursor diminish, growing points will remain in portions of the DNA for long periods
(Fig 11). If such growing points are particularly susceptible to nuclease action, scission of
DNA will result from prolonged incubation with inhibitor. The hypothesis requires

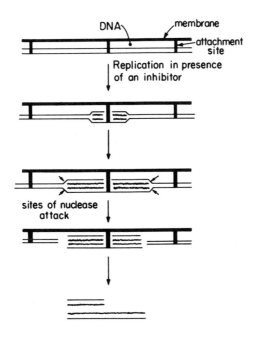

Fig 11. An interpretation of the origin of DNA fragments as a result of incubation with inhibitors DNA synthesis.

newly synthesized DNA to be attached to other materials in the cell and to precipitate or sediment in an aggregate under neutral but not alkaline (denaturing) conditions. In time, as additional breaks accumulate, or as the normal association of DNA with other cellular material breaks down, the DNA should be released from this aggregate. This is in accord with our observations. Precipitation of DNA in the Hirt pellet requires association with cellular material (6) and DNA synthesized in the presence of HU or after MMS treatment is first associated with the sedimenting pellet. After incubation of cells, much of this DNA is in the Hirt supernatant. Although the supernatant material obtained in the Hirt fractionation may be the end result of a series of degradative processes, we think that the presence of DNA fragments reflects real changes in the association of DNA in the cell.

SUMMARY

Our speculations can be summarized as follows: If excision-repair occurs before the replication complex for semiconservative synthesis reaches the MMS-damaged locus, the DNA replicates normally. However, if damage is induced during the S phase, so that the DNA still contains a lesion as the replication complex approaches, a double-strand break, irreparable by simple excision-repair is produced. Such "fixed" damage requires both recombination and excision-repair. DNA, newly synthesized from a damaged template, contains double-strand breaks yet the parts separated from the centromere remain associated. At some point the DNA fragments dissociate from the rest of the chromosomal material. Even if they are not lost at mitosis, the broken portions do not assemble at the initiation sites for the next S period.

As discussed above such an analysis also describes the mechanism of chromosome breakage by inhibitors of DNA synthesis. We, therefore, believe that the production of chromosome breaks by both alkylating agents and inhibitors of DNA synthesis is a consequence of the nature of DNA replication in procaryotic and eucaryotic organisms.

REFERENCES

1. Ayad, S., Fox, M. and Fox, B.: Non-semiconservative incorporation of labelled 5-bromo-2'-deoxyuridine in lymphoma cells treated with low doses of methyl methanesulfonate. Mutat. Res., 8:639, 1969.

2. Billen, D.: Replication of the bacterial chromosome. Location of new initiation sites after irradiation. J. Bact., 97:1169, 1969.

3. Borenfreund, E., Krim, M. and Bendich, A.: Chromosomal aberrations induced by hyponitrite and hydroxylamine derivatives. J. Nat. Cancer Inst., 32:667, 1964.

4. Cleaver, J.: Repair replication of mammalian cell DNA: Effects of compounds that inhibit DNA synthesis or dark repair. Radiat. Res., 37:334, 1969.

5. Comings, D.: The rationale for an ordered arrangement of chromatin in the interphase nucleus. Amer. J. Hum. Genet., 20:440, 1968.

6. Coyle, M., McMahon, M. and Strauss, B.: Failure of alkylated HEp.2 cells to replicate newly synthesized DNA. Mutat. Res., 12:427, 1971.

7. Coyle, M. and Strauss, B.: Cell killing and the accumulation of breaks in the DNA of HEp.2 cells incubated in the presence of hydroxyurea. Cancer Res., 30:2314, 1970.

8. Fjelde, A.: The establishment of mammalian cells in culture. In: Axenic Mammalian Cell Reactions. Edited by G. Tritsch. Marcel Dekker, New York, pp 1-29, 1969.

9. Hearst, J. and Botchan, M.: The eukaryotic chromosome. Ann. Rev. Biochem., 39:151, 1970.

10. Hirt, B.: Selective extraction of polyoma DNA from infected mouse cell cultures. J. Molec. Biol., 26:365, 1967.

11. Huberman, J. and Riggs, A.: On the mechanism of DNA replication in mammalian chromosomes. J. Molec. Biol., 32:327, 1968.

12. Kihlman, B.: Root tips for studying the effects of chemicals on chromosomes. In: Chemical Mutagens. Edited by Hollaender. Vol. 2. Plenum Press, New York, pp 489-514, 1971.

13. Kihlman, B.: Actions of chemicals on dividing cells. Prentice-Hall, Inc., N.Y., 1966.

14. McEwen, C.: Tables for estimating sedimentation through linear concentration gradients of sucrose solution. Anal. Biochem., 20:114, 1967.

15. Myers, T. and Strauss, B.: Effect of methyl methanesulphonate on synchronized cultures of HEp.2 cells. Nature, New Biology, 230:143, 1971.

16. Painter, R., Umber, J. and Young, B.: Repair replication in diploid and aneuploid human cells. Normal replication of repaired DNA after ultraviolet irradiation. Radiat. Res., 44:133, 1970.

17. Ris, H. and Kubai, D.: Chromosome structure. Ann. Rev. Genet., 4:263, 1970.

18. Rupp, W. and Howard-Flanders, P.: Discontinuities in the DNA synthesized in an excision defective strain of Escherichia coli following ultraviolet radiation. J. Molec. Biol., 31:291, 1968.

19. Smith, K., Hodgkins, B. and O'Leary, M.: The biological importance of ultraviolet light induced DNA-protein crosslinks in Escherichia coli 15 TAU Biochim. Biophys. Acta, 114:1, 1966.

20. Strauss, B. and Hill, T.: The intermediate in the degradation of DNA alkylated with a monofunctional alkylating agent. Biochim. Biophys. Acta, 213:14, 1970.

21. Taylor, J.: Replication and organization of chromosomes. Proc. XII Intern. Congr. Genetics Vol 3:177, 1969.

22. Taylor, J., Haut, W. and Tung, J.: Effects of flurodeoxyuridine on DNA replication, chromosome breakage and reunion. Proc. Nat. Acad. Sci. USA, 48:190, 1962.

23. Yu, C. and Sinclair, W.: Cytological effects on chinese hamster cells of synchronizing concentrations of hydroxyurea. J. Cell Physiol., 72:39, 1968.

THE REPAIR OF SUBLETHAL RADIATION INJURY AND THE REJOINING OF RADIATION-INDUCED DNA BREAKS BY CULTURED MAMMALIAN CELLS—ARE THEY RELATED?[1]

Glenn V. Dalrymple, A. J. Moss, Jr., Max L. Baker, John C. Nash, J. L. Sanders and K. P. Wilkinson

The Division of Nuclear Medicine, the Division of Biometry and the Department of Physiology and Biophysics, the University of Arkansas Medical Center and the Nuclear Medicine Service Little Rock Veterans Hospital, Little Rock, Arkansas

SUBLETHAL RADIATION INJURY

During the past decade, two important types of radiobiological injury to cultured mammalian cells were described and, to a degree, worked out in detail. The cell survival methods of Puck et al (1) were used by Elkind and Sutton (2) to demonstrate the repair of *sublethal*[2] radiation injury. They demonstrated the repair of sublethal injury by the split dose method. For this, they irradiated Chinese hamster cells with two doses of X-rays separated by different amounts of time. The results of their efforts showed the extrapolation number (N)[3] to increase from a value of 1.0 (when the doses were separated by 0 time, that is, a single dose) to a value characteristic of the cells irradiated with single doses. Although the extrapolation number varied to a considerable degree, the slope of the log-linear segment of the survival curve (as indicated by the D_0 value) remained essentially constant. For a given pair of doses, the cellular survival fraction increased from a minimum value to a maximum within a few hours. Since this increase in survival seemed more or less exponential repair, "half-times" of 1-2 hours were estimated.

The increase in survival, however, was not strictly exponential. As Elkind and Sutton (2) showed, the split dose survival curve possessed a degree of fine structure. Although a matter of speculation for several years (4,5), this fine structure seems to be a consequence of partial synchronization of the cells surviving the first dose. The progression of these cells in cohort fashion through different portions of the cell life cycle

[1] Supported, in part, by US AEC Contract No. AT-(40-1) 3884, and by Grant No. P-566, from the American Cancer Society.

[2] We use the nomenclature as expressed by Belli and Shelton (3). *Lethal* injury is registered when suppression of colony formation occurs under any circumstances. *Potentially lethal* injury may be repaired to nonlethal levels if suitable conditions are provided. If repair does not occur, conversion to a lethal state occurs and colony formation is suppressed. Cells *sustaining sublethal* radiation injury repair the damage and eventually form colonies.

[3] The terms N and D_0 refer to the familiar multitarget model from target theory:

$$S_f = 1 - (1 - e^{-D/D_0})^N$$

where S_f is the fraction of cells surviving a dose D; N is the extrapolation number and D_0 is the reciprocal of the slope of the log-linear segment. See Elkind and Whitmore (4) for more details of the application of the multitarget model in mammalian cell radiation biology.

(G_1, S, G_2, and M), resulted in wide differences in radiation response at the time of delivery of the second dose. This occurred because of differences in radiation sensitivity of the cells while in the different phases of the cell life cycle (6). On the idealized survival curve (Fig 1) this would be the period between t_1 and t_2.

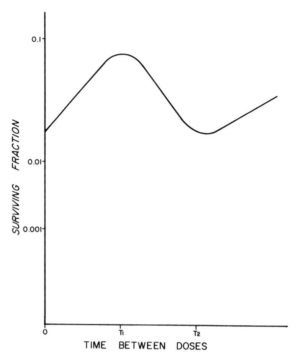

Fig 1. Hypothetical results from a paired-dose experiment with synchronous cells. (From Dalrymple et al, J. Theor. Biol., 21:368-386, 1968)

The increasing survival between t_0 and t_1 however, does not depend upon cell progression (4). Instead, it is a consequence of the actual repair of sublethal injury. This type of repair process is indeed very hardy. Only extreme treatments have been able to cause inhibition. Repair of this sublethal injury occurs in spite of such diverse treatments as hypoxia, low temperature, high temperature, FUdR, 5-FU, hydroxyurea, cycloheximide, puromycin, actinomycin-D, methotrexate and dinitrophenol (7-14). Only very drastic measures, such as prolonged treatment with methotrexate (7), extreme hypoxia (15) and treatment with actinomycin-D (11), seem to reduce the capacity of cells to repair sublethal injury.

Although a given dose of radiation, say at the levels used in clinical radiotherapy, causes massive cell killing, the cells that survive by repairing sublethal injury are very important. If we consider the cancer, these are the cells that may ultimately give rise to a recurrence of the lesion under treatment. If we consider the tumor bed of normal cells, the surviving cells will be needed to allow proper healing. Consequently, sublethal injury repair has been the subject of many investigations.

RADIATION DAMAGE TO DNA

A second large category of radiobiological injury concerns radiation induced DNA damage. Because of the biological importance of DNA, the repair of injury from any source (including radiation) has considerable interest. In 1965, McGrath and Williams published the report of an experiment with E. coli in which they found X-rays to produce large numbers of single-strand DNA breaks (16). Following appearance these breaks were rapidly rejoined; alkaline sucrose sedimentation methods provided the measurements. The studies of Kaplan, using E. coli, confirmed the findings of McGrath and Williams (17). In addition, he measured the production of double-strand DNA breaks; neutral sucrose sedimentation was used for the analysis. He found a dose-dependent increase in double-strand DNA breaks. Cells grown in BUdR had an increased yield of double-strand breaks on a per rad basis above cells grown in the absence of BUdR. In both instances (cells grown with or without BUdR), the double-strand breaks did not rejoin. Kaplan postulated that double-strand DNA breaks were principally responsible for the lethal effects of ionizing radiation. This postulate was based, in part, upon the findings of Freifelder (18) who related inactivation of T7 bacteriophage to double-strand breaks in the phage DNA. During the next few years the principle that single-strand DNA breaks represented reparable injury while double-strand breaks caused lethality provided the basis for a number of theoretical models to explain radiation effects at the molecular level (19-21).

In 1967, Lett et al reported the rejoining of single-strand DNA breaks by L5178Y cells after 30,000 rads of X-rays (22). Since then, other workers, using alkaline sucrose sedimentation, have shown several other lines of cultured mammalian cells to be able to rejoin single-strand DNA breaks (23-29). Also, this rejoining occurs during all portions of the cell life cycle (23,24,27).

Although rejoining of single-strand DNA breaks by cultured mammalian cells may be measured with moderate difficulty using alkaline sucrose methods, measuring double-strand breaks is considerably more complex.

The difficulties associated with measuring double-strand breaks in cultured mammalian cells stem largely from the contamination of the DNA by RNA and protein (30). In order to reduce the contribution by these factors, Corry and Cole isolated chromosomes from Chinese hamster cells (31). Lehmann and Omerod (32) summarized some of the technical considerations. Such factors as ionic strength (excessively high salt concentrations may cause improper sedimentation), rotor speed (excessively high rotor speeds may distort the sedimentation patterns) and radiation dose (apparently doses well above 30,000 rads are needed to produce the gaussian sedimentation patterns required to measure DNA). The experience of Lehmann and Omerod agrees with Kaplan in that postirradiation rejoining of double-strand breaks was not detected. Kitayama and Matsuyama (33), on the other hand, published results which suggest the bacterium M. radiodurans to be able to rejoin DNA breaks. Other data published by Lett et al (34) support these findings. As one would suspect, the whole question of double-strand breaks is associated with rather intense controversy. Certainly this area of investigation could benefit by clarification.

Another aspect of the problem concerns the quality of the DNA after rejoining of double-strand breaks (assuming for the moment that rejoining does occur). The probability seems low that the fragments would rejoin in exactly the proper manner (20). The result would be a "scrambling" of the genetic code which, in all likelihood, would be incompatible with survival.

At present, we have studies in progress to evaluate the question of the genetic code following rejoining.

Without question, ultracentrifuge studies have provided valuable quantitative information about the repair of radiation damage to DNA. Unfortunately, these studies do not concern themselves directly with molecular mechanisms. To help remedy this deficiency, we have used two enzymes, polynucleotide kinase (35-37) and DNA polymerase (38) to study the nature of radiation induced DNA breaks. Polynucleotide kinase labels DNA breaks characterized by 5' termini; under the proper assay conditions both end and internal 5' termini are labeled (39). DNA polymerase, on the other hand, adds labeled nucleotides to 3' OH termini of the DNA molecule (40). By using appropriate radioisotopic labeling we have shown that radiation produces a large number of DNA breaks which are characterized both by 5' and 3' OH termini. Following irradiation, the breaks are rapidly rejoined; the 5' and 3' OH termini decrease in number in a parallel fashion.

On the basis of these findings, we have suggested that DNA ligase may be responsible for at least part of the repair of radiation induced DNA damage (20,21,29,41-43). DNA ligase occurs widely in nature. It has been described both in microorganisms and in mammalian tissues (44,45). This enzyme, which requires a high energy co-factor, rejoins single-strand DNA breaks characterized by $5'PO_4$, $3'OH$ termini (37,44). Since we observe 5' and 3'OH termini after irradiation and since these termini disappear together, we believe the relationship to the action of DNA ligase is clear.

As more information emerges about DNA rejoining, several points seem very disturbing. First, the rate of rejoining of DNA breaks is much more rapid than the repair of sublethal injury. Where the rejoining half-time is of the order of a few minutes, the sublethal injury repair half-time is an hour or more. A second point concerned the ability of cells irradiated with supralethal doses (such as 10,000-20,000 rads for irradiating cultured mammalian cells) to rejoin DNA breaks. In other words, functionally dead cells were able to rejoin single-strand DNA breaks.

It was in view of apparently conflicting findings, such as these, that we conducted a series of experiments in which cells were irradiated under conditions of energy deprivation. In our view, this method of approach has clarified some of the questions about the relationship between the repair of sublethal injury and the rejoining of DNA breaks.

THE STATE OF ENERGY DEPRIVATION

A continuous source of energy in the form of high energy phosphate bonds (such as ATP) is required by virtually every living thing. Since rejoining of DNA breaks and the repair of sublethal radiation injury are biological activities, we felt that energy-rejoining processes should be involved. Our first step concerned the development of a means to

lower the intracellular ATP levels without causing cell killing. We found the classic un-
coupler of oxidative phosphorylation, 2,4-dinitrophenol (DNP), to produce a reduction
of intracellular ATP levels to 10% (or lower) of control (46). Cells under treatment with
DNP (5×10^{-5} M to 1×10^{-4} M) suffered no loss of viability even after treatment periods
of 24 hrs or longer (46).

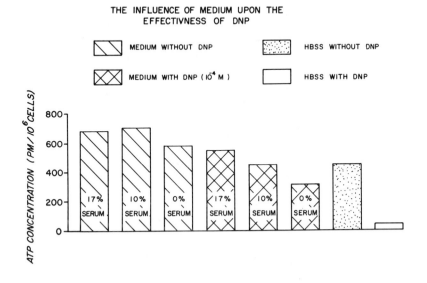

Fig 2. For this experiment L cells were suspended at a concentration of 10^6 cells/ml in the following:

   Complete medium (Eagle's MEM) + 17% calf serum
   Complete medium + 10% calf serum
   Complete medium without serum
   Complete medium + 17% calf serum + DNP (10^{-4} M)
   Complete medium + 10% calf serum + DNP
   Complete medium without serum + DNP
   Hanks balanced salts solution without glucose (HBSS) without DNP
   HBSS with DNP

The suspensions were incubated at 37°C for one hour. Perchloric acid (0.5N final concentration) was
added, the tubes chilled for 30 minutes, and then centrifuged. The ATP content of the acid soluble
fraction was measured by the firefly luciferase method (51). The results are given in units of picomoles
ATP/10^6 cells. (From Moss et al, Biophys. J., 11:158-174, 1971)

As Figure 2 shows, the method of applying the DNP to cultured mammalian
cells is critical. If the DNP is dissolved in medium (with or without added serum) the
components of the medium interfere with the action of the DNP. If the DNP is dissolved
in a balanced salts solution without glucose, however, extensive ATP depression occurs.
Consequently, for all of our studies we used cells suspended in (or treated with) Hanks
balanced salts solution without glucose (HBSS) as our "control" and DNP dissolved in
HBSS as our "treatment."

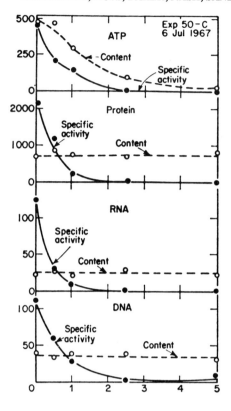

Fig 3. The effects of DNP on ATP, protein, RNA and DNA content and synthesis. The ordinate has the following units:

ATP$-$pm/10^6 cells (content) and cts/min per μM (incorporated radioactivity)
Protein$-\mu$g/10^6 cells and cts/min per mg protein
RNA$-\mu$g/10^6 cells and cts/min per μg RNA
DNA$-\mu$g/10^6 cells and cts/min per μg DNA

For this experiment L cells were suspended in HBSS (2×10^6 cells/ml) which contained varying concentrations of DNP. After a 15-minute incubation at 37°C, ^{14}C-glycine was added to the flasks (0.5 μCi/ml). Following a 30-minute incubation, the cells were extracted with perchloric acid. The ATP content was measured by the firefly luciferase method, and the ATP radioactivity was measured after Dowex column chromatography. The acid insoluble fraction was resolved into DNA, RNA and protein components by the Schmidt-Thannhauser method, the content of these macromolecules measured by the diphenylamine, orcinol and Lowry methods (respectively), and the radioactivity measured by gas flow methods (see reference 20 for details).

As the figure indicates, increasing DNP concentration depressed both ATP content and labeling. While macromolecular labeling was depressed, the contents remained fixed. (From Dalrymple et al, J. Theor. Biol., 21:368-386, 1968)

A second point concerned the ability of the DNP treatment to stop macromolecular synthesis (Fig 3). For this experiment, we measured the uptake of ^{14}C-glycine into ATP, DNA, RNA and protein as a function of DNP concentration. As Figure 3 indicates, 5×10^{-5} M DNP virtually obliterated the synthesis of these materials. Since DNP is known to be a potent inhibitor of the transport of many materials (including amino acids), we measured the incorporation of specific precursors into DNA, RNA and protein (14,47). Again, DNP produced evidence of a depression of macromolecular synthesis.

THE RELATIONSHIP OF ENERGY DEPRIVATION TO THE REJOINING OF DNA BREAKS

A. Ultracentrifuge Studies:

Figure 4 shows the rejoining of single-strand DNA breaks as measured by alkaline sucrose sedimentation. We should point out a variation in our methods as compared with other investigators (29). For our studies suspensions of L cells were irradiated with 10,000 rads of x-rays in HBSS and then incubated for the time periods shown. Following incubation, a detergent based lysing solution was added (2% TIPNS, 1% p-aminosalicylate

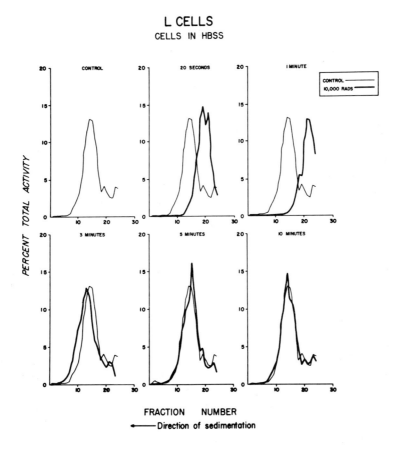

Fig 4. Alkaline sucrose sedimentation patterns of single-stranded DNA from L-cells suspended in HBSS. The suspension was given 10,000 rads and aliquots were withdrawn and lysed at the indicated times after irradiation. Rejoining of single-strand breaks is complete by 3 minutes (see text for details). (From Moss et al, Biophys. J., 11:158-174, 1971)

in 6% sec-butonal with 0.05 M EDTA; the pH was adjusted to 12.5 with NaOH). This caused immediate lysis. The lysates were held in the cold for 1 hr and then 50 λ portions of the lysate were layered onto 5%-23% isokinetic sucrose gradients (48) and then centrifuged in a SW 25.1 rotor for 4 hrs at 25,000 rpm. Each tube contained ^{14}C labeled T2 phage as a molecular weight marker. Following centrifugation, 10 drop fractions were collected and counted. As Figure 4 shows, a large number of DNA breaks were present at 0.3 and 1.0 minutes after irradiation. By 3 minutes, however, the molecular weight had returned to that of nonirradiated control.

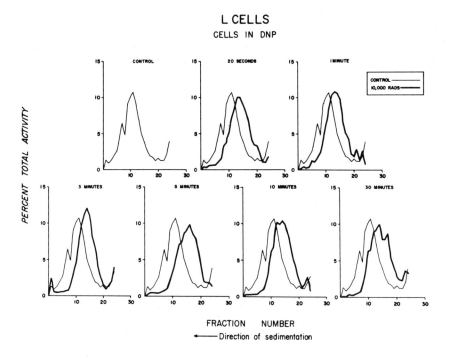

Fig 5. Alkaline sucrose sedimentation patterns of single-stranded DNA from L-cell suspensions in 10^{-4}M DNP in HBSS. The suspension was given 10,000 rads and aliquots were withdrawn and lysed at the indicated times after irradiation. In DNP there is no evidence of rejoining. (From Moss et al, Biophys. J., 11:158-174, 1971)

Figure 5 shows the influence of 1 x 10^{-4}M DNP on the rejoining of single-strand DNA breaks. This experiment was conducted in the same manner as that shown in Figure 4, except that the cells were suspended in DNP. A measurement indicated that ATP content of the cells to be less than 5% of control. As Figure 5 shows, immediately after irradiation the sedimentation pattern indicated a lowering of the DNA molecular weight because of DNA breaks. With time in DNP, however, no evidence of rejoining could be detected. Consequently, our ultracentrifuge studies indicate DNP to be a satisfactory inhibitor of DNA rejoining.

B. Polynucleotide Kinase and DNA Polymerase Studies:

Figure 6 shows the results of these experiments. L cells from the same culture were suspended either in HBSS or DNP; both control and irradiated suspensions were used. The cells were irradiated with 10,000 rads of X-rays as pairs; that is, a portion of the HBSS suspension was irradiated at the same time as the DNP suspension. At the appropriate times after irradiation the samples were quick-chilled and held at 0°C. Sham-irradiated controls paralleled all irradiated cells. After all cells were collected, and the DNA purified (29), a portion of the purified DNA was used for measurement of 5′ termini by the polynucleotide kinase method while another portion was used for measurement of 3′OH termini by the DNA polymerase method (29). The results are expressed as DNA specific activity (cpm/μg DNA). In the polynucleotide kinase reaction the 5′ termini are labeled with $^{32}PO_4$ while the 3′OH termini are identified by the incorporation of ^3H labeled trinucleotides.

For the cells in HBSS, immediately after irradiation, a large number of DNA breaks characterized by 5′ termini were identified by the elevated ^{32}P specific and activity. In a similar fashion an increased number of 3′OH termini were identified by an elevated ^3H specific activity. With time after irradiation, though, both specific activities fell toward control. In our opinion, this suggests rejoining of DNA breaks characterized by 5′PO_4, 3′OH termini very likely by DNA ligase.

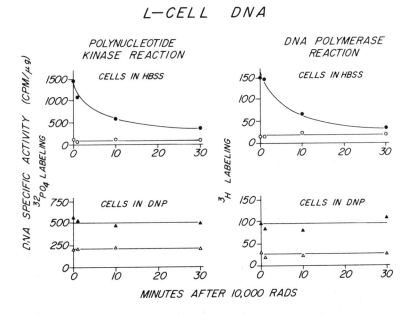

Fig 6. The left panels (upper and lower) show the results of the polynucleotide kinase assay. The right panels indicate the effectiveness of DNA to prime in the DNA polymerase reaction. The results are expressed as DNA specific activities; ^{32}P cpm/μg for the polynucleotide kinase assay and ^3H cpm/μg for the DNA polymerase reaction. As the lower panels show, the DNP prevented the decrease in ^{32}P and ^3H specific activity as seen for the cells suspended in HBSS. The closed symbols represent irradiated cells while the open symbols are the nonirradiated controls. (From Moss et al, Biophys J., 11:158-174, 1971)

For the cells in DNP, increased ^{32}P and ^{3}H specific activities occurred immediately after irradiation. There was no evidence, however, of rejoining of breaks as seen in the case of the cells in HBSS. Instead, the ^{32}P and ^{3}H specific activities remained at a constant level. In our opinion, these findings suggest that radiation produced DNA breaks characterized by 5'PO$_4$, 3'OH termini, but the rejoining was prevented because the action of DNA ligase was inhibited by the depressed ATP levels.

The final question concerned the rejoining of DNA breaks after the cells were held in DNP for a period of time. Figure 7 shows the results of experiments to investigate this point. For the experiment shown in the upper panel, L cells were irradiated with 1,000 rads of X-rays while suspended in growth medium. After a 30-second period, the cells were transferred to DNP and samples withdrawn over the next 2 hrs. After collection,

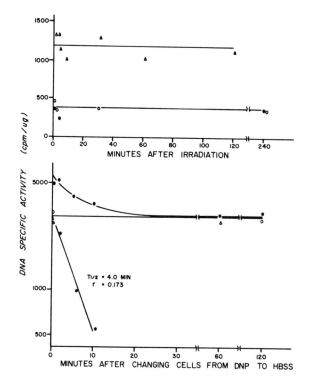

Fig 7. The influence of holding L cells in DNP upon DNA rejoining. The upper curve of the upper panel (△) shows the DNA specific activity of cells irradiated with 1000 rads in medium, held in medium for 0.5 min and then transferred to 10^{-4}M DNP. As this curve indicates, no DNA rejoining occurs while the cells are in DNP. The lower curves of this panel show nonirradiated cells in medium (o) and DNP (o). The lower panel shows the results of an experiment in which the cells were irradiated with 1000 rads while in medium, transferred to DNP at 0.5 min, held in DNP for 2 hr, and then suspended in HBSS. The DNA of the irradiated cells (o) contained more 5'PO$_4$ termini than the controls (△,o). Immediately after transfer from DNP to HBSS, the breaks rejoined rapidly, however. The lower points (o) were calculated by subtracting the control DNA specific activity (the horizontal line) from the DNA specific activities of the irradiated cells. The curve fitted to these points has half-time of 4.0 minutes. (From Dalrymple et al, J. Theor. Biol., 28:121-142, 1970)

the cells were chilled, the DNA purified and the number of 5′ termini measured by the polynucleotide kinase method. As Figure 7 shows, there was no evidence of rejoining as long as DNP was present. For the lower panel, the cells were suspended in medium, irradiated with 1,000 rads, transferred to DNP and held for 2 hrs. At the end of the holding period, they were transferred back to HBSS, samples collected and processed. In this instance the polynucleotide kinase assay shows a falling ^{32}P specific activity, which indicates rejoining of DNA breaks.

Other investigators have found energy inhibition to prevent DNA rejoining. Humphrey et al using alkaline sucrose sedimentation found that 1×10^{-4} M KCN prevented DNA rejoining by Chinese hamster (CHO) cells. Palcic and Skarsgard found that DNP (1×10^{-4} M) prevented rejoining of DNA breaks by Chinese hamster cells and mouse L-60 cells (49). Matsudaira and Furuno found that ATP is necessary for the rejoining of radiation-induced DNA breaks by Ehrlich ascites tumor cells (50). Swada and Okada treated L5178Y cells with DNP (dissolved in Fischer's medium); they did not observe inhibition of DNA rejoining (26). Possibly the influence of the components of medium upon DNP could have influenced the ability of their cells to rejoin DNA breaks.

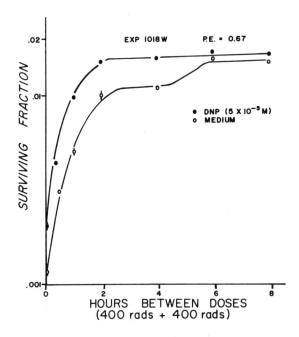

Fig 8. Paired-dose experiment with both initial and challenging doses delivered to cells in 5×10^{-5} M DNP. Thirty minutes before the initial 400-rad dose, the medium was removed from the DNP plates (closed circles) and replaced with DNP. The DNP remained in place for 10.5 hours after application and then was replaced with complete medium. The open circles show the response of the cells maintained in complete medium. The standard error bars are omitted unless they are larger than the plotted points. The colony average multiplicity (1.4 to 1.5) did not vary during the experiment. The plating efficiencies (0.67) were identical for the DNP and the medium-treated cells. (From Dalrymple et al, Radiat. Res, 37:90-102, 1969. Copyright held by Academic Press.)

THE EFFECT OF ENERGY DEPRIVATION ON REPAIR
OF SUBLETHAL INJURY

In 1966 Berry used split dose irradiations to show that HeLa cells treated with DNP could repair sublethal injury (7). Figure 8 shows the results of a similar experiment from our laboratory (14). For this L cells were seeded into plastic petri plates and the plates incubated overnight to allow attachment of the cells. Before irradiation the medium (Eagle's MEM with "nonessential" amino acids plus 17% calf serum) was removed from half the plates and replaced with warmed 5×10^{-5} M DNP. The cells of the other half of the plates remained in complete medium. After a 30-minute period, the plates (DNP and cells in medium) were irradiated with paired 400-rad doses of X-rays separated by 0-8 hrs. In the case of the DNP plates, the initial dose was delivered to the cells in DNP. The plates were incubated at 37°C between the doses. The DNP remained in place for a period of 10.5 hours. This meant that both initial and second doses were delivered while the cells were in contact with DNP. The DNP then was removed and replaced with medium. The plates were incubated for two weeks, after which the colonies were fixed, stained and counted.

As Figure 8 shows, the presence of DNP between doses did not prevent the repair of sublethal injury. If anything, the repair half-time is shorter than for cells maintained in complete medium (20). Consequently, these results indicate that the repair of sublethal injury occurs in spite of energy inhibition which is sufficient to prevent the rejoining of DNA breaks. In other experiments we have shown that if cells are irradiated in HBSS or complete medium and then DNP added after a period of time, an increased repair of sublethal injury occurs (14).

CONCLUSIONS

We believe that our results support the notion that radiation-induced single-strand breaks represent reparable radiation injury. The presence or absence of large numbers of single-strand breaks does not correlate with increased lethality. Treatments, such as dinitrophenol, which prevent rejoining, if anything, enhance the repair of sublethal injury.

The question of double-strand DNA breaks, however, still has not been completely settled. Whether cultured mammalian cells rejoin double-strand breaks or not, to us, is not the point at issue. As mentioned before, the *rejoining* of double-strand breaks by no means guarantees that normal DNA will result. Consequently, this point must remain an unanswered question. Hopefully, future efforts from our and other laboratories will clarify the problems.

ACKNOWLEDGMENTS

We thank Mrs. Anna G. Stewart and Mrs. Rowena Milliken for excellent technical assistance.

REFERENCES

1. Puck, T. T., Markovin, D., Marcus, P. I. and Cieciura, S. J.: Action of X-rays on mammalian cells. II. Survival curves of cells from normal human tissues. J. Exp. Med., 106:485, 1967.

2. Elkind, M. M. and Sutton, H.: Radiation response of mammalian cells grown in culture. I. Repair of x-ray damage in surviving Chinese hamster cells. Radiat. Res., 13:556, 1960.

3. Belli, J. A. and Shelton, M. J.: Potentially lethal radiation damage repair by mammalian cells in culture. Science, 165:490, 1969.

4. Elkind, M. M. and Whitmore, G. F.: The Radiobiology of Cultured Mammalian Cells. Gordon & Breach, New York, 1967, p 615.

5. Kallman, R. F.: Recovery from radiation injury; a proposed mechanism. Nature, 197:557, 1963.

6. Terasima, T. and Tolmach, L. J.: Variations in several responses of HeLa cells to x-irradiation during the division cycle. Biophys. J., 3:11, 1963.

7. Berry, R. J.: Effects of some metabolic inhibitors on x-ray dose response curves for the survival of mammalian cells in vitro and on early recovery between fractionated x-ray doses. Brit. J. Radiol., 39:458, 1966.

8. Kim, J. H., Eidinoff, M. L. and Laughlin, J. S.: Recovery from sub-lethal x-ray damage of mammalian cells during inhibition of synthesis of deoxyribonucleic acid. Nature, 204:598, 1964.

9. Phillips, R. A. and Tolmach, L. J.: Repair of potentially lethal damage in x-irradiated HeLa cells. Radiat. Res., 29:413, 1966.

10. Bacchetti, S. and Whitmore, G. F.: Actinomycin D and x-ray sensitivity in synchronized mouse L cells. Radiat. Res., 31:577, 1967.

11. Elkind, M. M., Whitmore, G. F. and Alescio, T.: Actinomycin D:suppression of recovery in x-irradiated mammalian cells. Science, 143:1454, 1964.

12. Elkind, M. M., Swain, R. W., Alescio, T., Sutton, H. and Moses, W. B.: Oxygen, nitrogen, recovery and radiation therapy. In: Cellular Radiation Biology, pp 442-466. Williams & Wilkins Co., Baltimore, Md., 1965.

13. Whitmore, G. F., Gulyas, S. and Botond, J.: Radiation sensitivity throughout the cell cycle and its relationship to recovery. In: Cellular Radiation Biology, pp 423-441. The Williams & Wilkins Co., Baltimore, Md., 1965.

14. Dalrymple, Glenn V., Sanders, J. L., Baker, Max L. and Wilkinson, K. P.: The effect of 2,4-dinitrophenol on the repair of radiation injury by L cells. Radiat. Res., 37:90, 1969.

15. Revesz, L. and Littbrand, B.: Culture age and cellular radiosensitivity. Exp. Cell. Res., 55:283, 1969.

16. McGrath, R. A. and Williams, R. W.: Reconstruction in vivo of irradiated Eschericia coli deoxyribonucleic acid; the rejoining of broken pieces. Nature (London), 212:534, 1966.

17. Kaplan, H. S.: DNA strand scission and loss of viability after X-irradiation of normal and sensitized bacterial cells. Proc. Nat. Acad. Sci, USA, 55:1442, 1966.

18. Freifelder, D.: Lethal changes in bacteriophage DNA produced by x-rays. Radiat. Res., Supp. 6:80, 1966.

19. Szybalski, W.: Molecular events resulting in radiation injury, repair and sensitization of DNA. Radiat. Res., Supp. 7:147, 1967.

20. Dalrymple, G. V., Sanders, J. L. and Baker, M. L.: Do cultured mammalian cells repair radiation injury by the "cut-and-patch" mechanism? J. Theor. Biol., 21:368, 1968.

21. Dalrymple, G. V., Baker, M. L., Sanders, J. L., Moss, A. J. Jr., Nash, J. C. and Wilkinson, K. P.: Do mammalian cells repair radiation injury by the "cut-and-patch" mechanism? II. An extension of the original model. J. Theor. Biol., 28:121, 1970.

22. Lett, J. T., Caldwell, I., Dean, C. J. and Alexander, P.: Rejoining of x-ray induced breaks in the DNA of leukemia cells. Nature, 214:790, 1967.

23. Lohman, P. H. M.: Induction and rejoining of breaks in the deoxyribonucleic acid of human cells irradiated at various phases of the cell cycle. Mutat. Res., 6:449, 1968.

24. Humphrey, R. M., Steward, D. L. and Sedita, B. A.: DNA-strand breaks and rejoining following exposure of synchronized Chinese hamster cells to ionizing radiation. Mutat. Res., 6:459, 1968.

25. Humphrey, Ronald M., Steward, D. L. and Sedita, B. A.: DNA-strand scission and rejoining in mammalian cells. In: Genetic Concepts and Neoplasia, pp 570-592. Williams & Wilkins Co., Baltimore, Md.

26. Sawada, S. and Okada, S.: Rejoining of single-stranded breaks of DNA in cultured mammalian cells. Radiat. Res., 41:145, 1970.

27. Lett, J. T. and Sun, C.: The production of strand breaks in mammalian DNA by x-rays: at different stages in the cell cycle. Radiat. Res., 44:771, 1970.

28. Elkind, M. M. and Kamper, C.: Two forms of repair of DNA in mammalian cells following irradiation. Biophys. J., 10:237, 1970.

29. Moss, A. J. Jr., Dalrymple, Glenn V., Sanders, J. L., Wilkinson, K. P. and Nash, John C.: Dinitrophenol inhibits the rejoining of radiation-induced DNA breaks by L Cells. Biophys. J., 11: 158, 1971.

30. Veatch, W. and Okada, S.: Radiation-induced breaks of DNA in cultured mammalian cells. Biophys. J., 9:330, 1969.

31. Corry, P. M. and Cole, A.: Radiation-induced double-strand scission of the DNA of mammalian metaphase chromosomes. Radiat. Res., 36:528, 1968.

32. Lehmann, A. R. and Ormerod, M. G.: Double-strand breaks in the DNA of a mammalian cell after x-irradiation. Biochim. Biophys. Acata, 217:268, 1970.

33. Kitayama, S. and Matsuyama, A.: Possibility of the repair of double strand scissions in *M. radiodurans* DNA caused by gamma-rays. Biochem. Biophys. Res. Commun, 33:418, 1968.

34. Lett, J. T., Caldwell, I. and Little, J. G.: Repair of x-ray damage to the DNA in *M. radiodurans:* the effect of 5-Bromodeoxyuridine. J. Molec. Biol., 48:395, 1970.

35. Richardson, C. C.: The 5'-terminal nucleotides of T7 bacteriophage deoxyribonucleic acid. J. Molec. Biol., 15:49, 1966.

36. Richardson, C. C.: Phosphorylation of nucleic acid by an enzyme from T4 bacteriophage-infected *Escherichia coli.* Proc. Nat. Acad. Sci., 54:158, 1965.

37. Weiss, B. and Richardson, C. C.: Enzymatic breakage and joining of deoxyribonucleic acid. I. Repair of single-strand breaks in DNA by an enzyme system of *Escherichia coli* infected with T4 bacteriophage. Proc. Nat. Acad. Sci., 57:1021, 1967.

38. Aposhian, H. V. and Kornberg, A.: Enzymatic synthesis of deoxyribonucleic acid. The polymerase formed after T2 bacteriophage infection of *Escherichia coli* a new enzyme. J. Biol. Chem., 237:519, 1962.

39. Weiss, B., Thompson, A. and Richardson, C. C.: Enzymatic breakage and joining of deoxyribonucleic acid. J. Biol. Chem., 243:4556, 1968.

40. Englund, P. T., Deutscher, M. P., Jovin, T. M., Kelly, R. B., Cozzarelli, N. R. and Kornberg, A.: Structural and functional properties of *Escherichia coli* DNA polymerase. Sympos. Quant. Biol., 33:1, 1968.

41. Dalrymple, G. V., Sanders, J. L., Moss, A. J. Jr., Baker, M. L. and Wilkinson, K. P.: Radiation produces breaks in L cell and mouse liver DNA characterized by 5' phosphoryl termini. Biochem. Biophys. Res. Commun., 35:300, 1969.

42. Dalrymple, G. V., Sanders, J. L., Moss, A. J. Jr., Baker, M. L. and Wilkins, K. P.: Energy dependent nucleolytic processes are responsible for the production of many post-irradiation breaks in L cell DNA. Biochem. Biophys. Res. Commun., 36:284, 1969.

43. Dalrymple, G. V., Sanders, J. L., Moss, A. J. Jr. and Wilkinson, K. P.: Radiation induced breaks increase the primary activity of rat sarcoma DNA in the DNA polymerase reaction. Biochem. Biophys. Res. Commun., 39:538, 1970.

44. Olivera, B. M. and Lehman, I. R.: Linkage of polynucleotides through phosphodiester bonds by an enzyme from *Escherichia coli.* Proc. Nat. Acad. Sci., USA, 57:1426, 1967.

45. Lindahl, T. and Edelman, G. M.: Polynucleotide ligase from myeloid and lymphoid tissues. Proc. Nat. Acad. Sci., USA, 61:680, 1968.

46. Dalrymple, G. V., Sanders, J. L. and Baker, M. L.: Dinitrophenol decreases the radiation sensitivity of L cells. Nature, 216:708, 1967.

47. Baker, M. L., Dalrymple, G. V., Sanders, J. L., Moss, A. J. Jr.: Effects of radiation on asynchronous and synchronized L cells under energy deprivation. Radiat. Res., 42:320, 1970.

48. Noll, Hans: Characterization of macromolecules by constant velocity sedimentation. Nature, 215: 360, 1967.

49. Palcic, B. and Skarsgard, L. D.: The effect of 2,4-dinitrophenol, temperature and O_2 on single strand breaks produced in DNA by ionizing radiation. Radiat. Res., (Abst.) (in press).

50. Matsudaira, H. and Furuno, I.: Requirement of adenosine triphosphate for the rejoining of x-ray-induced breaks in the DNA of Ehrlich ascites tumor cells. Fourth International Congress of Radiation Research, Evian, France, (Abst.) 541, 1970.

51. Addanki, A. S., Sotos, J. F. and Rearick, P. D.: Rapid determination of picomole quantities of ATP with a liquid scintillation counter. Anal. Biochem., 14:261, 1966.

THE IMPORTANCE OF REPAIR REPLICATION
FOR MAMMALIAN CELLS[1]

Robert B. Painter

Laboratory of Radiobiology, University of California
San Francisco, California

INTRODUCTION

The importance of repair replication after UV-induced damage to DNA in human cells has, I believe, been amply demonstrated by Cleaver who has shown that human cells defective in excision-repair are more sensitive (by a factor of at least three) to UV light than are normal human cells (1). Dr. Cleaver will present some of his data in this Symposium and therefore I will not discuss further any work with UV, except for comparison purposes.

The role of repair replication in the repair of damage to DNA induced by ionizing radiation is much more poorly understood. No good data for its action in bacteria have been forthcoming, although Billen et al (2), at least, have searched rather diligently for it. The great amount of DNA degradation that occurs after X-irradiation of bacteria probably obscures repair replication which, as I will show, almost certainly must occur.

Three groups recently have investigated the chemical nature of DNA single-strand breaks. Their data agree extremely well. The proposal of Krushinskaya and Shal'nov (3) that the $3'$-$4'$ group in deoxyribose was the main point of attack was confirmed by Kapp and Smith (4). Although Kapp and Smith (4) and Bopp and Hagen (5) both showed that the $5'$phosphate by far was the most frequent chain terminus formed, the failure of a polynucleotide ligase to rejoin the break showed that the single-strand break cannot consist of a simple rupture of the $3'$OH-$5'$PO$_4$ position (6). Previously, Hems (7) had shown that base elimination occurred with a G value of 0.228, very close to the value of 0.24 for sugar damage (production of malonic aldehyde) determined by Kapp and Smith (4). These data all suggest that single-strand breakage is usually accompanied by base loss from the DNA. It follows that single-strand rejoining must be accompanied by base insertion, which is synonymous with repair replication.

We reported (8) that repair replication occurred in HeLa cells after 100,000 R; this observation was received without much enthusiasm since this dose of radiation is supralethal, to put it mildly. In the intervening four years, I have attempted to detect repair replication at lower doses of X-radiation. This effort has met with a certain measure of success because it no longer is a problem to detect repair replication at zero dose. The problem has become that I cannot detect an increase in extent of repair replication over that occurring in unirradiated cultures until the dose administered to the cells exceeds 1000 R. I hope to convince you that this really is not surprising and that repair replication after X-irradiation is a real and necessary process in mammalian cells.

---

[1] Work performed under the auspices of the U.S. Atomic Energy Commission.

We obtained almost identical results with several mammalian cell lines, including human (HeLa, an aneuploid line, and WI-38, a diploid), Chinese hamster (Don and B14FAF), mouse L and another mouse line, P388F. Our results with the latter line differ from those reported by Ayad and Fox (9) and Fox et al (10) but are entirely consistent with the results from other cells we have investigated. I will present the data from mouse L cells because our experience with repair replication after X-irradiation is most extensive with this line.

METHODOLOGY AND RESULTS

The cells were grown in Eagle's medium supplemented with 15% fetal calf serum plus streptomycin (50µg/ml) and penicillin (50 units/ml). Irradiations were performed at about 2000 R/min, using 300 kVp, 20 ma, 2.0 mm Cu. Repair replication was demonstrated as described previously (8) with multiple rebandings when necessary (11). In this method, one seeks to show uptake of ^{3}H-bromouracil deoxyriboside (^{3}HBrUdR) into single strands of DNA at normal density regions of CsCl equilibrium density gradients. This is taken as evidence for repair replication because, under the conditions used for these experiments (in which incubation with unlabeled BrUdR is used before and after the ^{3}HBrUdR incubation), the incorporation of ^{3}HBrUdR by semiconservative replication causes exclusively the formation of heavy tritium-labeled DNA strands, which are

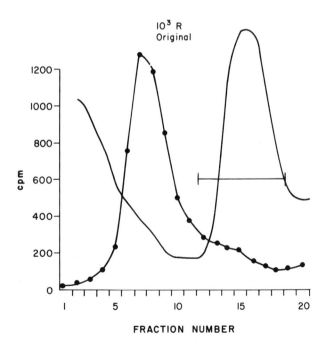

Fig 1. Original equilibrium density gradient profile of DNA from cells irradiated with 1000 R and incubated for three hours in the presence of ^{3}HBUdR. ●——● ^{3}H cpm. The line without data points is a reproduction of trace of transmittance at 260 nm automatically monitored during sample collection; the lower the transmittance, the higher the line. Normal density DNA lies between fractions 12 and 18. These fractions were combined and run in a second gradient (first reband, see Fig 2).

found at or near the bottom of the density gradients. Tritium is found at normal density regions only when ^{3}HBrUdR is present in segments of DNA which are so short, compared to the fragments isolated for gradient analysis, that they do not alter appreciably the density of those fragments.

Mouse L cells were irradiated with 0, 250, 1000 or 10,000 R. After the first centrifugation the equilibrium density gradient patterns from cells irradiated with 0, 250 or 1000 R were indistinguishable from one another and are typified by the results from the 10^3 R sample shown in Figure 1. No indication of a peak of radioactivity was seen in the normal density regions of three gradients. In the pattern from the cells irradiated with 10^4 R (not shown) a small peak of radioactivity was found in the normal density region. The normal density region of each gradient (shown by the enclosed bar in each figure) was rebanded into a second gradient. Figure 2 shows the results from the 0, 10^3 and 10^4 R gradients. Note that there are peaks of radioactivity of similar heights at densities slightly greater than normal in both the 0 and 10^3 R gradients. The results from the

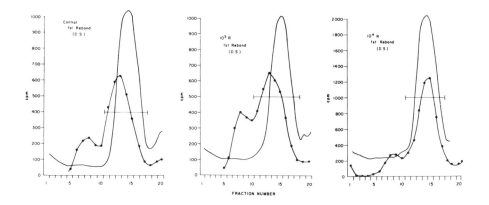

Fig 2. Profiles of first rebands from normal density regions or original equilibrium density gradients. Note change of scale for 10^4 R gradient. Fractions encompassed by the indicated bars were combined, dialyzed, heated to 90°C, treated with formaldehyde and run in a third (second reband) gradient (see Fig 3). Symbols as in Figure 1.

250 R gradient are not shown but were similar. The 10^4 R gradient, however, has a peak of radioactivity at normal density, and this peak contains more radioactivity than the peaks from the other gradients. The DNA at normal density regions of each of these gradients was collected again, converted to single strands by heating, and rebanded; the results are shown in Figure 3. Again the 0 and 10^3 R gradients are very similar with the greatest amount of radioactivity appearing near the bottom, at high density, of each gradient. The amount of radioactivity decreases through the normal density regions. The pattern from the 10^4 R gradient, while showing similar amounts of radioactivity at high density positions, also has a well-defined peak containing more radioactivity at a density slightly greater than that of normal DNA. The normal density region of each gradient was rebanded once more. This time (Fig 4) the patterns are very similar, but the 10^4 R gradient shows much more total radioactivity. The peaks of radioactivity in each case are very close to the density of normal DNA.

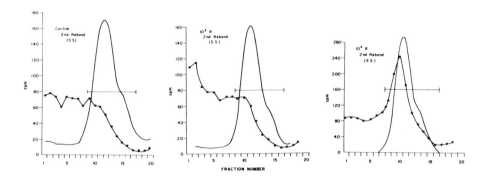

Fig 3. Profiles of second rebands, this time as single-stranded DNA. Note change of scale for 10^4 R gradient. Symbols as in Figure 1.

To quantify the results the specific activities of repaired DNA were determined. All fractions showing significant amounts of radioactivity or optical density at 260 nm were combined and dialysed. The A_{260} of 1 equals $50\mu g$ DNA. An aliquot of the solution was counted, the count corrected to cpm/ml and this value divided by DNA concentration to give the final specific activity in cpm/μg. The results, after the first

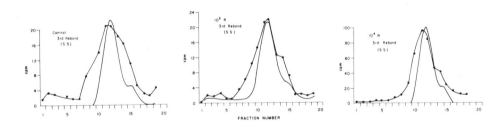

Fig 4. Profiles of third rebands (single-stranded DNA). Note change of scale for 10^4 R gradient. Symbols as in Figure 1.

reband (double-stranded DNA) and third reband (single-stranded DNA) are shown in Table I. In the single-stranded state DNA from cultures irradiated with 10^4 R has a significantly higher specific activity than the unirradiated control. Thus, irradiation with doses of 1000 R or less does not induce any more repair replication than that occurring (for whatever reason) in unirradiated cells.

The data from cultures irradiated with 10^4 R can be used to estimate the extent of base insertion that has occurred in these cells. The counting efficiency under the conditions used here (DNA on Whatmann 3 MM paper in PPO, POPOP, toluene) is about 10%, so that the specific activity of the DNA was about 500 dpm/μg. The decay constant (in minutes) for tritium is 10^{-7}, so that there were $\left(\dfrac{5 \times 10^2}{10^{-7}}\right) \simeq 5 \times 10^9$ tritium-labeled

TABLE I

Specific Activity of L Cell Repaired DNA (cpm/μg)

Dose to culture	After first reband (double-stranded)	After third reband (single-stranded)
0 (control)	163	15
250	150	19
1000	209	19
10000	249	51

BrUdR molecules per μg of this DNA. The specific activity of ^{3}HBrUdR (100 μCi/ml were used in this experiment) was 11 Ci/mmole, which is 0.38 of the specific activity of ^{3}HBrUdR in which each molecule has exactly one tritium atom. Therefore, 1.3 x 10^{10} BrUdR molecules existed in each μg of this DNA. Because FUdR was used in this experiment no endogenous DNA thymine was made. If base elimination is random, then 4.3 x 10^{10} bases were inserted per μg, since thymines make up about 0.3 of the total bases in mammalian DNA. The unirradiated cells, however, incorporated about 40% as much BrUdR as did the 10^4 R cells so that the amount induced by irradiation was about 2.6 x 10^{10} bases per μg DNA.

A dose of 10^4 R is roughly equivalent to 6 x 10^{11} ev/μg. The efficiency of single-strand production is about 60 ev/break (12,13) so 10^4 R produces about 10^{10} single-strand breaks per μg DNA. Therefore, about $\left(\dfrac{2.6 \times 10^{10}}{10^{10}} \right)$ = 2.5 bases are inserted by repair replication for each radiation-induced single-strand break that occurs in mammalian cell DNA. Since base damage probably exceeds break production (14), part of this repair may be associated with events other than single-strand breaks. It seems almost certain that fewer than three bases are inserted per radiation-induced break. These observations suggest that X-irradiation of mammalian cells causes single-strand DNA breaks which, although the majority are gaps due to the loss of one or more bases, are repaired without extensive widening of the gaps. This form of repair, therefore, does not involve the large-scale degradation of DNA that has been observed in X-irradiated bacteria (15,16) and explains the inability of previous investigators (17-19) to detect X-ray induced DNA degradation in mammalian cells.

These data also indicate why the extent of repair replication does not increase significantly above control values until the dose of radiation exceeds 1000 R. About 1.7 x 10^{10} bases per μg were inserted into control cell DNA. A dose of 1000 R induces 10^9 single-strand breaks/μg DNA and increases the total insertion only by about 3 x 10^9 bases, or 0.9 x 10^9 molecules of BrUdR, or 3.5 x 10^8 ^{3}HBrUdR molecules, or 35 dpm, or 3.5 cpm/μg which is within the range of the uncertainty of the method.

I would now like to compare the DNA damage induced by ionizing and ultraviolet (UV) radiations. The rad is the absorption by tissue of 100 ergs/gram, or 6×10^{13} ev/gram of ionizing radiation. The yield of ion pairs in tissue is somewhere between 30 to 60 ev/ion pair; we will use the former value to be safe. Thus, one rad will yield about 2×10^{12} $\left(\dfrac{6 \times 10^{13}}{3 \times 10^{1}} \right)$ ion pairs/gram. Because ionization is the only important means of energy release by this kind of radiation, the maximum number of primary lesions will not exceed appreciably the number of ion pairs.

For UV at 260 nm, the yield of thymine dimers in DNA in mammalian cells has been measured; about 0.05% of DNA thymines are converted to dimers per 100 ergs/mm^2 incident radiation (20,21). Therefore, 5×10^{-6} of DNA thymines are converted to dimers per erg/mm^2. (This value probably includes mixed dimers but not cytosine-cytosine dimers.) Thymines make up about 30% of the bases in mammalian DNA so there are about 6×10^{20} thymines per gm; thus one erg produces 3×10^{15} ($6 \times 10^{20} \times 5 \times 10^{-6}$) dimers per gm of DNA in mammalian cells. One erg/mm^2 of incident light at 260 nm, therefore, induces at least 1500 times as much damage to mammalian DNA as does one rad of ionizing radiation (damages other than thymine-containing dimers are not used for this estimate). Thus, the dose, 10,000 R, after which we can always demonstrate repair replication induced by ionizing radiation, is equivalent in terms of DNA damage to only about 7 ergs/mm^2 UV. It is not surprising, to me at least, that it is difficult to demonstrate repair replication in mammalian cells after ionizing radiation. First, the amount of DNA damage really is small, and second, in unirradiated cells there is a nonconservative replication that is phenomenologically identical to that induced by radiation.

The role of repair replication in unirradiated cells is unknown. We have hypothesized before (22) that this may result from DNA damage caused by "normal wear and tear," including thermal damage simply by existing at 310° Kelvin. I do not now believe, however, that this is correct. The specific activities of repaired DNA given in this paper are those measured in DNA from cells incubated with hydroxyurea. Recently, we have been looking at repair replication in unirradiated cells incubated with ^{3}HBrUdR in the absence of hydroxyurea. To our great surprise, we find that the extent of repair replication, again measured as tritium activity in normal density single-stranded DNA, is much greater in these cells. In fact, the effect of hydroxyurea is to suppress repair replication in these unirradiated cells to the same extent that it suppresses normal semiconservative replication. This result is both embarrassing and revealing. It is embarrassing because we have not observed it earlier -- our work has concentrated on hydroxyurea-treated cells in which *radiation-induced repair replication* is much easier to observe. It is revealing because it implies that repair replication observed in unirradiated cells is primarily, if not exclusively, a consequence or a component of normal semiconservative replication. This phenomenon is not correlated with unscheduled DNA synthesis. Unscheduled DNA synthesis induced by 200 ergs/mm^2 can be demonstrated easily either in the presence or absence of hydroxyurea. The extent of repair replication observed in unirradiated L cells is roughly equivalent to that induced by about 200 ergs/mm^2 but is not demonstrable autoradiographically. This nonconservative DNA synthesis seems to be a manifestation of a very important process and much of the work in our laboratory is now devoted to its study.

REFERENCES

1. Cleaver, J. E.: Int. J. Radiat. Biol., 18:557, 1970.
2. Billen, D., Hewitt, R. R., Lapthisophan, T. and Achey, P. M.: J. Bact., 94:1538, 1967.
3. Krushinskaya, N. P. and Shal'nov, M. I.: Radiobiology, 7:36, 1967.
4. Kapp, D. S. and Smith, K. C.: Radiat. Res., 12:340, 1970.
5. Bopp, A. and Hagen, V.: Biochim. Biophys. Acta, 209:320, 1970.
6. Kapp, D. S. and Smith, K. C.: Int. J. Radiat. Biol., 14:467, 1968.
7. Hems, G.: Nature, 186:710, 1960.
8. Painter, R. B. and Cleaver, J. E.: Nature, 216:369, 1967.
9. Ayad, S. R. and Fox, M.: Int. J. Radiat. Biol., 15:556, 1969.
10. Fox, M., Ayad, S. R. and Fox, B. W.: Int. J. Radiat. Biol., 18:101, 1970.
11. Painter, R. B., Umber, J. S. and Young, B. R.: Radiat. Res., 44:133, 1970.
12. Lett, J. T., Caldwell, I., Dean, C. J. and Alexander, P.: Nature, 214:790, 1967.
13. Elkind, M. M. and Kamper. C.: Biophys. J., 10:237, 1970.
14. Jung, H., Hagen, U., Ullrich, M. and Petersen, E. E.: Z. Naturforsch. [B], 24:1565, 1969.
15. Stuy, J. H.: J. Bact., 79:707, 1960.
16. Pollard, E. C. and Achey, P. M.: Science, 146:71, 1964.
17. Painter, R. B.: In: Effects of Radiation on Cellular Proliferation and Differentiation (IAEA, Vienna) p 91, 1968.
18. Looney, W. B. and Chang, L. O.: Radiat. Res., 37:525, 1969.
19. Hill, M., Int. J. Radiat. Biol., 15:483, 1969.
20. Trosko, J. E., Chu, E. H. Y. and Carrier, W. L.: Radiat. Res., 24:667, 1965.
21. Regan, J. D., Trosko, J. E. and Carrier, W. L.: Biophys. J., 8:319, 1968.
22. Rasmussen, R. E., Reisner, B. L. and Painter, R. B.: Int. J. Radiat. Biol., 17:285, 1970.

RESTORATION OF THE DNA STRUCTURE IN X-IRRADIATED EUCARYOTIC CELLS: IN VITRO AND IN VIVO[1]

J. T. Lett, C. Sun and K. T. Wheeler

Departments of Radiology and Radiation Biology, Physiology and Biophysics
Colorado State University
Fort Collins, Colorado

INTRODUCTION

There is little doubt that damage to the genetic apparatus is a principal cause of death following exposure of a cell to ionizing radiation. The obvious place to look for the lethal damage is in the chromosomal DNA. Given this basic precept the relevant question is, what is the nature of the fundamental radiochemical lesions in DNA which are ultimately responsible for cell death?

One well-known effect of ionizing radiations upon DNA is to introduce strand breaks into the twin helix (1,2). Two types of strand breaks have been observed which may be different in their biological expression. A single-strand break occurs when only one of the helices (strands) in the DNA duplex is broken. Such a break will not lead to a rupture of the duplex. A double-strand break occurs when both strands in the duplex are broken at adjacent, or nearly adjacent, sites. This type of break will result in the rupture of the twin helix.

Until about five years ago it was impossible to obtain a reliable measure of the extent to which strand breaks were produced by ionizing radiation in cells. The reason was quite simple. DNA is extremely susceptible to hydrodynamic shear and it is only too easy to produce more damage while extracting DNA from irradiated cells than is caused by the radiation itself (3). This difficulty was circumvented by McGrath and Williams (4). They introduced a technique which involved lysing cells on the top of an alkaline sucrose gradient in a centrifuge tube. Lysis is rapid at high pH (> 12). Under such conditions the DNA is released from the cell in a gentle fashion, the RNA and protein are removed and the twin helix dissociates into single strands. Subsequent to these processes the centrifuge rotor is accelerated and the single strands of DNA are sedimented through the alkaline sucrose gradient. The presence of the alkali in the gradient ensures that the single strands do not re-associate or form aggregates. From the changes observed in the sedimentation profiles after irradiation the molecular weights, and hence the number of strand breaks introduced into the DNA, can be measured. It is important to realize that this technique measures all the strand breaks that are present but does not distinguish between them. A *single*-strand break will appear as a *single*-strand break, a *double*-strand break will be seen as *two single*-strand breaks. The main experimental tool used in the experiments which we will describe utilizes a modification of the McGrath and Williams technique which is

[1] Supported by the Department of Health, Education and Welfare under NIH Grants NS08491 (NINDS) and CA 10714 (NCI); and also by Union Carbide Subcontract 3080 from the Oak Ridge National Laboratory (Dr. N. G. Anderson).

necessary for its fruitful application to mammalian cells, for as we shall see, the nature of mammalian chromosomal DNA is quite complex.

In principle, it is possible to measure double-strand breaks with neutral sucrose gradients; but the applications of such methods to date have been fraught with so many difficulties that is fair to say that the results are not reliable. We will not consider neutral gradients any further.

Most cells do not suffer the radiation insult passively since they possess the capacity to repair the damage (5) albeit to a limited extent. The next question then is, can cells rejoin all DNA strand breaks or only some of them? And further, can the cell restore the original structure and integrity to the chromosomal DNA? In order to achieve the latter the cell must be able to rejoin the strand breaks introduced by ionizing radiation into its DNA.

When unirradiated mammalian cells were lysed and then stored on the tops of alkaline sucrose gradients in alkaline EDTA[2] the sedimentation profiles exhibited by the DNA were found to depend upon the time of lysis plus storage, prior to centrifugation. The nature of the profiles suggested that the chromosomal DNA was being degraded through a series of well-defined components of decreasing size (6). This generated the idea that the molecular structure of mammalian DNA is based upon structural subunits of specific size which are joined together by links (or linkers) into multicomponent arrays (6). A very important member of such species is a single-stranded structural subunit which has a sedimentation coefficient of 165S and has been assigned a molecular weight of 5.5×10^8 daltons (6). This subunit is released from unirradiated cells at all positions of the cell cycle during 3-5 hours lytic-storage in alkaline EDTA. The actual time required, within those limits, does depend upon cycle position. Since these subunits are all of the same size they will exhibit a very narrow (monodisperse) sedimentation profile of the type shown in Figure 1.[3] Since X-rays deposit their energy at random it is to be expected that X-irradiation would result in the random formation of strand breaks in DNA so that DNA fragments extracted from X-irradiated cells should have random size distributions. A random distribution is also illustrated in Figure 1. Thus X-irradiation should cause damage which results in a characteristic change from the monodisperse distribution of the 165S subunit to a random size distribution. Such changes have been found to occur in cultured mammalian cells (7).

Now let us consider the converse. If DNA strand breaks are rejoined by irradiated cells then the DNA sedimentation profiles should undergo a change from random back to monodisperse. And if the sedimentation profile is completely restored to that exhibited by the subunits from unirradiated cells, then *all* the strand breaks within the subunits will have been rejoined, whether they were originally present as single-strand breaks or double-strand breaks. Most of the experiments we shall discuss have been carried out

[2]Ethylene diamine tetra-acetic acid.

[3]In actual fact this profile is not absolutely monodisperse but has a small tailing edge. The reason for this is that the subunits are probably themselves composed of subsidiary arrays of smaller units (6) and some further degradation does occur during extensive lytic-storage. However, these considerations are not pertinent to the present discussion.

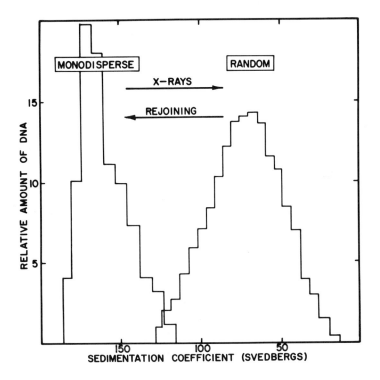

Fig 1. The closely monodisperse sedimentation profile associated with the 165S subunit and a profile indicating a random size distribution. The latter was obtained following a dose of 10.7 Krads.

with large X- or γ-doses (5-22 Krads) because the effects from such doses provide good illustrations of the phenomena which we wish to demonstrate.

The type of profile change to be anticipated during the rejoining of DNA strand breaks within the subunits from heavily irradiated cells, that is the return from a random distribution to the monodisperse distribution associated with the subunits, is shown in Figure 1. Now if the link(er)s between the subunits are also rejoined, molecules bigger than the subunits should also begin to appear in the gradients. Obviously, the two processes could proceed simultaneously or in some sequential fashion (8,9). How can they be visualized? The whole key to the situation lies in the lytic-storage time used in a particular situation and must be understood thoroughly before we can proceed further.

When unirradiated cells are lysed, 3-5 hours (of subsequent storage) are necessary to release the 165S subunit. However, after even low doses of X-rays (namely, 200 rads) the subunit profile is present following only a few minutes lytic-storage. An X-ray dose of 200 rads is so small that it will only break about 15% of the subunits so that the subunit profile is essentially intact (7). The most compelling interpretation of this phenomenon, and the one which we will employ, is that low doses of X-rays produce specific damage at or near the link(er) sites. Such a situation could occur if the link(er) sites were at exposed parts of the chromosome and subject to attack by indirect action, namely, the free radicals

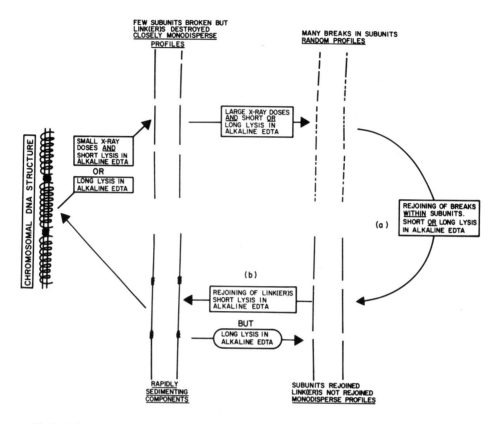

Fig 2. A diagrammatic representation of a possible breakdown scheme. It is important to note that there is no a priori reason why the single-stranded subunits should be aligned adjacently in the twin helical arrays as shown.

produced in water (7). The subunits would be protected against free radical attack by the chromosomal proteins. The basic experimental system and hypothesis are illustrated in Figure 2. If the link(er)s are open rejoining of the strand breaks within the subunit can be followed. Link(er)s which have been rejoined can be opened again by employing 3-5 hour lytic-storage times. However, if very short lytic-storage times are used (the shortest reproducible experimental time for the swinging bucket rotors is 6 min) both the rejoining of the breaks within the subunits and the rejoining of the link(er)s can be followed. Thus the experimental procedure is to compare 6 minute (short) lytic-storage with 3-5 hour (long) lytic-storage as incubation of the irradiated cells proceeds.

DIVIDING CELLS AND REJOINING IN VITRO: Chinese Hamster Ovary Cells

When Chinese hamster cells are heavily X-irradiated and then incubated, the cells do rejoin the strand breaks within the subunits (8,9) and the link(er)s between the subunits (9). Since these experiments have been described they will only be given in summary

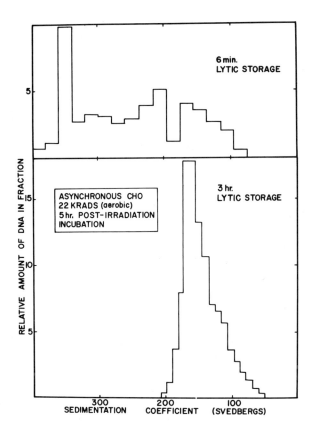

Fig 3. Comparison of 6 minute and 3 hour lytic-storage times. The DNA profiles were obtained from asynchronous cells following an X-ray dose of 22.1 Krads and 5 hours post-irradiation incubation in vitro. Chinese hamster ovary cells.

here.[4] The anticipated transition from a random distribution to a monodisperse distribution was observed when long lytic-storage times were used. Following a dose of 22 Krads about 97% of the strand breaks and hence about 60% of the subunits were rejoined. A typical comparison between short and long lytic-storage experiments is shown in Figure 3. After five hours post-irradiation incubation the majority of the subunits have been restored (5 hours lytic-storage) and presumably many of the link(er)s between them have been also rejoined (6 minute lytic-storage) because the latter profile indicates that rapidly sedimenting species ($> 165S$) are present. When the time course of the rejoining reactions is followed Figure 4(a) is obtained and the interpretation of these data would be that, to a first approximation, the two processes are occurring simultaneously.

The problem at this juncture is, is it possible to distinguish two separate rejoining processes? The answer is yes, because irradiated cells behave differently at different

---

[4]When this paper was delivered at the Symposium the material covered in all the references was also described so that complete continuity could be maintained.

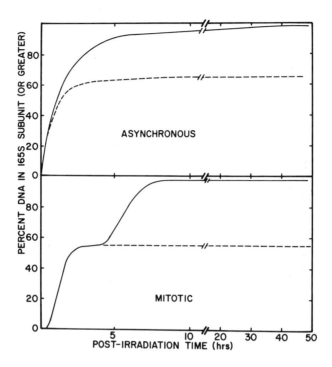

Fig 4. The percentage of subunit (or greater) reappearing in the profiles during post-irradiation incubation following an X-ray dose of 22.1 Krads. Chinese hamster ovary cells. Six minutes lytic-storage ————, 3 hours lytic-storage - - - - - - -. (a) Asynchronous cells, (b) Mitotic cells.

parts of the cycle. Irradiation of mitotic cell populations provides the best evidence that two distinct processes are operating. The evidence is presented in Figure 4 (b). In this figure it will be seen that there is no difference between the 6 minute experiments and the 3 hour experiments until at least about 4-5 hours of post-irradiation incubation have elapsed. In other words, the sedimentation profiles obtained from irradiated mitotic cells are identical under the two lytic-storage conditions for at least 4-5 hours after irradiation. Fast moving components, that is components larger than the subunit, only begin to appear in the 6 minute experiments after 5-6 hours post-irradiation incubation (Fig 5). Once the larger species do appear their size increases with increasing incubation time until they sediment as fast as those components which would have been obtained from unirradiated cells.

The next question is, what else occurs at *circa* 4-5 hours incubation? At least one answer to this question can be found very simply. DNA synthesis starts at that time, as can be seen from Figure 6. To sum up then, it is probably fair to say at this stage in our experiments that the rejoining of DNA strand breaks within the subunits and the rejoining of the subunits together are two distinct processes. Perhaps we can go a little further than this and conclude that:

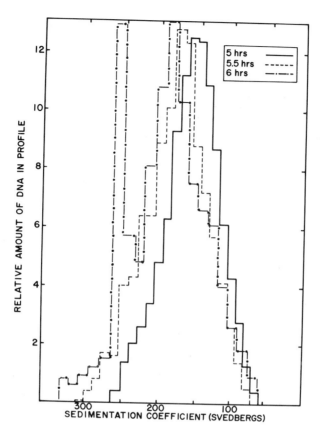

Fig 5. Sedimentation profiles obtained during the critical 4-6 hour post-irradiation period. Chinese hamster ovary cells. Mitotic cells irradiated with 22.1 Krads of X-rays. Incubation period, 5 hours ———— ; 5½ hours · · · · · ; 6 hours - - - - - - .

A tentative hypothesis for further work would be that cells can reconstitute the structural subunits anywhere within the cell cycle but can only put the subunits together and reconstitute the multicomponent arrays during S.

It is to be borne in mind however, that identification of the second process with DNA synthesis rather than another process which occurs concomitantly with DNA synthesis is preliminary at this time.

At present the fate of those DNA strand breaks within the subunits which are not rejoined following a dose of 22 Krads, that is to say, 3% of the breaks produced by that dose, is still unknown. The sensitivity of the present alkaline sucrose gradient method is such that we cannot tell unambiguously whether the fast-moving components incorporate the unrejoined fragments into larger components or whether the residual fragments are subsequently degraded.

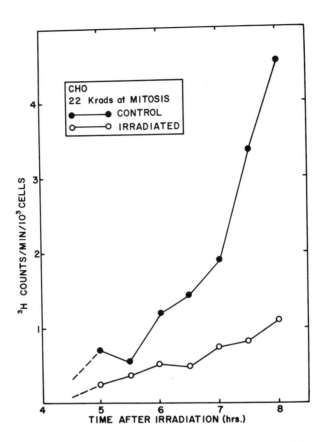

Fig 6. Thymidine incorporation profiles obtained by "flash" labelling for 10 minutes at the times indicated. Chinese hamster ovary cells. Mitotic cells: upper curve, unirradiated; lower curve 22.1 Krads of X-rays.

NONDIVIDING CELLS AND REJOINING IN VIVO: Cerebellar neurons

Thus far we have dealt with dividing cell populations. However, it is possible that radiation damage to nondividing cells can be critical, especially when the long-term effects of low incident environmental doses to mammals are considered. We are studying nondividing cells with a very specific idea in mind and it is an idea that has been referred to by Dr. Beers in his Introductory Remarks. We are attempting to determine whether DNA strand breaks accumulate with age in those nondividing tissues where cellular repopulation does not occur during the lifetime of the animal. We have chosen for our study the internal granular layer neurons in the cerebellum of the dog.

DNA strand breaks could accumulate in nondividing tissues with age, either because strand-break-rejoining mechanisms are absent from such tissues or else because strand-break-rejoining mechanisms may be present but deteriorate with age. It must be emphasized that the data to be presented are preliminary but have been introduced at this time to demonstrate to those workers who may be interested in this particular area that a decided breakthrough has been made. However, the experiments also introduce another feature which we wish to cover, namely the rejoining of DNA strand breaks in vivo. The cerebellar neuronal system has proven to be especially amenable to such a study.

The neurons were extracted from the internal granular layer of the cerebellum of the seven-week-old pup. In such animals the differentiation of the cerebellar neurons has virtually reached completion, so the tissue provides an ideal starting point for aging studies. The neuron preparations contained about 85% of differentiated granule neurons and *circa* 15% of glial, epithelial and Purkinje cells. This ratio was maintained or bettered when extractions were performed during post-irradiation incubation in vivo. Another point must be made at this time. It was necessary to develop a new alkaline sucrose gradient method for studying the DNA from nondividing tissue.

When swing-out rotors are used for sucrose gradient experiments the amount of DNA to be sedimented must be limited to microgram quantities (6). Otherwise anomalous sedimentation occurs. The detection of such small amounts of DNA is made possible by labeling the DNA with radioactive thymidine. Unfortunately, the DNA of nondividing cells cannot be made radioactive since DNA synthesis is dormant. In order to sediment the amounts of DNA necessary for chemical estimation of the gradient profile a large rotor was required. The only rotors big enough are zonal rotors. Therefore, we devised a zonal centrifuge method which used a titanium rotor, because of the high pH, and employed a reorienting gradient to obviate shearing the DNA (10). This rotor was especially

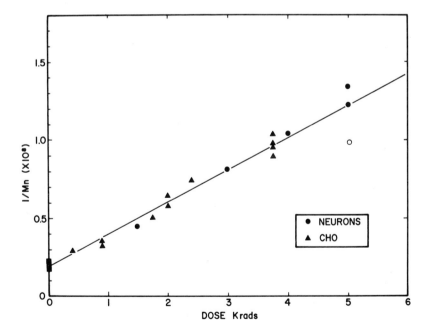

Fig 7. Change in reciprocal of the number-average molecular weight with X-ray dose. Chinese hamster ovary cells ▲, Canine cerebellar granule neurons ●. The experiment represented by the open circle is described in the text.

built for the purpose by Dr. Norman Anderson at Oak Ridge. With this method it is possible to use enough DNA so that the gradients can be analyzed by fluorometry. All the following data therefore, come from profiles determined by fluorometric measurements.

At the outset it was necessary to know whether X- or γ-rays produce strand breaks with the same efficiency in both dividing and nondividing cells. Data obtained with the neurons are compared with those from Chinese hamster cells (7) in Figure 7. It can be seen that within experimental error the changes in molecular weight observed in DNA of the two cell types are the same. For these experiments the neurons were irradiated in vitro because about 12 minutes are required to irradiate and extract the neurons from the brain. Therefore, some rejoining of strand breaks can occur during biopsy. A 12 minute "zero-time" experiment performed in this way gave rise to the open circle, shown in Figure 7.

During the initial stages of post-irradiation incubation in vivo the 165S subunit is rejoined in a manner similar to that exhibited by dividing cells in vitro. The same subunit is present in the DNA from both cell types because when the DNA from nonradioactive neurons and the DNA from radioactive Chinese hamster cells are sedimented in the same rotor the profiles overlap at 165S. The rejoining of the strand breaks within the subunit is shown in Figure 8. In these cases the canine cerebella received 5 Krads of collimated γ-rays. Five hours after irradiation the amount of subunit in the profile starts to decrease again and then a significant proportion of the profile is composed of slowly sedimenting species (Fig 9). After even longer post-irradiation incubation the slowly

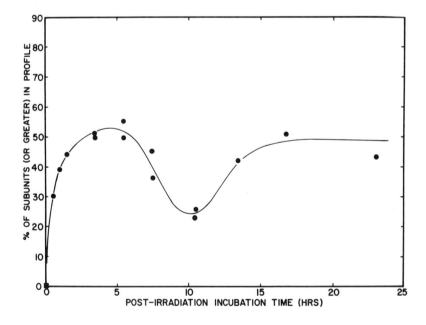

Fig 8. The percentage of subunit (or greater) reappearing in the profiles during post-irradiation incubation in vivo. Canine cerebellar granule neurons from the seven-week-old beagle. Collimated γ-ray dose of 5 Krads to the cerebellum.

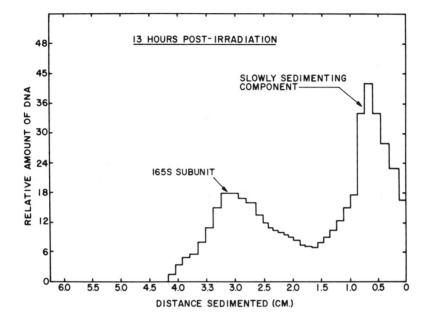

Fig 9. Typical profile obtained from a reoriented zonal gradient after 13 hours incubation following a collimated γ-ray dose of 5 Krads to the cerebellum, 30 minutes lytic-storage time. Profiles were measured by fluorometry. Cerebellar granule neurons from the seven-week-old beagle.

sedimenting species appear to be reincorporated into the 165S subunit or faster moving components.

The above data represent the essence of the preliminary story. In view of them, the immediate future could be very stimulating.

ACKNOWLEDGMENTS

Our thanks are expressed to Dr. R. J. Garner and his colleagues at the Collaborative Radiological Health Laboratory at Colorado State University for their help and advice with the beagle experiments. Some of the CHO cell experiments were performed by E. G. Siu.

REFERENCES

1. Lett, J. T., Stacey, K. A. and Alexander, P.: Crosslinking of dry deoxyribonucleic acids by electrons. Radiat. Res., 14:349, 1961.
2. Alexander, P., Lett, J. T., Kopp, P. and Itzhaki, R.: Degradation of dry deoxyribonucleic acid by polonium alpha-particles. Radiat. Res., 14:362, 1961.
3. Dean, C. J., Feldschreiber, P. and Lett, J. T.: Repair of X-ray damage to the DNA in *Micrococcus radiodurans*. Nature, 209:49, 1966.

4. McGrath, R. A. and Williams, R. W.: Reconstruction in vivo of irradiated *Escherichia coli.* deoxy-ribonucleic acid; the rejoining of broken pieces. Nature, 212:534, 1966.

5. Elkind, M. M. and Whitmore, G. F.: The radiobiology of cultured mammalian cells. Gordon & Breach, New York, 1967.

6. Lett, J. T., Klucis, E. S. and Sun, C.: On the size of the DNA in the mammalian chromosome: Structural subunits. Biophys. J., 10:277, 1970.

7. Lett, J. T. and Sun, C.: The production of strand breaks in mammalian DNA by X-rays: At different stages in the cell cycle. Radiat. Res., 44:771, 1970.

8. Lett, J. T.: In: Time and dose relationships in radiation biology. Brookhaven Nat. Lab. Report #50203:22-24, 1970.

9. Lett, J. T.: The formation and rejoining of strand breaks produced in mammalian DNA by X-rays: At different stages of the cell cycle. Proceedings of IV International Congress of Radiation Biology. Gordon & Breach (in press) 1971.

10. Klucis, E. S. and Lett, J. T.: Zonal centrifugation of mammalian DNA. Anal. Biochem., 35:480, 1970.

RECOVERY AND REPAIR IN CHINESE HAMSTER CELLS FOLLOWING UV-IRRADIATION[1]

R. M. Humphrey and R. E. Meyn

Section of Cellular Studies, Department of Physics
University of Texas M. D. Anderson Hospital
Houston, Texas

INTRODUCTION

Terasima and Tolmach (1) reported in 1960 the original observation that the lethal effect of X-rays on mammalian cells was highly dependent on the stage of the division cycle at the time the cells were exposed to the radiation. This phenomenon has since become known as the cell-age response function.

Subsequently, several groups of workers have demonstrated that all mammalian cells, thus far tested, display a characteristic age-dependent response to X-rays (2), ultraviolet light (UV) (3-5) and certain chemicals such as hydroxyurea (6), Actinomycin D (7) and N-methyl-N'-nitro-N-nitrosoguanidine (8). Several parameters, such as, survival, production of chromosomal aberrations and cellular progression have been measured to determine the cell-age response function.

Specifically with UV, a maximum response occurs during the DNA synthetic or S phase of the cell cycle (3,4,9-11), as measured by the previously mentioned parameters.

Several hypotheses have been advanced to explain the age response function. Some of the explanations advanced are: one, a quantitative difference in the amount of damage produced in critical-target molecules by a given dose of radiation; two, a change in the number and/or nature of the critical target molecules; and three, qualitative or quantitative differences in cellular repair capability.

On the basis of models presented by Elkind and Sutton (12) concerning the repair of X-ray induced sublethal damage, it appeared tenable to test for enhanced survival in mammalian cells following exposure to fractionated doses of UV. However, this approach appeared to be unfruitful on the basis of the report by Han et al (13) who failed to demonstrate enhanced survival with a fractionated UV dose schedule with mouse L cells. Also Trosko et al (14) and Klimek (15) were unable to demonstrate the removal of UV-induced pyrimidine dimers from the DNA of either hamster or mouse L cells. During this period Rasmussen and Painter (16) reported the discovery of UV-induced unscheduled DNA synthesis in the G_1, G_2 and M phase of the division cycle of HeLa cells. This finding implied that mammalian cells did have the ability to repair UV damage. Subsequently, several types of molecular repair have been demonstrated in mammalian cells and these are the subject matter of other papers in the present series.

[1] Supported in part by National Institute of Health Grants CA-04484 and CA-05099.

At the cellular level, Rauth (17) showed that the addition of caffeine, an inhibitor of dark-reactivation in bacteria, enhanced the UV sensitivity of L cells. He interpreted these results as indicating that L cells had a dark-reactivation system capable of acting on UV damage. Humphrey et al (18) have demonstrated the ability of Chinese hamster ovary (CHO) cell line to recover between fractionated doses of UV. They have also shown that another hamster cell line (B-14) could not recover. In an effort to correlate a repair process known to occur at the molecular level with survival at the colony forming level, these two rodent cell lines were tested also for their ability to bypass (19) UV-induced photoproducts in parental DNA during postirradiation DNA synthesis (20).

MATERIALS AND METHODS

Except for some brief details given below, the descriptions of cell lines, cell growth, UV-irradiation, synchrony and ultracentrifuge procedures have been summarized elsewhere (18,20).

The double mitotic synchrony method used to obtain the survival data shown in Figure 4 was developed by Mr. William Nagle (21). Cells are synchronized by the excess thymidine (TdR) method and as the population arrives at mitosis, the mitotic cells are selectively detached from the growth vessel, and stored at $4^{\circ}C$.

Large numbers of mitotic cells are obtained with a mitotic index of 95 to 98% and a plating efficiency (70%) similar to asynchronous populations. When mitotic cells are reincubated at $37^{\circ}C$ the cells divide and within 30 minutes the M. I. drops to 10% as the cells progress into the G_1 period (22). One hour after plating, the M. I. was 2% and one group of petri dishes was UV irradiated with different doses to determine the survival of cells in G_1. A second group received a single dose of ergs/mm² and was returned to the incubator for about 18 hours. This incubation period is equal to the time for normal progression from G_1 to M (12 hours) plus a radiation induced delay period (6 hours) (10). As cells move into mitosis they are re-selected, plated, incubated for 1 hour and reirradiated with different doses to determine the survival of second generation surviving cells.

RESULTS AND DISCUSSION

The survival curves of asynchronous populations of B-14 and CHO cells have similar slopes but they differ greatly in their shoulder regions (Table I). Since the shoulder

TABLE I

UV Survival Parameters for Asynchronous Populations of Hamster Cells

Cell Strain	D_o	Extrapolation Number	Dq
B-14FAF28	18 ergs/mm²	2	12
CHO	18 ergs/mm²	10	41

of a survival curve may represent the damage that must be accumulated for cell killing (12), the large shoulder of the CHO survival curve implies that these cells must be capable of tolerating more sublethal damage than B-14 cells.

This supposition was tested by performing a fractionated dose experiment, and Figure 1a shows the results for B-14 cells and Figure 1b for CHO cells. These data indicate that B-14 cells do not recover between fractionated doses whereas CHO cells exhibit a rather large recovery ratio (about 3X).

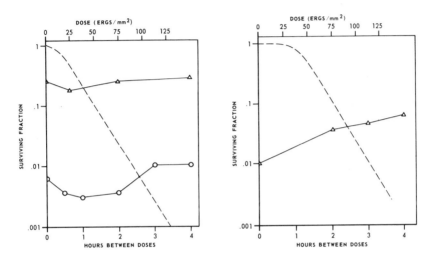

Fig 1a, b. (Reprinted from Ref. 18). Fig 1a - B-14 cells. First dose of 25 ergs/mm^2 plus a second dose of 25 ergs/mm^2 separated by time at 37°C. ($\triangle$) as above except with doses of 50 ergs/mm^2 (0). Dashed line represents survival of cells at time zero. Fig 1b - CHO cells. First dose of 50 ergs/mm^2 plus a second dose of 50 ergs/mm^2 separated by time at 37°C. Dashed line represents survival of cells at time zero.

The possibility existed that the increase in survival was due to a selection of the more radiation-resistant portion of the cell population by the first UV dose. This was eliminated by performing experiments on synchronized cells, in which the radiation was administered when the cells were either all in S phase or G_1 phase (Fig 2a, b). The conclusion reached from these experiments was that S phase cells were able to recover colony forming ability between fractionated UV doses, whereas G_1 phase cells could not. Additional experiments have been performed to confirm this conclusion.

In one experiment TdR synchronized cells were held at 5°C between fractionated doses (Fig 3a). The results can be compared with the data of Figure 2a. From Figure 2a it can be seen that at 37°C marked changes occur in the survival of the fractionated dose as well as the single dose schedule.

However, if the cells are kept at 5°C after removal of the TdR no significant recovery was observed. In a second experiment (Fig 3b) the cells were maintained in the

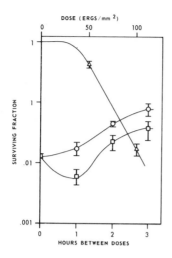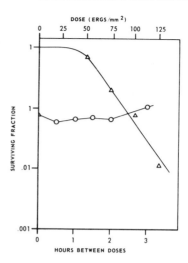

Fig 2a, b. (Reprinted from Ref. 18). Fig 2a - Recovery of synchronized population of CHO cells (S phase). Single dose of 100 ergs/mm^2 (3). First dose of 50 ergs/mm^2 plus a second dose of 50 ergs/mm^2 separated by time at 37°C. Single dose given at 0 hours (△). Fig 2b - as above except for G$_1$ phase cells.

presence of excess TdR during the single or fractionated dose schedule. Once again it can be seen that unless the cells are allowed to progress through S phase, neither recovery or cyclic associated changes in survival were observed.

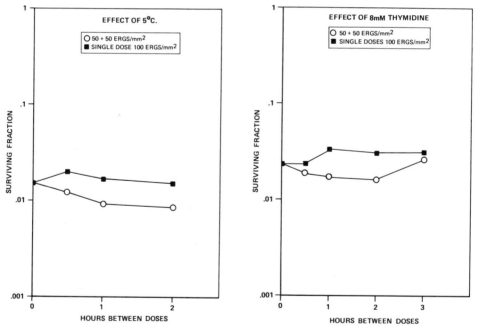

Fig 3a, b. Recovery of a synchronized population of CHO cells (S phase). Single dose of 100 ergs/mm^2 (5). First dose of 50 ergs/mm^2 plus a second dose of 50 ergs/mm^2 separated by time (o) a, cells maintained at 5°C; b, cells maintained in medium with 8 mm TdR.

Domon and Rauth (23) proposed a model for UV damage repair, in which they suggested that cells modify existing damage during replication of their DNA. This model was based on their finding that L cells irradiated during S phase and incubated in the presence of caffeine have a reduced survival when compared with noncaffeine treated controls. If the cells were allowed to progress through S before treatment with caffeine, then no caffeine enhancement of cell killing was observed. They further suggested that caffeine interferes with the S phase-specific modification process. The data on CHO cells presented here and time-lapse photography studies on L cells (11) are consistent with this model.

Fractionated dose experiments are complicated by synchrony decay since cells are progressing from one level of sensitivity to another in a rather short time. The following experiment was an attempt to overcome this problem. The design of these experiments was originally used to determine recovery capabilities in CHO cells following X-ray irradiation (21). Mitotic cells were plated and allowed to progress into the G_1 phase of the cycle. One group of plates was irradiated with different doses of UV in order to determine the survival of G_1 phase cells. Another group of plates received 75 ergs/mm^2 (41% survival) and were returned to the incubator. At the end of an 18-hour incubation at 37°C these cells which had progressed through S, G_2 and mitosis, were again mitotically selected, plated, incubated for 1 hour and irradiated in G_1. Figure 4 shows the results of this experiment. Curve I represents the survival for the original G_1 phase cells and has a D_o of 20 ergs/mm^2 and an n of 15. Curve II represents the survival for cells which had received 75 ergs/mm^2 in the previous G_1 phase. The D_o is similar to curve I and a shoulder

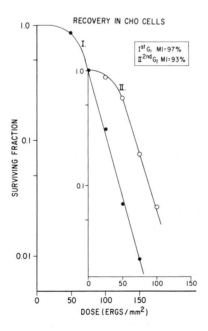

Fig 4. Curve I - Survival of CHO cells irradiated 1 hour after plating M cells (G_1 phase) (•). Curve II - Survival of cells irradiated to 41% survival level, allowed to progress to mitosis, selected, plated and irradiated with the second UV doses 1 hour after plating (o).

region is quite evident although reduced in width (n = 7). These data lend further support to the S phase modification model.

Dose fractionation experiments also were conducted utilizing four exposures of 25 ergs/mm^2, each separated by either 0.5, 1, 1.5, or 2.0 hour incubation periods at 37°C (Fig 5). For the CHO cells, the total dose of 100 ergs/mm^2 given over a period of six hours resulted in a factor 22 x increase in survival over that of this dose given as one single exposure.

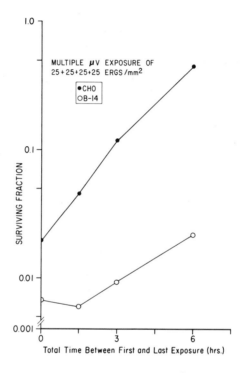

Fig 5. Cells irradiated with four exposures of 25 ergs/mm^2 each separated by 0.5, 1.0, 1.5, 2.0 hour incubation periods at 37°C. CHO - •, B-14 - o.

However, the increase in survival for B-14 cells is only about a factor of 3. This experiment again illustrates the relative lack of recovery capability in B-14 cells.

From the data presented thus far it would be expected that cells of rodent origin should possess some mechanism for recovery from UV damage. Although cells of human origin have been shown to be capable of excising of UV photoproducts (24), this aspect of repair has not been demonstrated in cells of rodent origin (14,15). One mechanism by which mammalian cells may recover involves the bypass of UV-induced photoproducts during DNA synthesis following irradiation, a process similar to that proposed for bacterial cells by Rupp and Howard-Flanders (19). The demonstration of gaps or discontinuities in newly synthesized DNA was performed as follows. Monolayers of CHO or B-14 cells

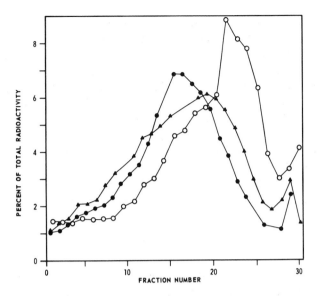

Fig 6. (Reprinted from Ref. 20). CHO cells. Sedimentation profiles of DNA synthesized immediately after irradiation. Controls (●); 50 ergs/mm^2 (▲); 100 ergs/mm^2 (o).

were irradiated with 0, 50, or 100 ergs/mm^2, incubated in medium containing H^{3}TdR for 1 hour, lysed on top of alkaline sucrose gradients and the DNA sedimented. The results of such an experiment on CHO cells is presented in Figure 6. As the dose of UV increases the sedimentation profile shifts toward a lower sedimentation coefficient. Similar results were obtained with B-14 cells. The synthesis of lower molecular weight DNA after UV-irradiation may be due to the bypass of a photoproduct which leaves a gap or discontinuity in the newly synthesized strand.

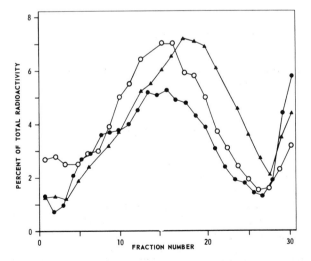

Fig 7. (Reprinted from Ref. 20). CHO cells. Sedimentation profiles of DNA synthesized 1 hour after irradiation with 50 ergs/mm^2 (▲) or incubated for an additional 2 hours (o); unirradiated control (●).

Furthermore, unless the gaps are sealed up a lethal event might result. CHO and B-14 cells were tested for the ability to seal up the gaps by performing the following experiment. Cultures were irradiated with 50 ergs/mm^2 and incubated for 1 hour in medium containing H^{3}TdR. At the end of the labeling period, the cultures were washed and incubated in normal medium for an additional 2 hours. At this time the cells were lysed and the DNA was sedimented on alkaline sucrose gradients. The results shown in Figure 7 illustrate that CHO cells are able to seal up gaps within 3 hours after irradiation.

The B-14 cell line, which does not show recovery between fractionated doses of UV was not expected to possess a bypass mechanism. However, these cells showed qualitatively the same results as the CHO cell line. Therefore, the bypass mechanism does not correlate with the enhanced survival observed in the fractionated dose experiments.

SUMMARY

Evidence has been presented indicating that recovery between fractionated doses of UV is both cell strain and cell cycle dependent. Since a cell-age response function is evident in a cell line, which does not exhibit recovery (B-14), it is probable that this particular form of recovery does not play an important role in determining the cell-age dependent response.

Data from experiments with synchronized populations support the model suggested by Rauth that for survival cells modify UV damage during the subsequent replication of their DNA.

CHO cells exhibit recovery between fractionated doses of UV and B-14 cells do not. However, both cell lines appear to have the capability to bypass UV-induced photoproduct. Therefore, the bypass mechanism does not correlate with recovery in these cells.

ACKNOWLEDGMENTS

The authors wish to thank Mrs. B. A. Sedita, Mrs. V. W. Willingham and Mrs. J. M. Winston for their expert technical assistance.

REFERENCES

1. Terasima, T. and Tolmach, L. J.: Nature, 190:1210, 1961.
2. Sinclair, W. K.: Radiat. Res., 33:620, 1968.
3. Han, A. and Sinclair, W. K.: Biophys. J., 9:1171, 1969.
4. Rauth, A. M. and Whitmore, G. F.: Radiat. Res., 28:84, 1966.
5. Djordjevic, B. and Tolmach, L. H.: Radiat. Res., 32:327, 1967.
6. Sinclair, W. K.: Science, 150:1729, 1965.
7. Elkind, M. M., Kano, E. and Sutton-Gilbert, H.: J. Cell Biol., 42:367, 1969.
8. Barranco, S. C. and Humphrey, R. M.: Mutat. Res., 11:421, 1971.
9. Humphrey, R. M., Dewey, W. C. and Cork, A.: Radiat. Res., 19:247, 1963.
10. Bootsma, D. and Humphrey, R. M.: Mutat. Res., 5:289, 1968.

11. Thompson, L. H. and Humphrey, R. M.: Radiat. Res., 41:183, 1970.
12. Elkind, M. M. and Sutton, H.: Radiat. Res., 13:556, 1960.
13. Han, A., Miletic, B. and Petrovic, D.: Int. J. Radiat. Biol., 8:187, 1964.
14. Trosko, J. E., Chu, E. H. Y. and Carrier, W. L.: Radiat. Res., 24:667, 1965.
15. Klimek, M.: Neoplasma, 12:459, 1965.
16. Rasmussem, R. E. and Painter, R. B.: Nature, 203:1360, 1964.
17. Rauth, A. M.: Radiat. Res., 31:121, 1967.
18. Humphrey, R. M., Sedita, B. A. and Meyn, R. E.: Int. J. Radiat. Biol., 18:61, 1970.
19. Rupp, W. D. and Howard-Flanders, P.: J. Molec. Biol., 31:291, 1968.
20. Meyn, R. E. and Humphrey, R. M.: Biophys. J., 11:295, 1971.
21. Nagle, W.: Ph.D. Dissertation, University of Texas Southwestern Medical School, 1971.
22. Barranco, S. C. and Humphrey, R. M.: Cancer Res., 31:191, 1971.
23. Domon, M. and Rauth, A. M.: Radiat. Res., 40:414, 1969.
24. Regan, J. D., Trosko, J. E. and Carrier, W. L.: Photochem. Photobiol., 8:319, 1968.

FACTORS WHICH INFLUENCE THE EXPRESSION OF RADIATION DAMAGE BY MAMMALIAN CELLS[1]

James A. Belli

Department of Radiation Therapy
Harvard Medical School
Boston, Massachusetts

An important biological expression of successful repair of radiation damage is survival. The latter is usually defined as a capacity for unlimited division measured by colony formation. Three levels of radiation damage may be defined. First, sublethal damage; cells having this level of damage eventually form colonies and, in order to test for its repair, a second or challenge stress must be applied. This second stress can take the form of radiation or drug. Second, lethal damage; when registered, suppression of colony formation occurs under any circumstance. Third, potentially lethal damage; this level of damage may be reparable to a nonlethal level if suitable conditions are provided; if repair does not take place, conversion to a lethal state occurs and colony formation is suppressed.

In this paper, I will show that mammalian cells in culture repair potentially lethal radiation damage if provided suitable conditions after a single exposure; that this repair capacity is found also in daughter cells into which "lethal" damage has been segregated at the time of the first postirradiation division; that this damage is segregated in a form which is probably similar to that registered in the parent; and that there is a post-irradiation subpopulation contained in developing colonies which have reached the end of their divisional history, presumably because of the "inheritance" of lethal damage, and this subpopulation can be rescued if provided suitable conditions.

Figure 1 shows the course of survival fluctuation as a function of time in Earle's balanced salt solution (EBSS) after a single dose of 900 R. The initial increase suggests that in the presence of buffer, mammalian cells repair damage which would have suppressed colony formation. The subsequent fall in survival suggests that, with continued repair, an unstable cellular state prevents unlimited division. This is a reasonable suggestion, since part of the repair process may be degradative, and, if interrupted at this point by an environment in which other cell functions (including division) must proceed, radiation damage will be expressed as a lethal event. The second survival increase is interpreted to mean that this unstable state exists transiently and is converted to a stable, nonlethal condition with further repair in buffer. The kinetics observed in this particular curve are similar to those observed by Boyle in bacterial systems incubated in minimal medium after irradiation and by Lett for single-strand rejoining of DNA in irradiated, nondividing cells (these proceedings).

A reasonable assumption is that the degradative portion of the repair sequence is temperature dependent. This assumption has been tested by incubating cells in buffer at 37°C for 2 hours; following this, buffer temperature was rapidly changed to 5°C.

[1] Supported by USPHS Grant CA 11264.

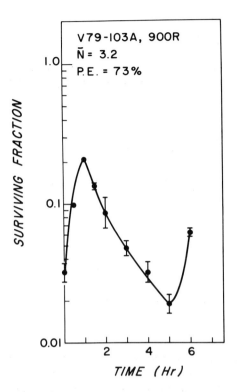

Fig 1. Survival of Chinese hamster cells after 900 R and as a function of time in Earle's balanced salt solution. $\bar{N}$: average number of cells per colony at irradiation (time-zero); P.E.: plating efficiency. Standard errors are shown except where smaller than the plotted points.

Figure 2 shows the results of this experiment. It is seen that the decrease in survival is suppressed during buffer incubation at low temperature supporting the suggestion that the repair sequence has a degradative component.

In other experiments (1), we have shown that the repair of potentially lethal damage by mammalian cells is cell-age dependent. Our results indicated that cells in DNA synthesis were able to repair potentially lethal damage; G_1 cells were not. Because repair of potentially lethal radiation damage is apparently accomplished most efficiently by cells in the process of replicating their DNA, it is not unreasonable to expect that this repair mechanism and the replication process are related. In more recent experiments, we have been able to show that cells irradiated during G_1 and allowed to progress into their first postirradiation synthetic period are able to repair potentially lethal radiation damage during that synthetic period if provided buffer at that time.

When a damaged cell experiences its first postirradiation division, the functional state of daughter cells, with respect to eventual colony formation, can assume one of three different combinations. First, both cells are reproductively viable and contribute progeny to the colony. Two, only one of the daughter cells is reproductively viable, but a colony is eventually observed. (Whether its nonviable sister experiences one or more divisions is

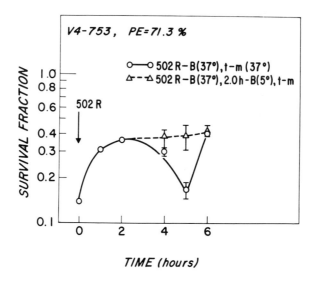

Fig 2. Effect of buffer temperature on survival after 502 R. m: Growth medium as final environment for colony formation.

not important, since the total contribution to the eventual colony by its progeny would be negligible.) Third, neither daughter cell is viable and a colony will not be observed. In the latter two cases, "lethal" damage has been sectored into one or both of the daughter cells. Experiments were designed to test whether this sectored damage is reparable.

Figure 3 shows the results of an experiment in which single Chinese hamster cells ($\bar{N}$ = 1.03) were irradiated with 756 R; 20.45 hours later these cells had reached a

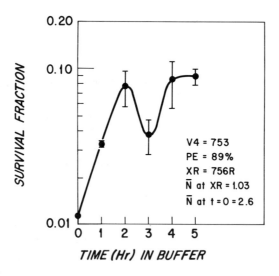

Fig 3. Survival of daughter cells from single cells exposed to 756 R.

multiplicity of 2.6 (time = zero in the figure). Growth medium was replaced with EBSS for intervals following which microcolonies were dispersed with dilute trypsin. The resulting single cells were provided growth medium for colony formation. The survival fraction for time = zero resulted when microcolonies were dispersed by trypsin without prior buffer treatment. Survival reached a maximum after two hours in buffer; this was followed by survival decrease and subsequent rise. These survival kinetics were similar to those observed with cells incubated in buffer immediately after X-irradiation (Fig 1). The degree of survival increase observed means that nonviable progeny from damaged parent cells had repaired their segregated damage to a level permitting expression of survival by colony formation.

If the trypsinization step is eliminated, survival increase will not be observed if nonviable cells must be associated with viable cells in a microcolony in order to accomplish repair of damage, that is to say, only one colony is eventually scored regardless of the contribution to the final population by cells which had repaired segregated damage. On the other hand, if repair capacity resides in one or more cells of a microcolony in which *all* of the progeny are nonviable, increased survival will be observed when buffer is provided and trypsinization omitted, which means successful repair by one or more of these cells will be reflected by eventual colony formation.

Figure 4 shows the results of an experiment in which single cells were irradiated with 800 R, allowed to grow to a multiplicity of 2.1 (time = zero in the figure), incubated in buffer for intervals and refed with growth medium for colony formation. When microcolonies were not dispersed with trypsin after incubation in buffer, survival kinetics were similar to those seen in Figure 3. An important implication of these findings is that when the level of damage registered in the parent cell does not suppress the first or second post-irradiation division, but is great enough to insure that *all* resulting progeny are nonviable,

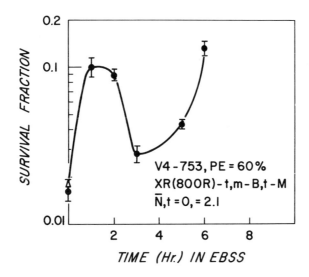

Fig 4. Survival of daughter cells from single cells exposed to 800 R. Microcolonies were not trypsinized after buffer (B) incubation for time (t).

a significant proportion of these progeny retain the capacity to repair their "inherited" damage. Therefore, the concept of potentially lethal damage can now be extended to daughter cells and, further, the repair system responsible for repairing this class of damage remains functional after division.

Figure 5 shows the results of an experiment to extend these findings. Single cells were irradiated with 504 R at time-zero. As a function of time after irradiation, the cell population was trypsinized and replated for colony formation. The open circles show the increase in relative survival when cells were grown in medium after irradiation. If before trypsinization and respreading for colony formation, microcolonies were exposed to

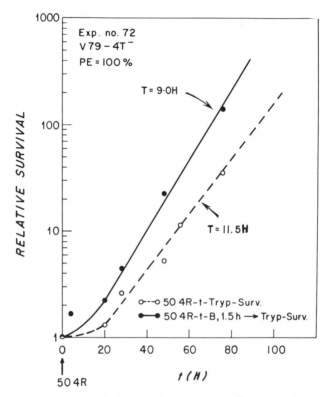

Fig 5. Rescue of nonviable cells by buffer (B) during colony formation after 504 R at time (t) = zero. Survival (surv.) is colony formation in complete medium. Buffer incubation for 1.5 hours.

Puck's saline F for 1.5 hours, the increase in relative survival was found to be that traced by the closed circles. This result indicates that at least through the 100 cell stage, there exists a subpopulation into which potentially lethal radiation damage had been segregated and that this damage is reparable if cells are incubated for a short time in buffer. Because the curves are divergent, we postulate that this cell population remains relatively constant during postirradiation growth.

In summary, mammalian cells in culture are able to repair potentially lethal radiation damage, if provided a minimum growth environment after a single exposure. When exposure to this environment is delayed until the first or second postirradiation division, nonviable daughter cells are also able to repair their segregated damage. During the development of a colony, there exists a subpopulation the members of which have reached the end of their divisional history and a substantial proportion of this population can be rescued if provided appropriate conditions.

REFERENCE

1. Belli, J. A. and Shelton, M.: Potentially lethal radiation damage: Repair by mammalian cells in culture. Science, 165:490, 1969.

UNSCHEDULED DNA SYNTHESIS AND CELLULAR RECOVERY IN VARIOUS MAMMALIAN CELL LINES[1]

James Shaeffer and Timothy Merz

Department of Radiological Science
The Johns Hopkins University School of Hygiene and Public Health
Baltimore, Maryland

Repair replication and unscheduled DNA synthesis are simply two different assay systems for the same basic event; namely, the replacement of precursors in excised regions of parental DNA strands damaged by ultraviolet irradiation, ionizing radiation, or by some radiomimetic compound. Whereas repair replication is measured by the incorporation of labeled DNA precursors into parental DNA strands separated by density gradient centrifugation techniques, unscheduled DNA synthesis is the autoradiographic measure of the incorporation of tritiated thymidine into the DNA of non-S phase cells; that is, cells that are not in the normal DNA replicative phase of the cell cycle.

Ever since the phenomenon of unscheduled DNA synthesis was first described by Rasmussen and Painter (1), several groups, ourselves included, have been attempting to shed some light on the possible relationships between X-ray induced unscheduled DNA synthesis and the Elkind recovery phenomenon (2) and between unscheduled synthesis and cell sensitivity.

One way of attacking this problem is to examine the relative extents of unscheduled DNA synthesis in many cell lines with the hope possibly of finding an unscheduled DNA synthesis-deficient line wherein a correlation could be made between the biochemical defect and alteration of function. This situation would be analogous to the correlation of sensitivity with lack of excision repair in E. coli B$_{s-1}$ (3,4) and also to the correlation of UV sensitivity with endonuclease deficiency in xeroderma pigmentosum (5,6).

We have made quantitative comparisons of the extent of X-ray induced unscheduled DNA synthesis in eight mammalian cell lines and have attempted to correlate X-ray induced unscheduled DNA synthesis with two survival parameters: cell sensitivity (D_o) and recovery ratio. Methods used for these assay systems are described elsewhere (7).

Figure 1 shows the dose response for unscheduled synthesis in the HeLa, L-929 and rat kangaroo kidney (RKK) lines. While the HeLa and L-929 lines had high and moderately high responses, respectively, it is noteworthy that the rat kangaroo kidney line exhibited no apparent unscheduled DNA synthesis.

[1] Supported by American Cancer Society Grant E 528 and by Project for Training in Radiological Health Grant 39896-03-68.

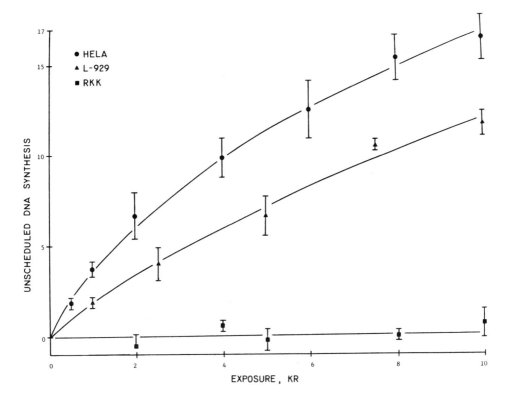

Fig 1. Dose responses for unscheduled DNA synthesis in three cell lines. Unscheduled synthesis was calculated by subtracting the mean number of silver grains over the non-S phase nuclei of unirradiated cells from the mean grain number of silver grains over the non-S phase nuclei of irradiated cells. Cells were kept in media containing $5\mu Ci/ml$ ^{3}H-thymidine (16-20 Ci/mM) for one hour following X-ray treatment. Autoradiographic slides were exposed for one week. Bars indicate standard errors of the mean for three replicate counts of 50 non-S phase cells per count.

The dose responses for the five other lines that we have examined is shown in Figure 2. They include mouse mammary adenocarcinoma (MAC), human laryngeal tumor (HLT), human embryonic kidney (HEK), G_1 phase phytohemagglutinin-stimulated human peripheral lymphocytes (HPL-G_1) and rat kangaroo liver (RKL).

Since the three lines shown in Figure 1 had a wide range of responses for unscheduled DNA synthesis, we decided to examine the survival and recovery curves of these lines. In Figure 3 are the single dose survival curves for the HeLa, L and RKK lines. A common feature in all three curves is the appearance of a shoulder. All three lines had approximately the same values of D_o: 110 R for the HeLa line, 130 R for the L-929 line and 100 R for the rat kangaroo kidney line. This can be seen more easily in Figure 4 where the three curves overlap. Also shown in Figure 4 is the survival curve for the mouse mammary adenocarcinoma line, which, although quite radiosensitive (D_o = 55 R), had a high response for unscheduled DNA synthesis (Fig 2). These data point to a non-relationship between X-ray induced unscheduled DNA synthesis and cell sensitivity.

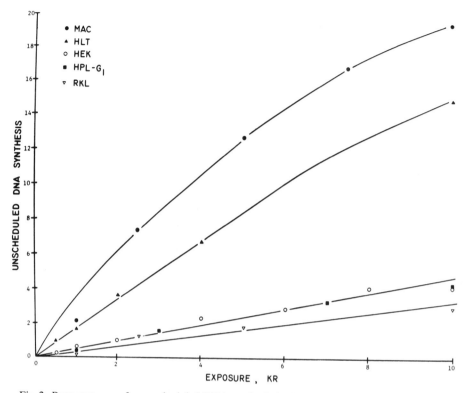

Fig 2. Dose responses for unscheduled DNA synthesis in five cell lines. Experimental conditions were the same as those described in Figure 1.

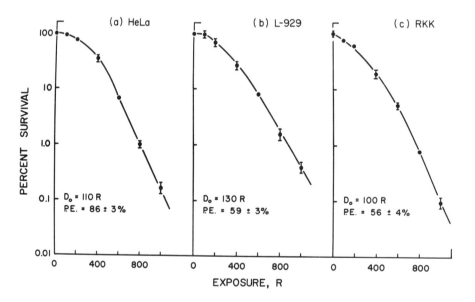

Fig 3. Survival curves of three cell lines following single exposures of X-irradiation. Bars indicate standard errors of three replicate plates.

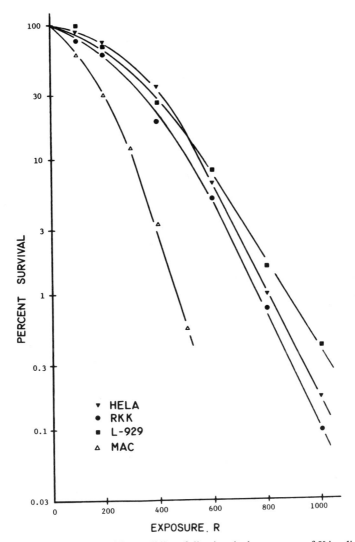

Fig 4. Survival curves of four cell lines following single exposures of X-irradiation.

With the HeLa, L-929 and rat kangaroo kidney lines, there were quantitatively different responses for unscheduled DNA synthesis yet comparable radiosensitivities. In the MAC line there is a high level of unscheduled DNA synthesis in a very radiosensitive line.

The recovery responses for the HeLa, L and RKK lines are shown in Figure 5. Split doses of 500 R were used, with the time interval between doses extending to 90 min. The fact that the rat kangaroo kidney line exhibits the usual recovery phenomenon, although it lacks unscheduled DNA synthesis, would indicate clearly dissociation of these two repair assay systems.

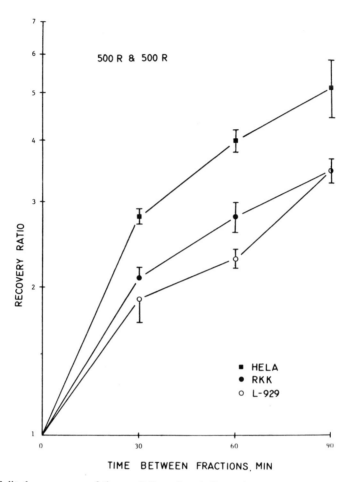

Fig 5. Split dose recovery of three cell lines. Bars indicate the standard errors of three replicate plates at each point.

TABLE I

Relationship Between Unscheduled DNA Synthesis, Modal Chromosome Number, DNA Content, D_o, and Recovery Ratio in Different Cell Lines

Cell Line	Relative Unscheduled DNA Synthesis (5KR)	Modal Chromosome Number	DNA/Cell, picograms	D_o, R	Recovery Ratio (60 min)
HeLa	11.2	79	15.0	110	4.0
L-929	6.7	66	15.1	130	2.3
RKK	0.2	11	14.4	100	2.8
MAC	12.6	86	-	55	-
HPL	2.2	46	6.5	-	-
HLT	8.3	46	-	-	-
HEK	2.6	46	6.0	-	-
RKL	1.5	13	-	-	-

Table I summarizes the data that we have accumulated on the eight cell lines at this time. There appears to be a direct relationship between unscheduled DNA synthesis and chromosome number (Fig 6) but this correlation does not hold between unscheduled synthesis and DNA content. The rat kangaroo kidney line contains quite a lot of DNA in only 11 chromosomes, yet exhibits virtually no unscheduled synthesis. The dotted line in Figure 6 is intended to indicate the directionality of the relationship between unscheduled synthesis and chromosome number. This is not meant to imply that the relationship is necessarily linear.

If the rat kangaroo kidney line is lacking in X-ray induced unscheduled DNA synthesis, we asked if it is also lacking in UV-stimulated unscheduled synthesis. Both UV and X-ray dose responses for unscheduled synthesis in the HeLa and rat kangaroo kidney lines are shown in Figure 7. It seems quite clear that the rat kangaroo kidney line is

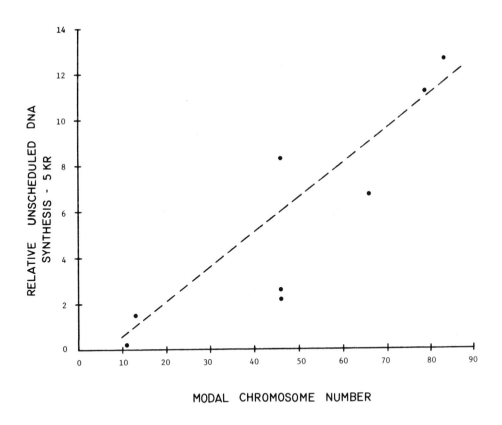

Fig 6. Relationship of X-ray induced unscheduled DNA synthesis to chromosome number in the eight lines examined in this study.

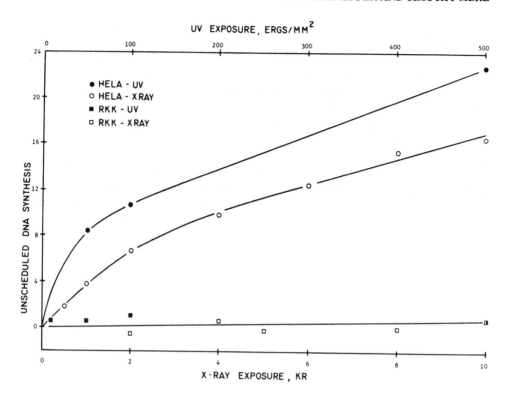

Fig 7. Comparison of dose responses for X-ray and UV-stimulated unscheduled DNA synthesis in HeLa and rat kangaroo kidney lines. Experimental conditions were the same as those described in Figure 1.

unresponsive, in terms of unscheduled synthesis, to both UV- and X-irradiation. The HeLa line, on the other hand, is responsive to both. In terms of grain production, 100 ergs/mm² in the HeLa line seems equivalent to approximately 5000 R of X-irradiation.

In summary, our results are as follows:

1. There appears to be no causal relationship between X-ray induced unscheduled DNA synthesis and cell recovery, based primarily on the lack of unscheduled synthesis in the rat kangaroo kidney line. Nor does there appear to be any relationship between X-ray induced unscheduled synthesis and cell sensitivity.

2. Unscheduled DNA synthesis appears to be related directly to chromosome number, while the relationship of unscheduled synthesis to DNA content per cell remains unclear.

3. The rat kangaroo kidney line exhibits neither UV nor X-ray induced unscheduled DNA synthesis, supporting the hypothesis (5) that, excluding the incision endonuclease needed for UV repair, both UV and X-ray stimulated unscheduled DNA synthesis involve common enzyme systems.

REFERENCES

1. Rasmussen, R. E. and Painter, R. B.: Radiation stimulated DNA synthesis in cultured mammalian cells. J. Cell Biol., 29:11, 1966.

2. Elkind, M. M. and Sutton, H.: X-ray damage and recovery in mammalian cells in culture. Nature, 184:1293, 1959.

3. Hill, R. F.: A radiation-sensitive mutant of E. coli. Biochim. Biophys. Acta, 30:636, 1958.

4. Ellison, S. A., Feiner, R. R. and Hill, R. F.: A host effect on bacteriophage survival after UV irradiation. Virology, 11:294, 1960.

5. Cleaver, J. E.: Xeroderma pigmentosum: a human disease in which an initial stage of DNA repair is defective. Proc. Nat. Acad. Sci. USA, 63:428, 1969.

6. Setlow, R. B., Regan, J. D., German, J. and Carrier, W. L.: Evidence that Xeroderma pigmentosum cells do not perform the first step in the repair of ultraviolet damage to their DNA. Proc. Nat. Acad. Sci. USA, 64:1035, 1969.

7. Shaeffer, J. and Merz, T.: A comparison of unscheduled DNA synthesis, D_0, cell recovery, and chromosome number in X-irradiated mammalian cell lines. Radiat. Res., 47:426, 1971.

DISCUSSION

Dr. Herriott
(Baltimore)

I might open by saying that I begin to detect consensus in the notion that there is repair of ionizing radiation in mammalian cells, at least at the single-strand level. If this is not so, I'd like to have some of you speak up and comment about it.

Dr. Humphrey
(Houston)

I would say there is consensus among those of us who have been doing alkaline gradients that there is rejoining in all stages of the cell cycle following ionizing radiation. It was rather surprising, at least to me, to find that mitotic cells rejoin single-strand breaks. Since mitotic cells are extremely X-ray sensitive, but still have the capability of rejoining breaks, it is very possible that single-strand breaks did not have any relationship to lethal events in the cell. But I think that Dr. Lett described this morning a very interesting facet in which subunits are not put back together again until an S phase. This means there is additional repair that requires at least the entrance of the cell into S phase. And this, I think, we also showed in the case of UV. So I think this supports the idea that there is a so-called S phase modification. No matter what sort of repair rejoining might go on in other phases of the cycle, it might require the entrance of the cell in the S phase, in order to effect survival.

Dr. Lett
(Fort Collins)

I think that I can follow that up a little. Three points should be borne in mind. Firstly, we only measured the rejoining of the strand breaks and can say little about the integrity of the rejoining. It may be that many of the breaks are rejoined incorrectly and give rise to lethal mutations. Secondly, we have the tendency to associate radio-resistance with bacteria and radio-sensitivity with mammalian cells. However, when you consider the efficiency with which mammalian cells dispose of DNA damage you should conclude that they are very radio-resistant. From an evolutionary point of view this is highly desirable. Finally, we are only looking at the gross DNA damage, and it may be that breaks cannot be rejoined in some chromosomes or in certain parts of them. Now, since the breaks that are liable to be lethal are only a very small fraction of those which are produced and rejoined, such a possibility would be beyond the resolution in our present experiments. So a break in one position could be lethal whereas the same type of break somewhere else need not be.

Dr. Dalrymple
(Little Rock)

The second side of the coin concerns the repair of sublethal radiation injury, which is equally as fascinating as the rejoining of DNA breaks. The repair of sublethal injury is very important from the clinical standpoint, because this is where we think in terms of how many cells will survive to allow a cancer to reoccur, or how many surviving bone marrow stem cells will be left in the patient so that he may be able to survive whole body doses. If one looks at the survival studies that are performed, to get good results with these studies, the surviving fractions are down at the order of one tenth of one percent to one percent, although this gives a ten-fold *relative* increase. We tend to lose sight of this giant vanished army of 99% killed cells. A question to throw out to the panel, particularly after hearing all those beautiful lectures about the UV lesions, what is the lesion in the DNA produced by ionizing radiation that is responsible for killing the cell? I don't have an answer, but maybe Dr. Painter might have one.

Dr. Painter   The unrepaired one, maybe.
(San Francisco)

Dr. Strauss   I think that it's worthwhile to comment about the simplicity
(Chicago)   of the UV-induced lesions, since there's a fair amount of work that indicates that UV induces crosslinks between DNA and protein. While we understand what happens to the thymine dimers, it's not at all clear that in the case of UV, the lethal lesion may not be something different. So simplicity can be found nowhere.

Dr. Herriott   It should also be added that there are other UV photo products in the DNA besides dimers.

Dr. Lett   I wonder also if I can make a comment about the magnitude of the problem in mammalian cells. Many of the previous presentations described experiments with viruses or bacteria. These are comparatively simple systems. Dr. W. C. Dewey, of Colorado State University, has found a strong correlation between one chromosome aberration and the death of a mammalian cell. In other words, the D_{37} coincides with one chromosome aberration per cell. If one chromosome aberration kills the cell, and one chromosome aberration can be related to one DNA break in the chromosome, then the sensitivity required to detect that break is enormous. Let's consider a simpler case; suppose we want to measure one DNA break per chromosome. The average size, in general, of the DNA in the chromosome is 10^{11} Daltons. If we used a railroad track as a model for the DNA of this chromosome, the ties, roughly speaking, would represent the base pairs, then the DNA would be 25,000 miles long, or stretch once around the earth. And we're looking for one break! This is where we have to get to, there's a big wilderness out there. We are just beginning to get to the 250 mile stage. So with bacteria you can design experiments, but with mammalian cells I'm afraid that Mother Nature still has a number of basic parameters to divulge.

Dr. Strauss   I have a question for Dr. Lett. Dr. Lindahl pointed out there might be as many as 100,000 apurinic sites produced per cell generation in mammalian cells. Now it's quite clear that apurinic sites hydrolyze very rapidly in alkaline. Therefore, I wonder what the relationships of any alkaline-sucrose gradient might be as far as the continuity of DNA in vivo, since any unrepaired apurinic site will serve as a site for a break in the surcose gradient, in any alkaline-sucrose gradient.

Dr. Lett   I don't really know how to answer this definitively; but if there were that number of apurinic sites, and they all gave rise to unrejoined strand breaks in the mammalian cells, then you would get much smaller DNA than we normally see in the sucrose gradients. Also, the DNA would degrade in alkali with time. We can store the 165S subunit on the top of the gradient for 12-15 hours (at 20°C) before significant strand breakage occurs. The only other answer would seem to be that loss of a purine does not necessarily result in a strand break. That's where I'll have to leave it at this time.

Dr. Painter   May I comment on that? If you take the total DNA in a mammalian cell, which is about 5×10^{12} Daltons, roughly, divided by Lett's subunits which is 5×10^8 you get 1×10^4 pieces, and so then you might argue that at the instant that lysis occurs, there are 10^4 apurinic sites which are responsible for this. I think that can be counteracted by Dr. Lett's demonstration that this is a monodisperse distribution and not a random one as one would expect. Maybe that's one of my problems, I'm not sure. I would expect those apurinic sites to be randomly distributed.

Dr. Strauss   I think it's impossible to assume that one has apurinic DNA that doesn't break in alkali, unless the DNA is arranged in some way, so that the alkali doesn't get to it. Once that happens then one has a conjugate of some sort, and the meaning of the gradient is not clear. I suspect that the question to be answered is the one that Dr. Painter proposed; that is, whether the distribution is monodisperse or not, and I can't answer that. That conclusion is either good or bad, depending on the physical chemistry, and I just don't know. I do have a question for Dr. Dalrymple. I wonder if I understood correctly, that you see repair in the presence of dinitrophenol.

Dr. Dalrymple   No, what we have shown is repair of sublethal radiation injury, the endpoint is survival. Now, in the presence of dinitrophenol, there is no rejoining of single-stranded DNA breaks, or of disappearance of five prime termini or three prime hydroxyl termini.

Dr. Humphrey   This is a question for Dr. Strauss. I understood from your hypothesis that in order to get from a single-strand break in the DNA to a chromatid break in the chromosome, that one might require DNA replication. The one problem in seeing how this might work, is that all agents I'm aware of, X-ray and alkylating agents and some others, cause extensive breaks in cells that are in the G-2 period, prior to mitosis. These cells do not undergo normal DNA replication prior to going into mitosis. How then, is a chromatid aberration produced in a G-2 phase cell?

Dr. Strauss   I would look at it in the following way: if there were a double-strand break in G-1, a chromosome aberration would occur if there were a single-strand break in G-1 or S, a chromatid aberration would result. A double-strand break in G-2 would also produce a chromatid aberration, two double-strand breaks in G-2 would be required in order to get a chromosome aberration. Incidentally, I think that the last papers describing work with Chinese hamster cells, were very much at variance with the hypothesis we proposed. I think that this afternoon Dr. Roberts may have some data to indicate that what happens in Chinese hamster cells, may be very different from what happens in HEP-2 cells or even HeLa cells, for reasons I don't understand.

Dr. Lett

I wonder if at this stage I could make an appeal to the audience. The big problem with the alkaline-sucrose, or any other sedimentation technique, is quantifying the size of the sedimenting molecules. The obvious way of confirming the sedimentation experiments is by electron microscopy. I have approached several good electron microscopists with the idea of having a look at the size of the subunit, to see if it really is as big as we think it is, and whether it's a single-strand. So far I have had little real success with my enquires. Is there anyone in the audience who would be prepared to take a good strong look at this thing to see if it really is as big as we think it is? It is essential that this be done. The only evidence that we have at the moment is the indirect evidence obtained from strand breaking efficiencies. We need a more definite answer.

Dr. Herriott

I'd like to ask one question of Dr. Painter. Were you suggesting that when you could not see a change produced by a thousand rads, that the system isn't sensitive enough to pick it up?

Dr. Painter

The induced repair from 1000 rads is not enough to increase significantly the specific activity that you see in the control. It turns out that the difference in this case would be 15 counts/minute/mcg and 18.5 counts/minute/mcg and the control will vary in that way.

Dr. Herriott

But that dose is sufficient to drop the viability of one log.

Dr. Painter

We were trying to show that the real problem no longer is finding repair replication at low doses, but the problem is to show stimulation of repair replication and I think it's just the fact that the repair event in mammalian cells is very localized and does not require a lot of degradation, as it does in bacteria (at least you get a tremendous amount of breakdown in your bacteria). You have this very localized repair and it is hard to show anything until you get to rather high doses. The DNA damage is just not enough to see.

Dr. Strauss

I wonder if Dr. Painter would agree that what causes repair replication in control cells is really an aspect of normal replication and is the material that has a density slightly shifted toward the hybrid and that repair synthesis is really that portion of the incorporated isotope that has a density equal to that of the unreplicated material.

Dr. Painter   I think the repair replication that we see, the nonsemicon-servative replication that we see in single strands of DNA in unirradiated cells in controls is not the same process as the repair replication induced by a damaging agent. I have no real idea what's causing the tritium to appear at normal density.

Dr. Herriott   Let's throw it open to the audience for discussion, and please identify yourself and your institution.

Dr. Lindahl (Stockholm)   I'd like to start by asking about calculation of 100,000 purine bases lost. This is what it would be in the solution during 20 hours at 37°. For the amount of DNA that is found in mammalian cells and if you allow repair processes in vivo, then obviously there would be very many fewer sites found at one specific time. You say the lesions can be repaired in ten minutes—you have less than a thousand breaks in the DNA isolated from the cells, and this would just allow the molecular weight to be as low as Dr. Lett finds. Then it's not necessarily a contradiction.

Dr. Strauss   No, that's correct. It's not a contradiction, but it would imply that there's no reason for supposing that this is a naturally existing subunit in the DNA, unless the formation of these apurinic sites are really the way nature makes subunits.

Dr. Lett   Dr. Painter's point is well taken. These are monodispersed, so that the apurinic sites are the very specific loci. I'd like to put the question back: does the nature of the ionic strength, or what have you, or ions in solution, affect the rate of apurination? Would you expect that the DNA surrounded by proteins to be less subject to this type of chemical reaction?

Dr. Lindahl   We have repeated and confirmed some data by Greer and Zamenhof on this point, and this is an ionic-strength-determined process, in that at low ionic strength you get proportionally more depurination at a certain temperature, well below the Tm. The measurements I showed are done at ionic strength of 0.15. So they are similar to physiological ionic strength.

Dr. Lett   Yes. Have you done it with isolated nucleo-proteins?

Dr. Lindahl   We have not done that, because it would be experimentally very difficult, in order to follow the depurination and measure it. You either have to heat it and go up to the high temperatures and go down in pH, and under both of these conditions see how it would affect the structure of nucleo-proteins.

Dr. Dalrymple   Given that the mammalian cell DNA can repair as easily as has been described, what do you feel is the biological importance of the depurination process? As it would happen in the mammalian cell.

Dr. Lindahl

I think this spontaneous type of damage that is of no obvious use to the organism, it has to cope with it somehow.

Dr. Brian Fox
(Manchester)

We have been interested in the sublethal level of radiation damage in mammalian cells. We've been working at levels around two and three hundred r. But I agree entirely with Dr. Lett's findings because I think Dr. Lett has changed his views about the high molecular weight in control materials. The control values which we had at the time, of course, have very high molecular weights, as he observed, and under certain circumstances we found that the control sedimented at 165 S or roughly in this region. We were unable to salt these two out, and we regarded the control features being of the order 150, 160 S. But since that time we have found all these other subunits at the bottom and we also concur with him that the 200 r radiation does produce an immediate drop of this 165 S, at the earliest time at which you can look after 200 r. We've been using the linear pulse accelerator, which can give the whole distortion in microseconds, and look at short time intervals, the shortest time interval we can look at, we find this 165 SP. But we find that on pulse incubation this goes through the series of molecular weights and by one hour it is almost completely at the base of the centrifuge tube, the high molecular weight region. Now at the same time, my wife and Dr. Myaze were engaged in work with the density labelling techniques also at these low levels with P38X. And the reference in which Dr. Painter, in fact, referred to in which we were able to show repair synthesis was in fact this first slide, which was taken now for granted, in which there is a light like peak in which there is a distinct repair synthesis. In other words, radioactivity due to IUdR following this similar sort of protocol to Dr. Painter's. We used IUdR instead of BUdR primarily because I have done some work with this material, and of course it is more dense. The survival of the BUdR doses is very similar to IUdR, and for all intents and purposes the use of IUdR parallels that of BUdR. As you see in the upper curve is cesium chloride density gradients of heavy IUdR treated cells, followed by IUdR in the presence of tritiated thymidine. The idea here is to use tritiated thymidine, I think this will be referred to later this afternoon, where you can introduce tritiated thymidine in that portion of the DNA, which is in fact in IUdR. You get exactly the same results as you would if you used tritiated IUdR. The top part is the control, the bottom is 250 r. As you see there's a marked amount of radioactivity in a light like peak. If you denature this, it appears with a light peak. Now clearly, there's a big difference between Dr. Painter's experiments and ours. I am sure that the facts in both cases are absolutely correct, so I can only assume that there must be something very different in the protocol. They haven't done what the Americans call, I think, a cookbook experiment, but we intend to do this. There are many differences. One is that the medium used is Fisher's medium, and it contains ten times the amount of folate that the medium that Dr. Painter uses. And also, that he uses other materials like FUdR and HU, which we do not. And there are also differences in isolation of the DNA. But I feel that we may have a form of incorporation of BUdR following x-rays which may be related to either very small mutants which for some reason are lost in the experiment which Dr. Painter has described.

Dr. Painter   I hadn't intended to bring this up but it's been brought up once and it will have to be. Fox and Fox have published two papers showing these kinds of data. The very interesting observation that at low doses, as low as 150 r, there is what I would call a massive amount of repair replication occurring in the cells. And as I said in my presentation I can't see this in any of the cells that I look at, until somewhere over a thousand r. That also includes this cell P388F. However, if one tries to do some quantitation on this system it gets a little hard to handle. The semiconservative replication which has gone on in this cell line, even in the control in the presence of the IUdR, is relatively low. This is the optical density trace here, and it comes up and only this far. Now these cells have been incubated with IUdR, a total of six hours. In our experiments in which we used BUdR, as Dr. Fox pointed out, but which should not make any great difference. I believe that the Foxes have actually done this experiment with BUdR as well. We get a peak of optical density which is almost as high as this one, not quite, in this six-hour incubation, indicating that our cells under the conditions that we use are growing much better. Now, considering this optical density peak and trying to figure out how much semiconservative replication did occur, you can come up with a figure which I think would probably be in order of about 10% of the genome might have been replicated at this time. Perhaps less, but certainly more than one percent. If you take the radioactivity measurements and compare the amount of radioactivity that's been incorporated by semiconservative replication in the control (or in the irradiated, since they are not different in this case) with the amount of radioactivity that has been incorporated by the nonsemiconservative mode in the parental DNA, and do some calculations with these data, it turns out that there would have to be about 10,000 tritium labelled IUdR molecules incorporated into each damaged site (using about 30 EV per damaged site in DNA) in the parental DNA. But if 10,000 IUdR molecules are incorporated into one site, they will form heavy DNA, and therefore that DNA should appear at intermediate density or probably at the same position as DNA made by semiconservative replication. So this finding of tritiated IUdR here is extremely difficult to understand, and that's the problem that we're having. Trying to figure out what is the meaning of incorporation into parental DNA when any kind of calculation, knowing the amount of damage that occurred, would indicate that this could not possibly be found. There is a possibility, I think, that there are two treatments, which in this case are IUdR at rather high concentrations and the insult by high radiation, which may cause a general metabolic breakdown, and so that you're having addition at every place in the molecule. You might have that, but at the damaged site only. You cannot explain these data; therefore, it remains very difficult (for me, at least) to interpret. Dr. Fox has also indicated that the extra DNA synthesis that goes on, after ionizing radiation, when looked at autoradiographically, shows no unscheduled DNA synthesis, which means that they don't see labelling of cells in the G-1 and G-2 period. But they do get an increase in S phase labelling, an increase in rate of synthesis. But that material is very strange, because it's extractable by cold perchloric acid, which means it can't be over 100 nucleotides long. That means this cannot be this material in the gradient because this material bands so sharply, you have to have a molecular weight in the order of few million to get that kind of banding, meaning the material they see autoradiographically as an increase, cannot be this material. I think a lot of problems remain at the present time as to what this phenomenon really is.

Dr. Bibek Ray (Raleigh)

My question is for Dr. Dalrymple. Treating freeze-dried urine salmonella we observed that repair can be inhibited by metabolic inhibitors, such as dinitrophenol. However, this repair is pH-dependent. At pH 6, we observed 100% inhibition. At pH 7, the quality was similarly pH-dependent in the dinitrophenol inhibition colony region on amino acid assimulation in bacteria. You will observe the repair of the sublethal injury offered in spite of the presence of dinitrophenol. This might be due to the effect of the pH we used. Thus at pH 6, 100% injury is repaired, while at pH 7, only 40% replication occurred.

Dr. Dalrymple

This is in bacteria. In all studies with dinitrophenal, one must be very careful to prevent conditions which interfere with its action, such as serum and other components of culture medium. Consequently, we do an ATP assay with all DNP preparations. If the ATP level has not been depressed to less than 10% of control, we will terminate the experiment at that point. As far as the pH is concerned, cultured mammalian cells have a difficult time maintaining very large shifts in pH. We have the pH of our medium adjusted to approximately 6.9. When we use Hanks Balanced Salts solution (with or without DNP) the pH is adjusted to 6.9.

Dr. Peter A. Cerutti (Gainesville)

After about two years we have found that among the major lesions which originated in the monomer, as well as in the model system poly dAT, and under in vivo conditions, in Micrococcus radiodurans, are five hydroperoxy- to six hydro-dihydrothiamine derivatives. There seems to be an awful lot of this formed when compared to the strand breakage. Also a second product which is formed under in vivo conditions seems to be a five hydroxymethyl thymine, and we have developed an assay with which we are now measuring certain repair spots, damage directly under in vivo conditions. So again I would like to make the plea that one should look at all these nucleotides and so some chemistry, as has been done in photochemistry of nucleic acids, just to get this really on a molecular level in order to talk about repair.

Dr. Dalrymple   You said you were measuring repair in some form, some system.

Dr. Cerutti   Yes, we have been doing studies on Micrococcus radiodurans with an assay, in a way you measure these products after release from the DNA, with an assay that you can compare to the thymine dimer assay. It is an assay in which the only difference is that here you measure a specific X-ray damage at the base, relative to photochemicals. The most important point is my plea to do some decent chemistry on these compounds.

Dr. Neal Brown   It's beginning to bother me a little bit the use of the word re-
(College Park)   pair replication. I would like to clarify what it means to me. And this would be replication concerning several nucleotides, in repairing the gap. Simply by showing that you are getting heavy labelling incorporated into parental density, and light densities in DNA samples, it is possible that this could happen by two different mechanisms, one by a random base insertion, this was originally meant for Dr. Strauss, if this has characterized his product, by phase on occasion. It's very dependent on the size of the molecules you're putting on the cesium chloride gradients. And so repair replication, is it repair replication, or is it merely random base insertion throughout the molecule? I think in getting at Dr. Painter's discussion of this, one must ascertain whether or not these are nucleotides clusters and what percentage in short strands they make up, or are they indeed randomly put through? Have any of you looked at your products of so-called repair replication to see whether these are in short strands? Dr. Strauss perhaps has done this.

Dr. Lett   The main difficulty in radiation chemistry is sensitivity. Most of the effects of X-rays result from direct action and, as Dr. Painter pointed out, there is no way at present to determine whether the DNA damage caused by OH radicals et cetera in solution is representative of that occurring in the cell. The DNA in the cell is protected against free radicals by proteins. Measurements of direct damage require very high experimental sensitivities. One break can be measured accurately, for example, in a subunit of 5×10^8 daltons, which is composed of approximately two million nucleotides. Although we have a sensitivity here of one in two million, we are still a factor of a hundred, at least, below the level at which we want to work. Similar sensitivities, say to one part in two hundred million, would also be necessary ultimately for biochemical or chemical assays.

Dr. Herriott   I sense that we're not going to get consensus on this, but Dr. Lindahl, you have one comment and then we must close.

Dr. Lindahl   This is a comment for Dr. Lett. The sedimentation of DNA is concentration dependent, and this leads to sharpening of the boundary. This very obvious and old experiment using schlieren optics are heterodispersed DNA (sediments like a very sharp peak) and this becomes more and more of a problem at higher molecular weights. So the very high molecular weights you are using even heterodispersed DNA population will sediment as a monomeric-like peak. So I'd like to suggest that your subunits might actually represent a random introduction of a small number of hits.

Dr. Lett   When T2 bacteriophage is irradiated with increasing X-ray doses the DNA distribution goes from monodispersed to random. Mammalian DNA seems to parallel this exactly. That's all I can say until electron microscopy can be done, except that we sediment DNA at concentrations one thousand-fold below those necessary to perform schlieren optics.

Dr. Lindahl   Yes, but your mammalian system is one order of magnitude higher molecular weight than your T2 model system.

Dr. Strauss   In reply to Dr. Brown, all material is sheared before being put on the gradient, which should break off clusters or added bases at the end. On the other hand, I do not know how many bases are inserted at each lesion although I do know the lesions are necessary for the insertion. However, Dr. Painter does have real data on this point.

Dr. Painter   We have examined the product DNA caused by repair replication after a dose to HeLa cells of 100,000 R. We measured the rate of loss of its acid insoluble radioactivity after treatment with an exonuclease (snake venom phosphodiesterase) and compared this rate with 1) a DNA specifically labeled only at the ends with a terminal transferase and 2) a uniformly labeled DNA. The kinetics of loss of acid insoluble radioactivity were like the uniformly labeled DNA but not at all like the end-labeled DNA; the rate of loss of the latter was extremely high compared to the others. Thus the labelling of the "repaired" DNA was within fragements of DNA, not just at their ends. (This work was published in Proceedings of the M. D. Anderson Symposium for 1969, "Genetic Concepts and Neoplasia," Williams and Wilkins 1970, Baltimore, p. 593.) It is difficult to see how base insertion *within* a parental DNA molecule can occur by a process other than repair replication.

Part IV

CELLULAR REPAIR-PROCESSES II

EXCISION REPAIR: OUR CURRENT KNOWLEDGE BASED ON HUMAN (XERODERMA PIGMENTOSUM) AND CATTLE CELLS[1]

J. E. Cleaver

Laboratory of Radiobiology, University of California
San Francisco, California

Xeroderma pigmentosum (XP) is a human disease that is inherited as an autosomal mutation in which the major clinical symptoms are a high level of actinic skin cancer, namely, squamous carcinomas, sarcomas, melanomas (1,2). Cancer eye in Hereford cattle is an inherited disease that appears in inbred strains of cattle with varying frequencies up to almost 100% in the animals of a strain (3). The major characteristic is epithelial malignancy of sunlight-exposed skin around the eye and on the cornea (3). Therefore there is some superficial similarity in these two hereditary diseases; both show high levels of actinic skin cancer. We discovered xeroderma pigmentosum by chance; cancer eye was the result of a deliberate search for an animal analogue to the human disease. As the result of a number of years' work, we now know that XP cells are defective in the repair of ultraviolet (UV) radiation damage to DNA (4-12) whereas cells from cattle with cancer eye have no detectable defect in DNA repair (13). Both human cells and cattle cells have been useful in studying the nature of DNA repair, but at present it is only the work with XP cells that has produced evidence for the functional significance of one pathway for DNA repair. XP now appears to be the human analogue of the E. coli UVR⁻ HCR⁻ mutants (4,6,7,10-12).

DETECTION OF EXCISION REPAIR

Once I had made the hypothesis (4) that a UV-sensitive skin disease might be an analogue of UV-sensitive bacteria and have a defect in excision repair, the experiments that had to be done with cultured fibroblasts were self-evident. A model of the excision repair pathway in bacteria had been available for many years (Fig 1) (14-16) and the following experimental tests were made of the model:

(a) Are individual cells sensitive to UV light?
(b) How well do fibroblasts support the growth of UV-damaged viruses?
(c) Are thymine-containing dimers formed and removed from DNA?
(d) Are single-strand gaps made and joined during excision?
(e) Are short regions of new bases inserted into DNA to replace excised dimers?
(f) Are short regions of new bases inserted to repair single-strand breaks?

There is a danger, however, that in attempting to detect excision repair we allow the heuristic model to become a Procrustean bed into which we crop or stretch data that

---

[1] Under the auspices of the U.S. Atomic Energy Commission.

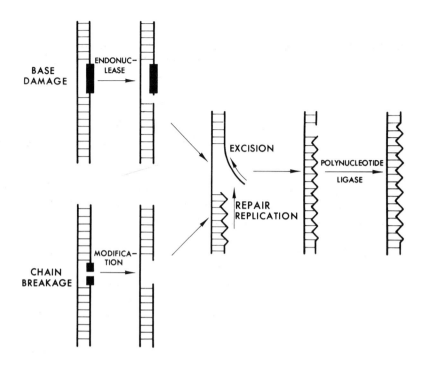

Fig 1. Heuristic scheme for the operational steps in excision repair of damaged bases (namely, pyrimidine dimers) and broken strands (namely, ionizing radiation damage) by a common pathway. Initial step for each kind of damage has some unique features but the excision, replication and ligase steps can be common.

do not truly fit. We want to see excision of dimers, strand breakage and repair replication, even when techniques are not adequate. We need to view published claims critically and determine whether the evidence really substantiates the claims because excision repair in mammalian cells might be subtly different from excision repair in bacteria. With this caution in mind, I believe that definite answers to all of these questions except (d) are now available. An answer to (d) is still in doubt because attempts to demonstrate single-strand breaks during excision have been equivocal and inconsistent due to the complications in techniques and extreme variability in published profiles (7,17).

SENSITIVITY OF XERODERMA PIGMENTOSUM
AND CATTLE CELLS

The manifestation of xeroderma pigmentosum and cancer eye is a high incidence of UV-induced skin cancers, but this could be due to a variety of systemic factors other than the inherent properties of individual cells (9). It is important to demonstrate that the genotype has some phenotypic expression in individual cells. The main method at our disposal is colony formation by single cells, but unfortunately primary fibroblasts have a low plating efficiency, a maximum of 10 to 20% (11,18,19). Use of this method presupposes

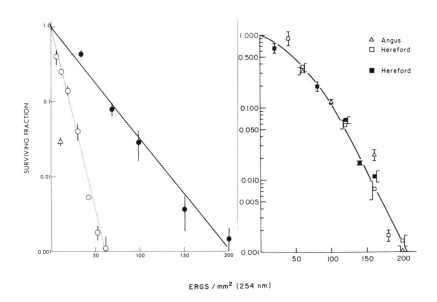

Fig 2. Left–Single cell survival curve for normal and XP fibroblasts irradiated with UV light at 14 ergs/mm^2 (mainly 254 nm). Plating efficiency of unirradiated cells was between 9 and 18%. Normal fibroblasts ●. XP6 ○, XP7 △. Bars denote 95% confidence limits and lines are drawn by regression analysis using all data points, except those for XP7. Normal cells n = 1.0, D_0 = 29 ergs/mm^2. XP6 n = 0.9, D_0 = 9 ergs/mm^2. (From the International Journal of Radiation Biology (11))
Right–Single cell survival curve, n = 11, D_0 = 23 ergs/mm^2, for high cancer Hereford and cancer-free Angus cattle. Plating efficiencies between 20 and 25%. Hereford, ▫, ■ (two different inbred strains), Angus △.

that the cells which form colonies are a random sample of the population and are typical of the whole population in terms of their UV sensitivity. Granted these presuppositions, XP fibroblasts are much more sensitive than normal cells, as shown in Figure 2 (11,19). The sensitivity of cattle cells, however, is independent of the incidence of cancer (Fig 2), and this disease is clearly not analogous to XP.

EXCISION OF PYRIMIDINE DIMERS FROM HUMAN CELLS

The number of dimers formed in the DNA of human cells increases linearly with UV dose if the cells are fixed immediately after irradiation (Fig 3). When cells are allowed to grow for a time after irradiation before fixation and measurement, normal cells excise some (50 to 75% at low doses) of the dimers from their DNA, whereas xeroderma pigmentosum cells apparently do not (Fig 3) (7,9,10,20). This assay, however, is not sufficiently precise to distinguish between a low and a completely negligible excision level. Other studies make it likely that low levels of excision occur in xeroderma pigmentosum cells (4,8,9,11,12).

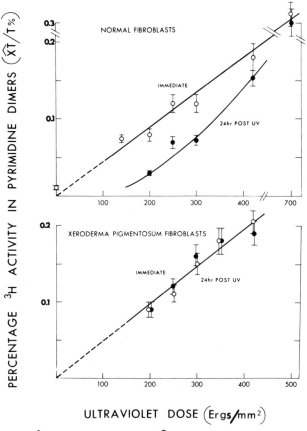

Fig 3. Percentage of ^{3}H in pyrimidine dimers ($\widehat{TT}$/T) as a function of UV (254 nm) dose. o, value immediately after irradiation; •, value 24 hours after irradiation. Top, normal fibroblasts; bottom, XP fibroblasts. Bars denote standard errors for 3 or more determinations or a standard deviation of 10% for a single determination. (From the Journal of Photochemistry and Photobiology (10))

Cattle fibroblasts similarly excise pyrimidine dimers from DNA and there is no difference in the excision from either strain (Fig 4). These results are quite different from those obtained with established cultures of other nonprimate mammalian cells (21-23). Established strains of mouse and Chinese hamster do not excise dimers from their DNA, at least in a form that is acid soluble and distinguishable from cellular DNA by the acid fixatives commonly employed in dimer assays (21-23). But cells of all species do perform excision repair, as determined by observation of the insertion of new bases into DNA (24-27). The excision step in some cells, therefore, may not produce acid soluble dimers even though the dimers may be excised from DNA. In view of the results from primary cultures of cattle, dimer excision should be looked for now in primary mouse and Chinese hamster cells to find out if the alterations that lead to the establishment of cell cultures affect the excision of dimers.

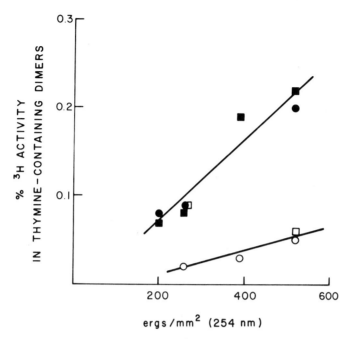

Fig 4. Percentage of ^{3}H in pyrimidine dimers ($\widehat{TT}$/T) as a function of UV (254 nm) dose. Values immediately after irradiation—o Hereford, □ Angus. Values 24 hours after irradiation—o Hereford, □ Angus.

STRAND BREAKAGE AND REUNION DURING EXCISION

The method used to study single-strand breaks in DNA of mammalian cells involves lysis of cells at high pH on the top of alkaline sucrose gradients and subsequent sedimentation to determine sedimentation rate and molecular weight distributions (28-31). Lysis of mammalian cells to release alkali-denatured single-stranded DNA is a complex process depending on the nature of the cells, the time, temperature, salt concentration, pH and the presence of chelating agents (EDTA) and detergent and other unspecified factors (28-31). In studying irradiated cells one must discriminate between the effects of radiation dose on the lysis rate and on the molecular weight of DNA strands. The interdependence of these two effects is unknown, but in general it seems that both ionizing radiation (31) and UV light (Fig 5) enhance the rate of cell lysis and the release of DNA. Lysis conditions that are too short for control cells result in DNA sedimenting rapidly as a gel (28), whereas the same conditions may release DNA completely from irradiated cells (Fig 5). Such conditions recently were used unwittingly to detect molecular weight changes in HeLa cells during excision (17). In primary human cells (normal and XP), however, the only data thus far published show profiles that are so variable[2] that they constitute no evidence at all for strand breakage and reunion (7).

[2]Quantitative analysis of the published alkaline sucrose gradients indicate that the irradiated profiles have a consistently smaller M_w than control profiles for *both* normal and XP cells. Thus, though the profiles give equivocal evidence for the repair defect in XP, the radiation effect observed may be related to the enhanced lysis rate discussed above (Cleaver, unpublished calculations).

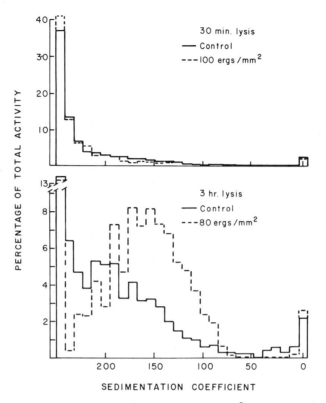

Fig 5. Influence of lysis time in 0.5 M NaOH, 0.1 M EDTA, 25°C on top of 5 to 20% alkaline sucrose gradient on sedimentation of DNA from control (———) and UV-irradiated (————) Hereford cattle cells.

To avoid the complications of radiation effects on lysis rates, my own studies in cattle cells have been done by lysing cells for extended periods of three to six hours before sedimentation. In unirradiated cells a reproducible profile of DNA then is obtained in which weight (M_w) and number (M_n) average molecular weights are almost the same, at approximately 5×10^8 daltons. In irradiated cells the molecular weights initially are smaller than in controls and M_w is greater than M_n, corresponding to the introduction of a small number (approximately 1 per 5×10^8) of random breaks (Fig 6). When cells are allowed to grow for various times after irradiation the molecular weights gradually return to control values (Fig 7). These results illustrate the breakage and reunion which occur during excision of dimers from cattle cell DNA. Since the initial number of breaks at 100 ergs/mm² is about 5×10^3 per cell whereas the number of dimers per cell is about 10^6, less than 1% of the dimers are associated with breaks at any one time.

The data on M_n changes after irradiation do not tell the whole story, however. After irradiation the gradient profiles show the formation of molecules which sediment at a molecular weight position which corresponds roughly to twice the control value (Fig 7). Although the nature of these molecules is unknown, some of their characteristics can be described (13). They consist exclusively of DNA present at the time of irradiation and

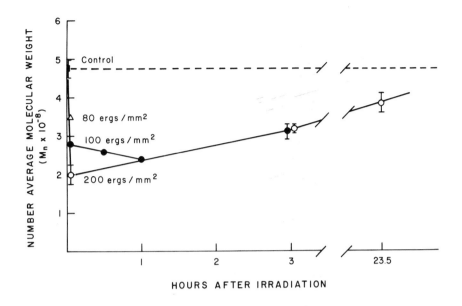

Fig 6. Changes in M_n (number average) as a function of time after irradiation of cattle fibroblasts with various UV doses. Initial drop in M_n represents introduction of approximately 0.3 breaks (80 ergs/mm^2), 1 break (100 ergs/mm^2), or 1.4 breaks (200 ergs/mm^2) per 4.75×10^8 daltons. These breaks presumably represent action of an endonuclease acting in vicinity of UV photoproducts.

make up about 20 to 30% of the DNA by 24 hours after irradiation; their formation requires time, is retarded by reduction in temperature, but is unaffected by hydroxyurea which inhibits semiconservative but not repair replication (32,33), and they are stable for up to 12 hours lysis in alkali. At first sight these larger molecules could be involved in recombinational processes, but since they consist exclusively of DNA present at the time of irradiation, this would exclude a simple application of a recombination model (34). The larger molecules, however, may be formed by errors in repair replication by which the irradiated molecules are abnormally linked together. Since these alkaline gradients reveal a control DNA molecular weight of about 5×10^8 as a reproducible size (24,31), this might be the size of DNA subunits which are linked by alkali labile regions. Errors in excision repair may modify these links to make them alkali stable.

INSERTION OF NEW BASES INTO DNA: REPAIR REPLICATION

Replacement of excised dimer-containing regions requires synthesis of small amounts of DNA in short regions, that is, repair replication (4-6,8,9,11,12,16,24-27,32, 33). This has to be detected in the presence of the relatively large amounts of semiconservative DNA replication that occurs during the cell cycle.

A method to detect repair replication was devised by Pettijohn and Hanawalt (16). This takes advantage of the difference between the short pieces synthesized during

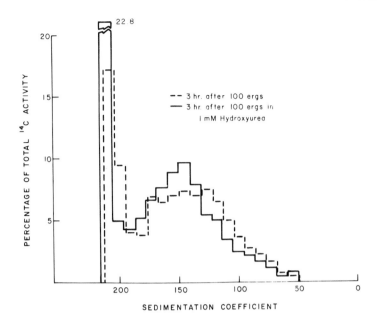

Fig 7. Radioactivity profiles for ^{14}CTdR-labeled cattle fibroblasts irradiated with 100 ergs/mm^2 UV, grown for 3 hours in nonradioactive medium with or without 2mM hydroxyurea, before lysis for 5 hours in 0.5 M NaOH, 0.1M EDTA and sedimentation in alkaline sucrose gradients.

repair and the long strands synthesized by semiconservative replication. Tritiated bromodeoxyuridine (^{3}HBrUdR, molecular weight 308) is used as a heavy analogue of ^{3}HTdR (molecular weight 242) and is incorporated into DNA in its place. The long chains formed by semiconservative replication are denser than normal and ^{3}H-labeled. The pieces synthesized by repair replication are such small patches in long molecules that the density of the molecules is unchanged, but they too will be ^{3}H-labeled. Thus, the presence of ^{3}H-labeled molecules of normal density is an indication that repair replication has occurred. DNA can be fractionated on the basis of its density by means of centrifugation through cesium chloride gradients (Figs 8-10). In these experiments we routinely use hydroxyurea to suppress semiconservative replication preferentially, with no quantitative effect on repair replication (24,32,33). This improves resolution to the extent that only a single isopycnic centrifugation is required to give quantitative measurements of repair replication that are precise (± 20%) at low UV doses (Figs 9, 10) (11,24) and in XP cells that still retain a low capacity for repair replication (Table I). Unscheduled synthesis, the autoradiographic equivalent of repair replication (27), is a similarly precise assay method and this has been used to demonstrate a correlation between the severity of clinical symptoms in XP and the reduction in excision repair (8). Recently, several XP patients have been discovered in which repair replication seems to be normal, though the clinical symptoms are unambiguous (XP13, 14, Table I). The status of these patients in the general picture now developed for the biochemical basis of XP is enigmatic.

An estimate of the average size of the patch made during excision repair can be made from the kinetics of repair replication (Fig 10) and of dimer excision (Fig 4). At

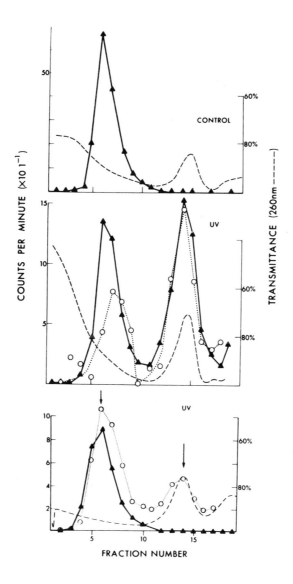

Fig 8. Equilibrium density gradients from normal and xeroderma pigmentosum cells irradiated with 200 ergs/mm^2 ultraviolet light and labeled for 4 hours with ^{3}HBrUdR. Arrows mark positions of normal density (1.698 gm/cc) and bromouracil substituted density (1.751 gm/cc). Dashed line indicates the total amount of DNA in the gradients (high values in the first few fractions are an artefact). Top, unirradiated normal cells. Center, normal (▲) and heterozygous xeroderma pigmentosum (○) fibroblasts irradiated with 200 ergs/mm^2. Note the large peak of radioactivity at a density of 1.698 gm/cc which indicates repair replication. Bottom, two different fibroblast cultures, from unrelated homozygous xeroderma pigmentosum patients, irradiated with 200 ergs/mm^2 UV. Note the low repair replication peak at 1.698 gm/cc in one case (○) and the absence of the other case (▲). (From the International Journal of Radiation Biology (11))

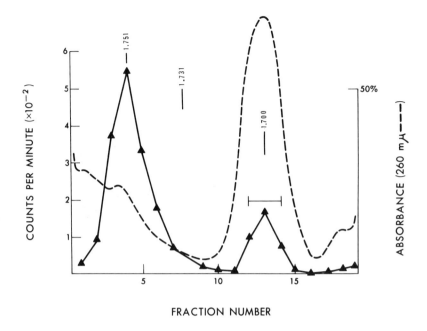

Fig 9. CsCl isopycnic gradient of Chinese hamster V79 cells grown in BrUdR (5 μg/ml) plus 10^{-6}M FUdR for 1 hour, irradiated with 35 ergs/mm^2 UV (254 nm) and labeled for 4 hours with ^{3}HBrUdR (20 μCi/ml, 5 μg/ml) plus 10^{-6}M FUdR and 4 x 10^{-4}M hydroxyurea. Bar denotes peak of ^{3}H labeled normal density DNA labeled by repair replication. (From the Journal of Photochemistry and Photo-biology (24))

100 ergs/mm^2 the proportion of thymine radioactivity in dimers is 0.04% and most of this is excised in 24 hours; a large proportion of the repair replication occurs in the first four hours and the total amount over a 24 hour period represents only about twice that in the first four hours and the BrU molecules incorporated are about 0.32% of the bases in DNA. Thus, for each dimer excised on the average of about 25 BrU bases are inserted, or about 80 bases altogether. This estimate agrees well with previous estimates of 200 bases or less in HeLa cells (12) and 14 to 25 BrU bases in primary human fibroblasts (39).

Damage from ionizing radiations (6,35) and chemical mutagens (36) is repaired to normal extents by XP fibroblasts. These agents appear to cause nonenzymatic break-age of the DNA strands (37,38) and repair of the breaks presumably bypasses the initial enzymatic steps required for repair of UV damage (pyrimidine dimers) (Fig 1).

In different cell types there is no simple correlation between amounts of repair replication and their UV sensitivity (Table II). This does not indicate that excision repair has no relevance to cell survival. Rather, there must be many factors contributing to sur-vival, of which excision repair is one. Only when all other factors are similar, as in XP and normal cells, will differences in excision repair show a simple correlation with sur-vival.

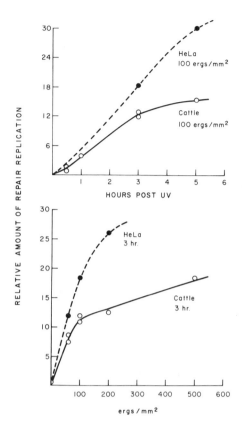

Fig 10. Relative amounts of repair replication in cattle (Hereford) and HeLa cells as a function of UV dose and time after irradiation. Repair replication amounts based on specific activities of repaired DNA isolated from isopycnic gradients (Figs. 8, 9).

Repair replication levels are not, however, direct measurements of activity of repair enzymes. Until we have some direct measurements similar to those available for the UV specific endonuclease of M. luteus (34-36), these observations are only suggestive of differences amongst XP patients and cells of various species.

PRENATAL DIAGNOSIS OF XERODERMA PIGMENTOSUM

As with any hereditary disease that can be diagnosed biochemically or cytologically, the possibility of a fetal XP genotype can be assessed by testing amniocentetic cells. Amniocentetic cells from normal pregnancies have the same repair replication levels as do normal adult skin and HeLa cells (11,12) and either of the latter can also serve as valid controls in a prenatal test. All of the methods described for study of excision repair could be used for XP prenatal diagnosis within the available time, though not all have equal precision. Probably the least reliable methods would involve colony survival (11,19), dimer excision (7,10) and alkaline sucrose gradients (7). Repair replication in isopycnic

TABLE I

Relative Levels of Excision Repair (Measured during 4 hours after 220 ergs/mm^2
UV light, 254 nm).* (11,12)

			Percent
Normal skin fibroblasts			100
Normal skin fibroblasts (SV40 transformed)			121
Fibroblasts (amniocentetic, 3 pregnancies)			103, 72, 99
HeLa (cervical carcinoma)			94
Xeroderma pigmentosum			
Heterozygote	♀	HPH1	67, 84, 87
	♀	XPHK §	100
	♂	XPH11M	44, 48
	♀	XPH11F	47, 42
Homozygote		XPJ	6
		XP6	5.1, 5.3
		XP7	5
		XP10	75
		XP11	< 4
(SV40 transformed)		XP7	< 16
		XP13†	100
		XP14†	100
Homozygote		XP1 §†	9
		XP2 §†	25
		XP1W §	0
		XPKM §†	0
		XPKF §†	0

*Standard deviation is 20 percent of quoted value. Upper limit cited when no distinct normal density
^{3}H peak was detectable in the isopycnic gradient. Diagnosis of XP10 was uncertain because of few
malignancies.
§deSanctis Cacchione syndrome. XP1,2 diagnosed by E. Klein, Roswell Park Institute. XP1W, KM,
KF diagnosed by W. B. Reed, UCLA. This form of XP has mental abnormalities in addition to skin
symptoms.
†Siblings.

gradients (4,9,11,12), unscheduled synthesis in autoradiographs (4,6,8,9,11,12) and
photolysis of BrU-containing repaired regions (39,40) are all suitable methods.

At present there is a pregnancy in a family with one XP child, which is under
test in The Johns Hopkins Department of Pediatrics. The amniocentetic cells from this
pregnancy will be tested simultaneously at both Oak Ridge National Laboratory and our
laboratory with different methods to obtain the fullest information on the fetus. Trial

TABLE II

Relative Levels of UV Sensitivity and Repair Replication in Mammalian Cells

Cells	D_o*	N*	Repair replication level† (Relative to human) Percent
Primary human (skin)	22-29	1-4	100
WI-38	24	1.3	100
Amniocentetic	23	4.0	100
HeLa	108	2.0	100
Xeroderma, XP6	9	1.0	5
Xeroderma, XP1,2	2	1.0	9-25
Primary mouse (fetal)	–	–	100
L cells (wild)	70-80	4-5	60 (34 to 38.5°C)
L cells (temperature-sensitive mutants)	–	–	65 (permissive 34°C) 23 (restrictive 38.5°C)
Chinese hamster V79	43-50	4-5, 1-6	100
B14FAF	60	3	10-20
Primary cattle (skin)	23	11	60

*Survival parameters (from references 11,19,47,48)
†Measured near to plateau of repair replication–3 to 4 hours after dose of 200 to 250 ergs/mm^2 (Fig 11). Standard deviation 20% of cited relative level.

experiments on cells from both parents and the XP daughter (XP11M, F and XP11, Table I) (11,12) gave us complete repair replication and unscheduled synthesis results in 10 days from receipt of the cells, which is adequate speed, consistent with accuracy for prenatal diagnosis. Of particular interest in this family, a normal, heterozygote or homozygote fetus could be identified by repair replication measurements (Table I) (Fig 11). In both parental heterozygotes repair replication levels are normal at low doses (below 100 ergs/mm^2) but reach a plateau at about half the level of control cells at higher doses. There are, however, known instances of XP homozygotes with repair replication levels as high as the heterozygotes described above (8) (Table I). At present, repair replication or unscheduled synthesis measurements would resolve accurately the genotype of a fetus in this family under study, only if a wide range of doses were used.

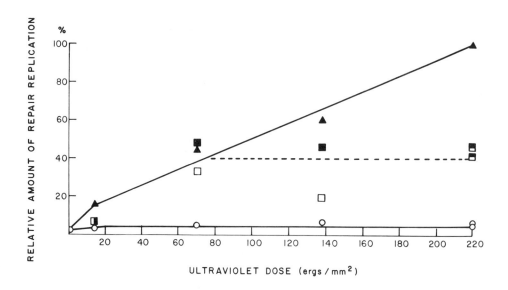

Fig 11. Relative repair levels in normal, heterozygous and homozygous XP fibroblasts. Normal ▲, heterozygous XP □ (mother), ■ (father), homozygous XP6 ○ (daughter). Levels based on specific activities in isopycnic gradients (Figs 8, 9 and Table I).

CHARACTERISTICS OF XERODERMA PIGMENTOSUM AND SITE OF ENZYMATIC DEFECT

We now can make a fairly comprehensive list of the functional and biochemical characteristics of xeroderma pigmentosum.

(a) XP is caused by an autosomal recessive mutation, but the karyotype is normal (1,2).

(b) Homozygotes are UV-sensitive and show enhanced pigmentation and actinic carcinogenesis (1). Some patients also show characteristic mental retardation, skeletal defects and gonadal and glandular disfunction (the de Sanctis Cacchione syndrome). Death often results from metastasis early in life.

(c) XP cells in vitro are sensitive to killing by UV light (11,19) and have reduced ability to support the reproduction of UV-inactivated viruses (41,42).

(d) XP cells fail to excise UV photoproducts (pyrimidine dimers) from their DNA in contrast to normal cells (7,10).

(e) XP cells insert fewer bases into DNA during repair of UV damage than do normal cells (4-6,8,9,11,12).

(f) XP cells repair damage from ionizing radiation (6,35), monofunctional alkylating agents (36) and bromouracil photosensitization (6) to normal extents.

From the above evidence, it is reasonable to assume that an enzyme involved in excision is affected in XP cells. The enzymes involved in repair have only been isolated from some bacteria, notably M. luteus (L. Grossman (43-45)). In this organism three

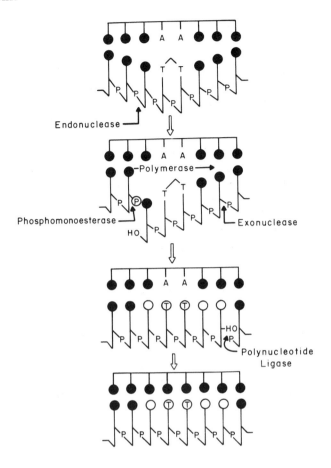

Fig 12. Scheme for the biochemical steps in repair of pyrimidine dimers in DNA (redrawn from Grossman et al (45)).

enzymes are involved in excision of dimers (Fig 12): 1) an endonuclease which cleaves the chain near a dimer to leave 3′phosphoryl and 5′hydroxyl termini, the latter adjacent to the dimer, 2) a 3′phosphomonoesterase to remove the terminal phosphate, 3) an exonuclease to degrade the dimer-containing sequence. At least two more enzymes are required for completion of repair—a polymerase to lay down a new strand to replace the excised region, and a ligase to make the final link to complete the repair patch. In E. coli the exonuclease and polymerase functions seem to be on a single enzyme (46).

A similar sequence seems to occur in human cells and the enzyme affected in XP is probably the endonuclease (6,7,9). At the present time, however, there is no direct evidence based on enzyme isolation studies for the nature of the defective enzyme, and the few patients with normal repair replication raise the possibility of other biochemical defects which may not necessarily be involved in DNA repair.

CONCLUSIONS—EXCISION REPAIR IN MAMMALIAN CELLS

It appears that mammalian cells, human and cattle in particular, have a repair pathway similar to excision repair in bacteria. In some established cell lines the excision step has yet to be detected and the role of pyrimidine dimers is still a mystery, though much evidence suggests that excision in some form occurs. In XP cells the defect in excision repair is similar to that in UVR⁻HCR⁻ bacterial mutants (4-12) and the discovery of the basis of this disease has been invaluable in proving the existence and importance of excision repair in higher organisms. Similar mutations in animals, if they became available, would be invaluable in studying all aspects of excision repair and its relationship to radiation carcinogenesis. Little work has been done on the isolation of any enzymes associated with excision repair in mammalian cells and this may be the next step to anticipate. We hope that such studies will be as instructive as those of the research groups of Grossman on M. luteus (43-45) and Kornberg on E. coli (46). Whether the human DNA polymerase will prove as versatile as its bacterial counterpart remains to be seen.

ACKNOWLEDGMENTS

Three groups of people deserve acknowledgment for their invaluable assistance to my own part in this work. First and foremost, the XP patients and their parents who have cooperated with little hope of immediate benefit; second, the many dermatologists who have aided me in my trespass into their field; and third, the research staff and assistants of the Laboratory of Radiobiology, whose contributions in ideas and hard work have been invaluable. Among the latter, Mr. G. H. Thomas deserves special mention for performing the major portion of our own technical work.

REFERENCES

1. Wilkinson, D. S., Rook, A. and Ebling, F. J.: Textbook of Dermatology, Vol 1, Blackwell, Oxford and Edinburgh, p 62, 1968.
2. El-Hefnawi, H., Smith, S. M. and Penrose, L. S.: Ann. Hum. Genet., 28:273, 1965.
3. Kainer, R. and Cleaver, J. E.: Amer. J. Vet. Res, in preparation.
4. Cleaver, J. E.: Nature, 218:652, 1968.
5. Reed, W. B., Landing, B., Sugarman, G., Cleaver, J. E. and Melnyk, J.: J.A.M.A., 207:2073, 1969.
6. Cleaver, J. E.: Proc. Nat. Acad. Sci. USA, 63:428, 1969.
7. Setlow, R. B., Regan, J. D., German, J. and Carrier, W. L.: Proc. Nat. Acad. Sci. USA, 64:1035, 1969.
8. Bootsma, D., Mulder, M. P., Pot, F. and Cohen, J. A.: Mutat. Res., 9:507, 1970.
9. Cleaver, J. E.: J. Invest. Derm., 54:8, 1970.
10. Cleaver, J. E. and Trosko, J. E.: Photochem. Photobiol., 11:547, 1970.
11. Cleaver, J. E.: Int. J. Radiat. Biol., 18:557, 1970.
12. Cleaver, J. E.: In: Nucleic Acid-Protein Interactions—Nucleic Acid Synthesis in Viral Infection. Edited by D. W. Ribbons, J. F. Woessner and J. Schultz. North Holland, Amsterdam, 1971.
13. Cleaver, J. E., Lett, J. T., Thomas, G. H. and Trosko, J. E.: Exp. Cell Res., in press, 1972.
14. Setlow, R. B. and Carrier, W. L.: Proc. Nat. Acad. Sci. USA, 51:226, 1964.
15. Boyce, R. P. and Howard-Flanders, P.: Proc. Nat. Acad. Sci. USA, 51:293, 1964.
16. Pettijohn, D. and Hanawalt, P. C.: J. Molec. Biol., 9:395, 1964.
17. Ben-Hur, E. and Ben-Ishai, R.: Photochem. Photobiol, 13:337, 1971.
18. Goldstein, S., Littlefield, J. W. and Soeldner, J. S.: Proc. Nat. Acad. Sci. USA, 64:155, 1969.

19. Goldstein, S.: Proc. Soc. Exp. Biol. Med., 137:730, 1971.
20. Regan, J. D., Trosko, J. E. and Carrier, W. L.: Biophys. J., 8:319, 1968.
21. Trosko, J. E., Chu, E. H. Y. and Carrier, W. L.: Radiat. Res., 24:667, 1965.
22. Klimek, M.: Photochem. Photobiol., 5:603, 1966.
23. Horikawa, M., Nikaido, O. and Sugahara, T.: Nature, 218:489, 1968.
24. Cleaver, J. E.: Photochem. Photobiol., 12:17, 1970.
25. Rasmussen, R. E. and Painter, R. B.: Nature, 203:1360, 1964.
26. Rasmussen, R. E. and Painter, R. B.: J. Cell Biol., 29:11, 1966.
27. Painter, R. B. and Cleaver, J. E.: Radiat. Res., 37:451, 1969.
28. Lett, J. T., Caldwell, I., Dean, C. J. and Alexander, P.: Nature, 214:790, 1967.
29. Lett, J. T., Klucis, E. S. and Sun, C.: Biophys. J., 10:277, 1970.
30. Lett, J. T. and Sun, C.: Radiat. Res., 44:771, 1970.
31. Elkind, M. M. and Kamper, C.: Biophys. J., 10:237, 1970.
32. Djordjevic, B. and Tolmach, L. J.: Radiat. Res., 32:327, 1967.
33. Cleaver, J. E.: Radiat. Res., 37:334, 1969.
34. Rupp, W. D. and Howard-Flanders, P.: J. Molec. Biol., 31:291, 1967.
35. Kleijer, W. J., Lohman, P. H. M., Mulder, M. P. and Bootsma, D.: Mutat. Res., 9:517, 1970.
36. Cleaver, J. E.: Mutat. Res., 12:453, 1971.
37. Dean, C. J., Ormerod, M. G., Serianni, R. W. and Alexander, P.: Nature, 222:1042, 1969.
38. Strauss, B. B. and Hill, T.: Biochim. Biophys. Acta, 213:14, 1970.
39. Regan, J. D., Setlow, R. B. and Ley, R. D.: Proc. Natl. Acad. Sci. USA, 68:708, 1971.
40. Setlow, R. B. and Regan, J. D.: Proc. 15th Ann. Mtg. Biophys. Soc., 1971.
41. Rabson, A. S., Tyrell, S. A. and Legallais, F. Y.: Proc. Soc. Exp. Biol. Med., 132:802, 1969.
42. Aaronson, S. A. and Lytle, C. D.: Nature, 228:359, 1970.
43. Kaplan, J. C., Kushner, S. R. and Grossman, L.: Proc. Natl. Acad. Sci. USA, 63:144, 1969.
44. Grossman, L.: Proc. IVth Int. Congress Radiation Research, Evian, France, in press, 1970.
45. Grossman, L., Kaplan, J., Kushner, S. and Mahler, I.: Ann. Ist Super. Sanita, 5:318, 1969.
46. Kelley, R. B., Atkinson, R. B., Huberman, J. A. and Kornberg, A.: Nature, 224:495, 1969.
47. Painter, R. B.: Photophysiology, 5:169, 1970.
48. Cleaver, J. E.: Int. J. Rad. Biol., 16:277, 1969.

RECOMBINATIONAL REPAIR IN UV-IRRADIATED ESCHERICHIA COLI[1]

Paul Howard-Flanders and W. Dean Rupp

Department of Radiology
Department of Molecular Biophysics and Biochemistry
Yale University, New Haven, Connecticut

The existence of a repair process associated with genetic recombination was suspected following the isolation of recombination-deficient mutants of E. coli. It was noted that these mutants are sensitive to ultraviolet light (UV) (2) and that their sensitivity is not due to any failure in the excision-repair system, since it is expressed even in excision-defective mutants. Indeed, double mutants carrying mutations affecting both excision and recombination are so highly UV sensitive that they are frequently killed by the induction of a single pyrimidine dimer in the DNA of their genome (6).

Recombinational repair may be defined as the mechanism by which wild type cells are more resistant to radiation than recombination-deficient mutants. This repair process appears to act after DNA replication in cells exposed to UV and is therefore sometimes called postreplication repair. However, since mechanisms for survival after other radiations may act before as well as after DNA replication, the term recombinational repair may be preferable.

The experiments to be described were carried out in collaboration with V. N. Iyer and R. S. Cole. They will be concerned firstly, with the replication of DNA containing damaged bases and the properties of the newly synthesized DNA; secondly, with the changes that take place after UV-irradiation in the bacterial DNA, as judged by the availability of templates for DNA synthesis; thirdly, with evidence for exchanges between sister duplexes in UV-irradiated cells and studies on the molecular weight of the exchanged segments; and fourthly and finally, the possible mechanisms and structures involved.

MOLECULAR WEIGHT OF DNA SYNTHESIZED AFTER UV-IRRADIATION

In studies on DNA metabolism in UV-irradiated cells, it has been found that DNA synthesis is slowed and that the newly synthesized strands are of lower than normal molecular weight. At UV doses ranging between 15 and 100 ergs/mm^2, the measurements indicate that the molecular weight is inversely proportional to the UV dose. Several examples of molecular weight values determined by sedimentation in alkaline sucrose gradients, are shown in Table I. Whereas the number-average molecular weight of DNA from controls is usually over 100 million, exposure to a UV dose of 90 ergs/mm^2, reduced the molecular weight of the newly synthesized DNA to about 5 million. This is to be compared with the mean molecular weight between dimers of 6 million, as calculated from

[1] Supported by United States Public Health Service Grant CA-06519, GM-11014 and AMK-69397.

TABLE I

Molecular Weight of DNA Synthesized after UV-Irradiation

	UV dose 254 nm	Newly Synthesized DNA from UV'd cells MW_n x 10^{-6}	Calculated MW_n between dimers x 10^{-6}
E. coli*	15	25	36
	30	17	18
	60	8.6	9
	90	4.7	6
Mouse**	110	12	9.5
lymphoma	220	5.6	5.6

*From Figure 3 and from Howard-Flanders, P. et al (8).
**Lehmann, A. R. (11).

published values for the yield and adjusted to allow for dimer containing cytosine as well as thymine (14).

Experiments of this type have also been carried out on mammalian cells in tissue culture. In spite of the technical difficulties associated with applying sedimentation methods to mammalian systems, several studies have indicated that the same relationship may also hold (3,9,11,16). Thus, in both prokaryotic and eukaryotic cells, the molecular weight of newly synthesized DNA chains is apparently limited to the molecular weight of the intact template between photoproducts.

The simplest interpretation of these results is that only the undamaged portions of the DNA between photoproducts is replicated. Each newly synthesized chain is terminated at a dimer in the template strand, and a new chain is initiated at some point beyond.

Experiments on excision-defective mutants have the advantage that the dimers remain in position and the template strands are not cut during dimer excision. These conditions favor accurate molecular weight determination. However, similar results are obtained in wild type cells provided measurements are made before a significant fraction of dimers has been excised (17). Photoreactivation by visible light also has been shown to reduce the numbers of dimers that remain in the template and so affect synthesis (17). Thus, the removal of photoproducts from the bacterial DNA can be observed by investigating the changes in the molecular weight of the DNA synthesized.

ARE THE GAPS BETWEEN NEWLY SYNTHESIZED STRANDS OPPOSITE DIMERS?

The gaps between the ends of the newly synthesized chains appear to be opposite dimers in DNA strands transferred between mating bacteria. This conclusion is based upon the need in excision-repair for an intact complementary strand (19). Bacterial or F factor DNA transferred from UV-irradiated donors during mating is not subject to repair by excision in the recipient; the genetic activity of the transferred DNA being identical in normal and excision-defective recipients. However, continuity along the transferred DNA must be maintained, as exposure of the recipient to visible light results in photoreactivation. These results indicate that the pyrimidine dimers remain in single-stranded regions after transfer, and that excision enzymes do not cut single strands containing dimers (4,7).

WIDTH OF THE GAP BETWEEN STRANDS OPPOSITE DIMERS

To investigate the width of the gaps between the DNA chains synthesized in UV-irradiated cells, Iyer and Rupp (10) have taken advantage of the preferential binding of single-stranded over native DNA to benzylated naphthoylated DEAE cellulose columns. After allowing DNA solutions to absorb to these columns, native DNA is eluted by 1 M salt, while denatured DNA remains bound and requires the addition of caffeine for elution. The columns were calibrated with phage DNA rendered partially single-stranded by digestion to the extent of from 1 to 5% with phage λ exonuclease, and exhibited a linear relationship between the degree of single-strandedness and the concentration of caffeine. Judging from the amount of caffeine required to elute newly synthesized DNA from irradiated bacteria, as compared to controls, they concluded that about 3% of the DNA replicated after exposure to a UV dose of 60 ergs/mm^2 appears to be single-stranded. Since this UV dose would induce 1.5 pyrimidine dimers in a single strand of the molecular weight of the extracted bacterial DNA, it was estimated that the single-stranded regions were about half a million daltons in length. Although this result must be treated with reserve, because overhanging chains unable to pair would affect binding just as much as single-stranded regions, the results make it unlikely that these gaps are limited to just the two nucleotides opposite each pyrimidine dimer. A more plausible interpretation is that the chain being synthesized is terminated at the pyrimidine dimer and a new chain is initiated hundreds or thousands of bases beyond.

INTEGRATION OF LOW MOLECULAR WEIGHT DNA SYNTHESIZED IN UV-IRRADIATED BACTERIA INTO HIGH MOLECULAR WEIGHT CHAINS

Although the newly synthesized chains from UV-irradiated bacteria are of molecular weight low in comparison to that from control unirradiated cells, this new DNA becomes integrated into high molecular weight chains during subsequent incubation. The newly synthesized DNA remains of low molecular weight for about 15 minutes, but increases and approaches the molecular weight of control DNA during the subsequent 45 minutes (14). Similar increases in the molecular weight during subsequent incubation have been observed in mammalian cells (3,9,11,16).

MOLECULAR WEIGHT OF DNA SYNTHESIZED AT VARIOUS TIMES
AFTER UV-IRRADIATION

A diagram of the replicating fork in a UV-irradiated bacterium is shown in Figure 1. As seen at B, DNA synthesized in UV-irradiated cells is formed only on the undamaged chains between pyrimidine dimers. With further incubation, the newly synthesized chains join into high molecular weight molecules (14), possibly as seen at C. If most of the dimers remain in the original template strand, then these joined strands may form good templates for the synthesis of high molecular weight chains. At the same time, the original growth fork will advance and continue to generate DNA of low molecular weight.

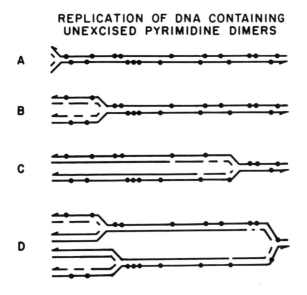

**REPLICATION OF DNA CONTAINING
UNEXCISED PYRIMIDINE DIMERS**

Fig 1. Diagram of the replication of DNA in UV-irradiated excision-defective bacteria, showing a replication fork moving from left to right. Newly synthesized DNA is of length limited to the spacing between pyrimidine dimers, as seen at B. Later this material is joined into high molecular weight chains as seen at C. New growth forks are formed and follow behind the first, synthesizing high molecular weight DNA on the reconstructed daughter strands and low molecular weight DNA on the template strands still containing pyrimidine dimers, as seen at D.

As new rounds of replication are initiated, the new growth forks may advance behind the first, as shown in line D of Figure 1. It is to be expected that both high and low molecular weight chains will be synthesized at this time. Since four damaged and only two reconstructed daughter strands are now being replicated, about twice as much low molecular weight as high molecular weight material would be synthesized.

We have carried out a series of experiments to test the predictions of this model, and have determined the molecular weight distributions of the DNA synthesized at times between one and three hours after irradiation. The plan for these experiments is to expose excision-defective mutants to 60 ergs/mm^2 of UV-irradiation, and then to incubate the cells for a varying period before pulse labelling for ten minutes with ^{3}H-thymidine. The sedimentation profiles in alkaline sucrose gradients of the ^{3}H-thymidine labelled DNA synthesized after UV-irradiation are shown in Figure 2; sedimentation being from right to left. At times between 0 and 40 minutes after exposure to this UV dose, DNA molecular weight about 10 million is synthesized, while at 70 and 120 minutes, the newly synthesized DNA has a broad distribution of molecular weight extending from about 10 to 200 million daltons. Thus the prediction that both high and low molecular weight chains will be synthesized is borne out by these findings.

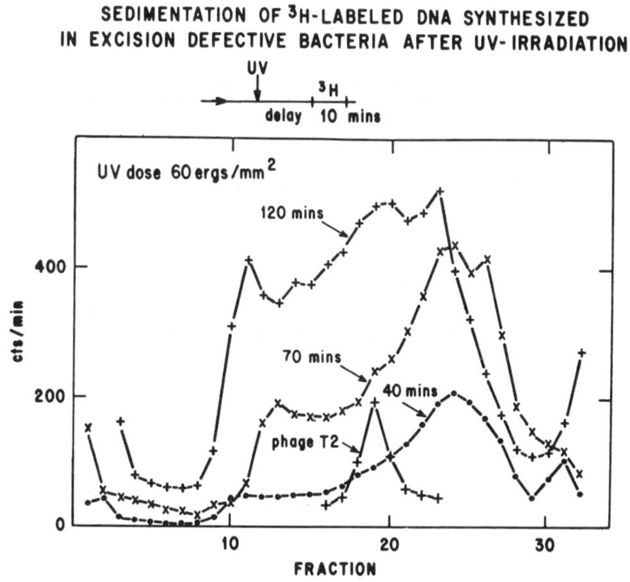

Fig 2. Distribution of ^{3}H-labelled DNA synthesized in UV-irradiated excision-defective bacteria in alkaline sucrose. Sedimentation is from right to left. Exponentially growing bacteria were exposed to 60 ergs/mm^2, incubated for 40, 70 or 120 minutes, and then labelled with ^{3}H-thymidine for 10 minutes, before being converted to spheroplasts and lysed in surface layer of the gradient. The 5 to 20% sucrose gradient at pH 12.3 was centrifuged at 40,000 rpm for 60 minutes at 20° in a SW65 rotor. The gradients contained 0.7 M NaCl, 1 mM EDTA and enough NaOH to bring the pH to 12.3. (15)

The breadth of the distribution of molecular weights in the DNA synthesized during the ten minute pulse starting 120 minutes after irradiation further is illustrated in Figure 3, which also shows the distributions for unirradiated controls and for cells exposed to a UV dose of only 15 ergs/mm^2. The 120 minute distribution extends from molecular weights as low as those obtained after 15 ergs/mm^2, all the way up to molecular weights as high as those obtained in the unirradiated controls which peak at about 200 million daltons. Evidently high molecular weight strands are present and act as

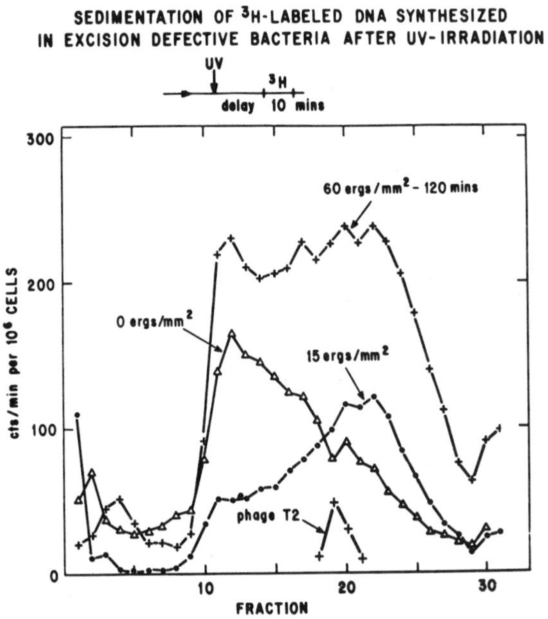

Fig 3. Distribution of ^{3}H-labeled DNA synthesized after UV-irradiation in excision-defective bacteria. Comparison of DNA from unirradiated controls, cells exposed to 15 ergs/mm^2, incubated for 10 minutes, and then labeled for 10 minutes, or cells exposed for 60 ergs/mm^2, incubated for 120 minutes and then labeled for 10 minutes. Conditions are as for Figure 2.

templates for DNA synthesis in the irradiated cells at 120 minutes, in spite of the fact that the pyrimidine dimers are not excised and must remain in the DNA in which they were formed.

Our interpretation of these results is twofold. First, they accord with the model in which the newly synthesized DNA joins into high molecular weight strands which can then serve as new templates. Second, they indicate that some growth forks advance along some templates which contain many pyrimidine dimers and other templates that contain too few dimers to be detected by this method. It can be concluded that the pyrimidine dimers tend to remain in the original strands as in Figure 1 and not to become distributed equally among all the progeny strands.

CHANGES IN THE RATE OF SYNTHESIS OF HIGH AND LOW MOLECULAR WEIGHT DNA AFTER UV-IRRADIATION

The upper part of Figure 4 shows a summary of the rates of synthesis of high and low molecular weight DNA as a function of time after UV-irradiation, the amount of radioactivity in the high molecular weight DNA 70 million daltons or more, or in low molecular weight DNA between 5 and 70 million daltons. The effect of exposure to 60

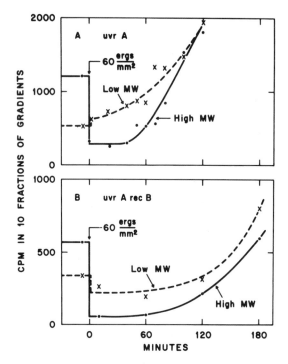

Fig 4. Rate of synthesis of high (70-200 x 10^6) and low (5-70 x 10^6) molecular weight at various times after exposure to 60 ergs/mm^2, in *E. coli uvrA* (top) and *uvrA recB* (bottom) strains.

ergs/mm^2 is to depress the synthesis of high molecular weight DNA to a low level from which it starts to recover only after one hour. The synthesis of low molecular weight DNA, however, is less affected by the irradiation and the increase occurs relatively soon after exposure. By one hour after irradiation, the excision-defective mutants have reconstructed high molecular weight templates that can serve for the direct synthesis of high molecular weight material.

EFFECT OF REC MUTATIONS ON THE INCREASE IN MOLECULAR WEIGHT OF NEWLY SYNTHESIZED DNA

It is interesting that no increase in molecular weight of the daughter chains has been observed in bacteria carrying a *recA* mutation while cells carrying *recB* retain the capacity to reconstruct high molecular weight templates, although they do so more slowly than wild type. As seen in the lower part of Figure 4, it takes two hours instead of one hour before high molecular weight templates start to become available. Mutants carrying *recB* are not as radiosensitive as *recA* mutants, and presumably can perform the steps of recombinational repair at reduced efficiency.

DETECTION OF SISTER EXCHANGES BY MEANS OF DENSITY LABELS

We have suggested that the increase in molecular weight of the daughter strands may be due to recombination between the sister duplexes formed by the replication of DNA containing pyrimidine dimers. These sister exchanges could provide the transfer of information between duplexes needed for the reconstruction of chains carrying the entire base sequence of a functional chromosome. It is visualized that this may take place even though pyrimidine dimers remain in the DNA (14).

To test for such exchanges we have developed an experiment involving the use of density labels in which bacteria were grown so as to contain DNA molecules of hybrid density with one light and one heavy strand. The idea underlying these experiments is that if continuity is maintained in a 3′ to 5′ direction along the chains in the hybrid duplexes, then any exchanges that involve cutting and rejoining strands in a new configuration will

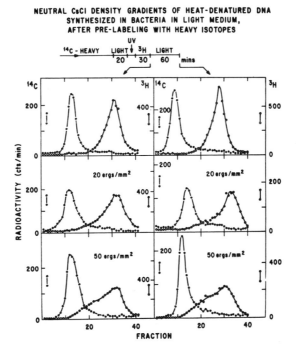

Fig 5. Distribution of heavy $^{13}C^{15}N$ ^{14}C-labeled and light ^{3}H-labeled phenol extracted heat-denatured DNA strands in neutral CsCl equilibrium density gradient. The heavy and light strands from unirradiated cells separate cleanly, while material from UV-irradiated cells contains ^{3}H-labeled molecules of intermediate density.

Excision-defective mutants of *E. coli* were uniformly labeled by growth for many generations with heavy isotopes and ^{14}C-thymidine. They were transferred to light growth medium for 20 minutes and exposed to 0, 20 or 50 ergs/mm^2 before labeling with ^{3}H-thymidine for 30 minutes. Right hand panels: cells were incubated in nonradioactive medium for a further 60 minutes.

lead to heavy strands becoming linked to light. When this DNA is extracted and denatured by heat or alkali, the resulting shear degradation will produce molecules of intermediate density that can be detected in a CsCl density gradient.

Bacteria were grown for several generations in heavy medium containing heavy isotopes and ^{14}C-thymidine. The cells were washed, incubated in a nonradioactive light medium for 20 minutes to flush the heavy isotopes from the precursor pools. The cells were divided into three fractions and exposed to 0, 20 or 50 ergs/mm^2 of UV light and then incubated in medium containing light isotopes and ^{3}H-thymidine for 30 minutes. The DNA was denatured by heating at 98° for five minutes, quickly cooled and centrifuged in CsCl gradients. The heavy and light strands separate cleanly as seen at the top of Figure 5. Following exposure to 20 or to 50 ergs/mm^2, however, the ^{3}H-labeled material is broadened to the left indicating that a fraction of the strands, increasing with increasing UV dose, contain heavy as well as light isotopes, as seen in the lower panels of Figure 5.

FREQUENCY OF SISTER EXCHANGES

A substantial fraction of the ^{3}H-labeled molecules are of intermediate density. It can be estimated from the curves in Figure 5 that 45% of the ^{3}H-radioactivity from cells exposed to 50 ergs/mm^2 is present in molecules of intermediate density. We have determined the molecular weight of these molecules by sedimentation in alkaline sucrose and calculate that one intermediate density molecule is detected for every 1.7 pyrimidine dimers in the DNA replicated in the ^{3}H-containing medium. This comes very close to showing that one sister exchange is induced for every pyrimidine dimer that undergoes replication. These sister exchanges may provide for the transfer of information between the sister duplexes that is needed for recombinational repair (15).

LENGTHS OF HEAVY CHAIN FRAGMENTS INCORPORATED INTO INTERMEDIATE DENSITY CHAINS

To investigate the lengths of the heavy isotopes labeled segments incorporated into the strands of intermediate density, a second experiment of this type was performed. However, to improve the sensitivity with which molecules of intermediate density could be detected, the ^{14}C-label was omitted from the heavy medium. Cells were grown in heavy medium for many generations, transferred to light medium, exposed to various doses of UV light and then incubated with ^{3}H-thymidine. Lysates made from these cells were centrifuged in alkaline CsCl gradients with the results shown in Figure 6.

The graph on the left shows that the ^{3}H-radioactivity is associated with a single light peak for the control cells. After UV-irradiation, however, although the amount of radioactivity incorporated is reduced fourfold at the peak, there is far more radioactivity in the heavy shoulder. Fractions 9, 10 and 11 marked by the rectangles B and D were collected, pooled and recentrifuged. The fractions from the peaks marked A and C also were collected and recentrifuged. The results are shown in the upper high hand panels of Figure 6.

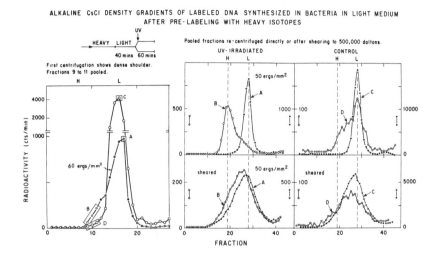

Fig 6. Density distributions in alkaline CsCl equilibrium density gradients of acid insoluble ^{3}H-thymidine labeled DNA synthesized in bacteria in light medium, after pre-labeling with heavy isotopes. This experiment is similar to that of Figure 5, except that the cells were lysed and centrifuged in alkaline CsCl without phenol extraction, and the ^{14}C label was omitted to increase the sensitivity with which intermediate density molecules could be detected. The light strands from unirradiated cells band in a single light peak, while those from UV-irradiated cells band in a peak with a shoulder towards higher densities.

The panels in the middle show the distributions obtained when the pooled fractions 9, 10 and 11 from the left hand gradient were recentrifuged with or without shearing to 500,000 molecular weight.

Right hand panels show the same from unirradiated cells (15).

The top panels show the density distributions for the material from irradiated cells taken from the peak A and from the left shoulder B. Fraction A from the peak again bands in a single light peak, while the pooled fractions 9 to 11 marked B from the heavy shoulder are mostly of high density. The dotted lines indicate the positions of marker heavy and light ^{32}P labeled DNA.

When the fractions C and D from the unirradiated cells are recentrifuged, material from the peak C again is found in a single peak, while the material from the heavy shoulder D exhibits a slight shoulder of perhaps one tenth of the magnitude found for the irradiated cells. This confirms that molecules of intermediate density are readily detected in the irradiated cells, while there is relatively little in control cells.

To investigate the lengths of the labelled segments incorporated into the recombinant molecules, the pooled fractions from the heavy shoulder B and D were sheared by passing through a French pressure cell. As seen in the lower panels after shearing from about 10 million to 500,000 molecular weight, the heavy parts of the chains largely are broken away from the radioactive segments which now band more nearly at the light position. This shows that the segments of heavy and light DNA are frequently long enough to be disrupted by shearing to 500,000 and are frequently longer than this and may be a few million molecular weight in length. Relatively little heavy DNA is seen in the material from unirradiated controls (right hand panels).

Our interpretation of the material in the dense shoulder is that it is due to exchanges between the heavy and light strands and that these exchanges frequently involve segments of length in excess of one million molecular weight.

The intermediate density material could be due to the insertion of short segments of heavy DNA into relatively long segments of light ^{3}H-labeled DNA as shown at A in Figure 7. Alternatively it could be due to the insertion of short lengths of light ^{3}H-labeled DNA into relatively long lengths of heavy DNA. After shearing to about 10 million molecular weight during extraction, the long molecules from the cell would be

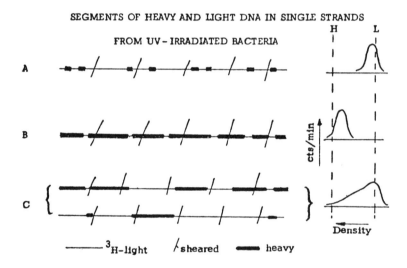

Fig 7. Diagram of possible structures in DNA strands in UV-irradiated cells showing segments of heavy DNA alternating with ^{3}H-labeled light DNA. The distributions of radioactivity produced by denatured DNA after shearing in CsCl density gradients are shown on the right. A, insertion of short regions of heavy label, as in repair synthesis after excision. B, exchanges resulting in the insertion of short regions of light DNA into predominantly heavy strands. C, exchanges produce segments of varying length and a sloping distribution in the density gradient. Compare with the distribution in the lower panels of Figure 5.

broken by shearing as indicated by the arrows, and distributions of denatured molecules in CsCl density gradients would be as seen on the right hand side. It is not clear that either A or B or a combination of the two would generate distributions comparable to those seen in the lower panels of Figure 5, and indicated at C. Instead we suggest that there is a distribution in the sizes of ^{3}H-labeled light and heavy DNA segments, possibly as shown on the left at C.

EVIDENCE FOR LOCAL REPAIR AT THE JOIN IN RECOMBINATIONAL REPAIR

Local repair replication may occur in sister exchanges and contribute to filling the gaps. Repair synthesis would escape detection in these experiments on E. coli, as it would carry the same labels as other light DNA.

A new method recently was devised by Regan, Setlow and Ley (13) which permits the detection of short regions of repair between polynucleotide chains. This method depends upon the photolysis by 313 nm wavelength light of any regions of DNA repair that contain bromodeoxyuridine. Some evidence for repair synthesis in joining the newly synthesized fragments has already been obtained in mouse leukemia cells (11).

POSSIBLE STRUCTURES FORMED IN RECOMBINATIONAL REPAIR

Various DNA structures that might result from possible mechanisms for recombinational repair are illustrated in Figures 8 and 9. The template strands, which in our experiments are labeled with heavy isotopes prior to irradiation, are represented by heavy lines, while the light daughter strands synthesized after irradiation and including any possible regions of repair are represented by narrow lines. The UV-induced pyrimidine dimers are represented by small circles. DNA repair synthesis may occur locally in the joins, but would carry the same labels as other light DNA and is not detected in these experiments.

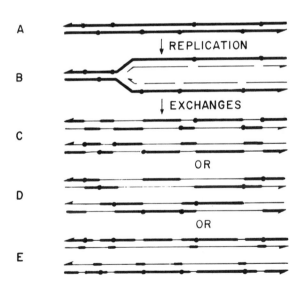

Fig 8. Diagram of hypothetical structure in the DNA of UV-irradiated excision-defective cells, showing the replication of twin helical DNA-containing UV-induced pyrimidine dimers, after replication the newly synthesized strands are represented by narrow lines and are of lower than normal molecular weight. C, D and E alternative possible structures formed by sister exchanges of various types. C, dimers cause exchange in all four strands. D, only the strand opposite the dimer is exchanged, and the exchanges are of indefinite length. E, only the strand opposite the dimer is exchanged, but the exchanges are of limited length.

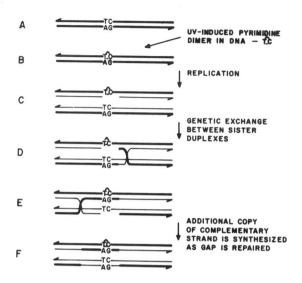

Fig 9. Hypothetical scheme for recombinational repair by sister exchanges following DNA replication. Duplex DNA seen at A is exposed to UV light which produces a T̂C dimer seen at B. Replication results in a gap in the daughter strand opposite the dimer. This is filled in by a sister exchanges and repair synthesis as seen at D, E and F.

The model at Figure 8E involving single-strand exchanges of short but variable lengths, is in best accord with our results, while the models C and D are less likely because the dimers become distributed among the strands.

Figure 9 shows how information may be transferred between damaged sister duplexes by a single-strand exchange, an extra copy of the undamaged base sequence being synthesized, much as in gene conversion.

THE NEED FOR EXCISION-REPAIR AND RECOMBINATIONAL REPAIR

Why do bacteria need two mechanisms for dark repair after UV-irradiation? Why is the UV-resistance of wild type cells many times higher than that of excision-defective or recombination-deficient mutants? To answer these questions we may consider what happens when several thousand pyrimidine dimers are induced in the DNA of wild type cells. The majority of these products are excised in advance of DNA replication. However, a minority not excised in time, may pass through the growth fork. After replication, the dimers would be opposite gaps and no longer subject to excision, since this process requires an intact complementary strand. Only when the gap has been filled by sister exchanges, will the dimers again be subject to excision. Thus in growing cells, dimers passing through the growth fork are excised only in cells able to make sister exchanges.

In excision-defective mutants, recombinational repair may be able to overcome the effects of dimers in any part of the chromosome. However, recombinational repair is far more complex than excision-repair, and has a correspondingly limited capacity when expressed in the numbers of damaged bases than can be tolerated. Cell survival, which requires the reconstruction of an intact chromosome, may be achieved with 50 or a 100 dimers per chromosome rather than several thousand as in wild type.

CONCLUSION

In conclusion, we have detected molecules of intermediate density in the sheared single-stranded DNA obtained from UV-irradiated, but not control bacteria. These intermediate density molecules may be due to UV-induced genetic exchanges between sister duplexes formed when DNA containing damaged bases is replicated. To judge from the fraction of molecules that are of intermediate density, one single-strand sister exchange occurs for every one to two pyrimidine dimers in the DNA that undergoes replication. These exchanges may underlie the reconstruction of high molecular weight templates that become available for DNA synthesis one to two hours after irradiation and provide a basis for the survival of colony-forming ability.

ACKNOWLEDGMENTS

We would like to thank Mrs. Sophia Mroczkowski, Mrs. Donna Reno and Charles Wilde III for performing some of these experiments.

REFERENCES

1. Brunk, C. F. and Hanawalt, P. C.: Science, 158:663, 1967.
2. Clark, A. J. and Margulies, A. D.: Proc. Nat. Acad. Sci. USA, 53:451, 1965.
3. Cleaver, J. E. and Thomas, G. H.: Biochem. Biophys. Res. Comm., 36:203, 1969.
4. Cole, R. S.: J. Bact., 106:143, 1971.
5. Cooper, P. K. and Hanawalt, P. C.: Photochem. Photobiol., 13:83, 1971.
6. Howard-Flanders, P. and Boyce, R. P.: Radiat. Res. Suppl., 6:156, 1966.
7. Howard-Flanders, P., Rupp, W. D., Wilkins, B. M. and Cole, R. S.: Cold Spring Harbor Symp. Quant. Biol., 33:195-207, 1968.
8. Howard-Flanders, P., Wilkins, B. M. and Rupp, W. D.: In: Molecular Genetics, p 161. Edited by Wittmann, H. G. and Schuster, H. Springer-Verlag, New York, 1968.
9. Humphrey, R. M. and Meyn, R. E.: This Symposium, p 159, 1971.
10. Iyer, V. N. and Rupp, W. D.: Biochim. Biophys. Acta, 228:117, 1971.
11. Lehmann, A. R.: Personal communication.
12. McGrath, R. A. and Williams, R. W.: Nature, 212:534, 1966.
13. Regan, J. D., Setlow, R. B. and Ley, R. D.: Proc. Nat. Acad. Sci. USA, 68:708, 1971.
14. Rupp, W. D. and Howard-Flanders, P.: J. Molec. Biol., 31:291, 1968.
15. Rupp, W. D., Wilde, C. E., Reno, D. and Howard-Flanders, P.: J. Molec. Biol., 61:25, 1971.
16. Rupp, W. D., Zipser, E., von Essen, C., Reno, D., Proznitz, L. and Howard-Flanders, P.: In: Time and Dose Relationships in Radiation Biology as Applied to Radiotherapy, p 1. Edited by Bond, V. P., Brookhaven National Laboratory, Upton, New York, 1970.
17. Smith, K. C. and Meun, D. H. C.: J. Molec. Biol., 51:459, 1970.
18. Wilkins, B. M. and Howard-Flanders, P.: Genetics, 60:243, 1969.
19. Yarus, M. and Sinsheimer, R. L.: J. Molec. Biol., 8:614, 1964.

REPAIR OF ALKYLATED DNA IN MAMMALIAN CELLS

J. J. Roberts

Chester Beatty Research Institute
London, England

An interest in the potential repair of alkylated DNA has been stimulated for two reasons. The first is that resistance to the cytotoxic action of certain chemotherapeutically useful alkylating agents may be a function of the ability of cells to repair DNA damage, since it is currently believed that the cell-killing action of these compounds is due to a reaction with DNA, probably cross-linking of twin strands, which thereby inhibits DNA synthesis. The second is that it is becoming increasingly apparent that a large number of carcinogenic compounds either are alkylating agents per se or can be metabolized to alkylating species or to compounds which can react as carbonium ions, that is, in the same way as alkylating agents. In the first category are compounds such as β-propiolactone (1), N-methyl-N-nitrosourea (2), or 7-bromomethyl-12-methylbenzanthracene (3), which can react directly with macromolecules, while in the second are dimethylnitrosamine, methyl hydrazine and certain cycasin derivatives such as methylazoxymethanol acetate which are almost certainly converted by oxidative metabolism to methyl carbonium ions in vivo (2). Evidence has accumulated that aromatic hydrocarbons such as dibenz a,h-anthracene are metabolized to epoxide derivatives (4) shown recently to be capable of transforming hamster embryo cells in culture more readily than the parent hydrocarbon (5) and that certain carcinogenic aromatic amines such as acetylaminofluorene are metabolized to arylhydroxylamines (6). These metabolites can react with DNA as carbonium ions.

There are many possible ways in which DNA repair could be involved in carcinogenesis. The initiating action of these various carcinogens is probably associated with their reaction with DNA leading possibly to somatic mutation, the subsequent promotional stage of carcinogenesis being associated with the stimulation of cell division. If this interpretation is correct then the ability of a cell to repair lesions in DNA before the ultimate expression of this damage may be of more significance than the initial event. An alternative and appealing possibility, since it could form the basis of a unifying hypothesis for chemical carcinogenesis is that faulty repair may introduce new and common mutational errors into the variously chemically-modified DNAs. If chemical agents act by inducing oncogenic viruses then it is conceivable that this is a consequence of chemical damage to DNA which results in liberation of virus from cellular DNA during an abortive repair process. Finally one could speculate on the possibility that there is a deterioration of cellular repair processes with age which upsets a normal balance between damage and repair.

In order to be certain that so-called DNA repair phenomena are involved in the recovery of cells from the effects of alkylation it is necessary to establish that alkylation of DNA results in a particular biological effect on cells. The ideal would be to find that repair of DNA is accompanied by the elimination or modification of specific mutagenic effects of alkylation in mammalian cells. Mammalian cell genetics is only beginning to approach this degree of sophistication. As discussed earlier alkylation of DNA is probably involved in carcinogenesis but there is no precise definitive evidence to support this view at present. If quantitative measurement of carcinogenesis in vitro can be achieved, one might hopefully have a system in which the relevance of DNA repair processes could be studied. We, therefore, are left with the role of reactions with DNA in producing cell death, which now seems well established on a number of counts. Thus, at concentrations of mustard gas permitting high survival of cells in culture the only detectable biochemical effect is an inhibition in the rate of DNA synthesis, and this inhibition is a consequence of alkylation of DNA per se and not due to the inhibition of enzymes involved in DNA synthesis. Inhibition of DNA synthesis leads to an extended S phase and subsequent mitotic delay (Fig 1). That the mitotic delay is the result of the inhibition in rate of DNA

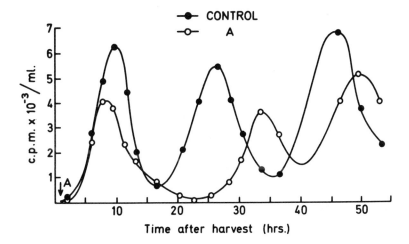

Fig 1. The effect of treatment with mustard gas during the G_1 phase of the cell cycle (arrowed A) on subsequent DNA synthesis in a synchronous population of HeLa cells. The cells were treated with mustard gas (0.075 μg/ml in ether 0.05%) and the extent of DNA synthesis in treated and untreated cells measured at various times thereafter by the uptake of [^{3}H] TdR into cold TCA insoluble material in a 1 ml aliquot of cells.

• - • , Control; o - o , 0.075 μg/ml mustard gas.

synthesis following alkylation of DNA was confirmed by showing that G_2-treated cells divide normally and then, following a depression in DNA synthesis in the succeeding cell cycle, exhibit a mitotic delay (8). A scheme which represents diagrammatically these events is shown in Figure 2 which depicts the state of the DNA at various times during the cell cycle and the presence of cross-links in the DNA. The existence of mustard gas-induced cross-links presumably prevents separation of the two strands of DNA as is required during semiconservative replication. Thus, cells become blocked in the S phase and continue to synthesise DNA at a reduced rate. Since RNA and protein synthesis are unaffected cells enlarge to form giant cells. Eventually some of these cells, which have been treated with low concentrations of mustard gas, divide. Measurement of levels of alkylation of DNA, RNA and protein molecules support this view on target theory. At the D_0 dose of mustard gas for HeLa cells less than 1 molecule of protein (mol wt 1×10^5) in 2000 but every molecule of DNA of mol wt 3×10^8 daltons was alkylated (7).

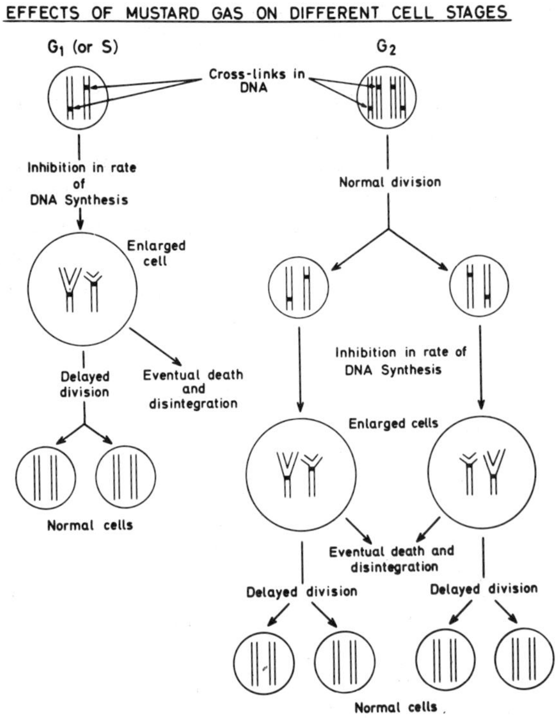

Fig 2. Scheme showing the effect of treatment with mustard gas or half mustard gas during different phases of the HeLa cell cycle on subsequent DNA synthesis and cell division.

Chemical, biochemical and biological observations indicate that cells recover from the otherwise lethal effect of DNA alkylations thus implying the existence of a mechanism(s) for repairing lesions in DNA. As can be seen in Figure 1 (and also in Figure 6 which shows the effects of half mustard gas on DNA synthesis) those cells which divide after the initially extended S phase and subsequent mitotic delay do not exhibit any extension of the S phase or mitotic delay in the following cell cycle but divide thereafter with a normal generation time. This implies that the damage which resulted in the depression of DNA synthesis has been repaired during the delay period.

Cells given a pulse-treatment of mustard gas early in the G_1 phase of the cell cycle showed less subsequent depression of DNA synthesis than those treated just prior to the onset of DNA synthesis and this was interpreted as being due to the repair of DNA lesions during the G_1 phase (8). Variations in the colony-forming ability of cells treated at different times during the cell cycle accorded with this view. Maximum sensitivity was at the G_1/S interphase while early G_1- and G_2-treated cells were the least sensitive.

The chemical evidence for repair comes from measurements on the extent of reaction of ^{35}S labelled mustard gas with HeLa cell constituents and in particular from a consideration of the number of cross-links in DNA. At the D_o dose of this agent for HeLa cells it can be calculated that there are approximately 1500 DNA interstrand cross-links per cell. Since theoretically one cross-link could be regarded as adequate to stop replication of DNA these cross-links must have been circumvented or eliminated. Indeed we have found that the products of alkylation are partially excised from DNA of mustard-treated HeLa cells (7) while Reid and Walker observed a time-dependent removal of cross-links from mustard-resistant mouse L cells (9). The nature of the initially excised material is not yet known but by analogy with the established mechanism of removal of UV-induced lesions it is reasonable to suppose it consists of oligonucleotides containing alkylguanine residues. It should be stressed, however, that loss of chemical groups from DNA is not necessarily indicative of an enzyme-mediated repair mechanism since it is known that alkyl purines are lost hydrolytically from alkylated DNA and this occurs at a rate which is similar to the observed loss of radioactivity from cells (10).

Further biochemical support for the concept of repair of chemical damage to mammalian cell DNA came from the demonstration of nonsemiconservative ("repair") DNA synthesis in HeLa cells (11) and P388 cells (12), following alkylation with a variety of agents. It thus appears that a mechanism analogous to the well-established "cut and patch" repair of UV-irradiation-induced lesions exists for the removal of alkylation damage from the DNA of mammalian cells.

In order to establish whether these indications of repair truly were related to the recovery of cells from the effects of alkylation or constituted merely nonspecific responses to damage of cells we have attempted to answer the following questions:

1. Is the amount of "repair synthesis" dependent on the initial level of DNA alkylation?
2. Are the kinetics of "repair synthesis" related to those of removal of alkyl groups from DNA, and is the latter an enzyme-mediated reaction?
3. How much "repair synthesis" is associated with the loss of each alkyl group from DNA?
4. What DNA precursors are incorporated during "repair replication"?
5. Are differences in the various manifestations of "cut and patch" repair associated with differences in the sensitivity of cell types to a particular agent (such as, drug resistance, susceptibility to carcinogens)?
6. If not, are there other mechanisms of DNA repair?
7. Can "repair synthesis" be inhibited?

There are certain problems associated with the study of quantitative aspects of alkylation repair which do not apply to the study of repair of UV-damaged DNA. For example, it can be presumed that a given dose of UV-irradiation always produces a certain number of pyrimidine dimers in DNA during a given time. The extracellular concentration of a chemical agent, however, gives no indication of the true extent of DNA reaction. Even closely related alkylating agents, capable of introducing the same groups into DNA, may require very different concentrations to produce the same extent of DNA reaction. Furthermore, the rate of reaction of apparently similar compounds can be very different. The extent and nature of the reaction with DNA may be the same for two compounds but differ markedly with other cellular constituents. Last, but probably not least, while the major product of reaction may be the same for a variety of compounds the

REACTION OF MMS, MNU AND MNNG WITH

HAMSTER CELL DNA

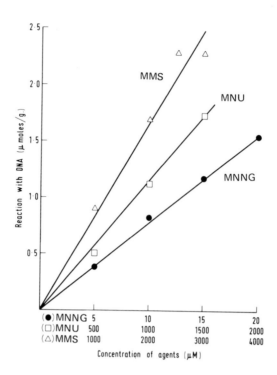

Fig 3. Extent of methylation of DNA isolated from Chinese hamster V79-379A cells following treatment for 1 hr in suspension at 37° with various concentrations of [3H] MNNG (•), [3H] MNU (□) and [14C] MMS (△). The concentrations of the three compounds at any one point on the abscissa were chosen to give approximately equal effects on cell survival as determined by colony forming ability of treated cells.

minor products which are formed simultaneously may be very different for one compound compared with another, and it may be these minor products which constitute the significant biological lesion. Thus, mustard gas and its monofunctional analogue, half mustard gas, react with DNA to produce predominantly 7-hydroxyethylthioethyl-guanine but it is the ability of mustard gas to produce a small proportion of cross-linking reactions which confers its higher cytotoxic effect in comparison with that of the half mustard (8). MMS, MNU and MNNG[1] all react with DNA to give predominently 7-methylguanine. MNU unlike MMS is a potent mutagen for T2 phage (13) and it has been suggested by Loveless (14) that this difference might reside in the ability of MNU to react with guanine residues at the extranuclear 0-6 atom to a greater extent than does MMS. When, therefore, a

[1] Abbreviations: MMS, methyl methanesulphonate; MNU, N-methyl-N-nitrosourea; MNNG, N-methyl-N'-nitro-N-nitrosoguanidine.

particular biochemical manifestation of repair is being followed, be it excision or repair replication, it is important if possible to ensure that it relates to the significant lesion. Some of these aspects are illustrated by the finding that the concentrations of the methylating agents MMS, MNU and MNNG which are equitoxic to Chinese hamster V79-379A cells differ by nearly 200-fold (15), (Fig 3). However, when the fraction of cells surviving treatment was plotted as a function of reaction with DNA essentially the same plot was obtained for all three compounds (Fig 4).

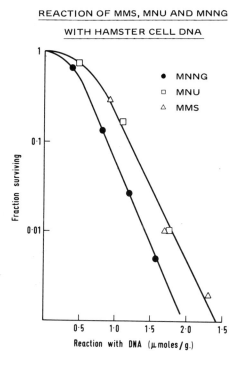

Fig 4. Relationship between the survival of Chinese hamster V79-379A cells and the extents of methylation of their DNA by [^{3}H] MNNG (●), [^{3}H] MNU (□), [^{14}C] MMS (△).

Repair replication was determined in hamster cells following treatment with these same compounds by following the incorporation of [^{3}H] BUdR[2] (or a mixture of BUdR and [^{3}H] TdR[2] which was shown to be equivalent to [^{3}H] BUdR) into light single-stranded DNA (16). The specific activity of this DNA gave a measurement of repair replication and was plotted against dose to give a linear relationship, although this did not hold at higher concentrations when the repair mechanism either was inhibited by other cellular reactions or became saturated. Again it was found that for the three methylating agents, at equitoxic concentrations, resulting in an equal extent of DNA binding, there was an equal amount of repair replication (Fig 5). This approach was extended to other cell lines and to other cytotoxic compounds and it was apparent that in every case examined the extent of repair replication was broadly speaking directly proportional to the amount of reaction occurring with DNA. This was so despite the fact that in these situations equal extents of DNA reaction did not always elicit the same cytotoxic effect, as I shall mention later.

[2] Abbreviations: BUdR, 5-bromo-2'-deoxyuridine; TdR, thymidine.

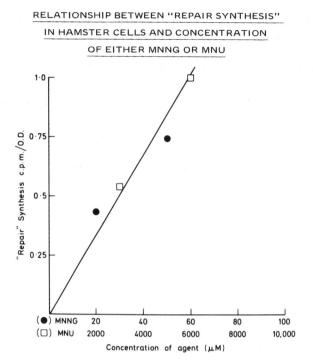

Fig 5. Relationship between amount of "repair synthesis" in Chinese hamster V79-379A cells and the concentration of MNNG or MNU.

Repair replication was shown to occur for many hours following alkylation of hamster cells with MNNG or of HeLa cells with mustard gas (16). Loss of labelled methyl groups from DNA of hamster cells alkylated with [^{3}H] MNNG was also followed over this period. It was found that both these events proceeded at comparable rates, suggesting that one was a consequence of the other. This is consistent with the biochemical evidence indicating that recovery of cells from low concentrations of drugs which permit high survival occurs during a period of several hours (Fig 1).

From a knowledge of the actual number of methyl groups lost from DNA in a given time and of the number of thymidine molecules incorporated into DNA by repair replication during the same period and under the same conditions it was possible to arrive at a rough estimate of the number of nucleotides inserted into DNA per methyl group lost. The calculation, which assumes that the DNA polymerase(s) used for normal and repair DNA synthesis does not discriminate differently as between BUdR and [^{3}H] TdR, suggests that 100 nucleotides are inserted into DNA for every methyl group lost.

The method used for repair replication permits us to examine the fourth question posed, namely, what precursors can be used for DNA repair? We have reported that a mixture of [^{3}H] TdR or [^{3}H] CdR and BUdR is equivalent to [^{3}H] BUdR for the detection of repair replication (16). Initially we failed to detect repair replication using a mixture of [^{3}H] deoxyguanosine or [^{3}H] deoxyadenosine and BUdR. We have now found that by using more highly labelled purine nucleosides and by repeated rebanding of the "light" DNA to remove any contaminating labelled "heavy" DNA and labelled RNA that both these purines as well as the pyrimidine can be utilized for repair replication.

These quantitative and kinetic aspects of repair replication clearly indicate that it is related to the level of DNA alkylation produced by these various agents. Furthermore, it would seem that it is involved in the recovery of cells containing damaged DNA by a process related to the "cut and patch" repair of UV-induced thymine dimers (18). It would not appear to be a nonspecific response to cell death possibly involving end-addition of nucleotides (12). This latter view was fostered by the apparent need for supralethal doses of agents in order to detect repair replication as was the case following treatment of HeLa cells with X-rays (19) or mustard gas (11). With the relatively non-toxic monofunctional compounds such as MMS and "resistant" cells like P388 lymphoma or Chinese hamster V79-379A and improved methods for detecting "repair synthesis," this can now be observed at concentrations resulting in nearly 100% survival.

If we accept that repair replication is involved in the recovery of cells from alkylation we may now ask the question, why do cells differ in their response to a particular agent? Do sensitive cells lack excision enzymes or the ability to undergo repair replication? Comparison of these two manifestations of repair in sensitive and resistant Yoshida sarcoma cells showed that this was not the case. Despite a nearly 20-fold difference in the level of alkylation at equitoxic doses both cell types exhibited the same rate of excision of mustard gas and the same extent of repair replication (20).

HeLa cells and hamster cells differ markedly in their response to MNNG and MMU, less so to MMS while mustard gas and half mustard gas affect both cell lines to the same extent (15). We, therefore, have considered whether hamster cells can repair lesions introduced by MNNG or MNU more readily than can HeLa cells. Again it was found that at equal levels of DNA reaction both cell types showed the same amount of "repair synthesis" (16) suggesting that the greater sensitivity of HeLa cells to MNNG or MNU did not reside in their inability to repair lesions introduced by these compounds by a "cut and patch" mechanism. This prompted us to consider that a difference in the efficiency of some other mechanism for repairing DNA lesions existed as between the two cell lines. Some evidence for this was obtained from a comparison of the effects of mustard gas, half mustard gas and MNU or DNA synthesis in synchromous populations of either HeLa or hamster cells at equitoxic concentrations of these agents. Treatment of HeLa cells with low concentrations of MNU leads to effects on DNA synthesis and progression through the cell cycle quite different from those previously observed after treatment with mustard gas (Fig 1) or half mustard gas (Fig 6). Both these latter agents caused an immediate dose-dependent depression of DNA synthesis in the S phase of the cycle in which treatment occurred and a subsequent mitotic delay. However, MNU failed to produce any immediate effect on the rate of DNA synthesis. Treated cells divided without delay but in the following cell cycle showed a clear dose-dependent depression in the rate of DNA synthesis (Fig 7) and commensurate mitotic delay. Thus it appears that DNA alkylated by MNU is required to undergo replication in order that a lesion be produced which constitutes a block to DNA synthesis (21). Substantiation of this view came from the fate of G_2-treated cells. These cells divided twice before exhibiting a like depression in the rate of DNA synthesis. Figure 8 depicts schematically this alkylation of DNA and its consequences for cells treated during the G_1 or G_2 phases of the cell cycle. The additional lesion could be a

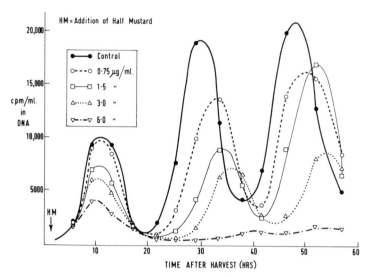

Fig 6. The effect of treatment with half mustard gas during the G_1 phase of the cell cycle (arrowed HM) on subsequent DNA synthesis in a synchronous population of HeLa cells. DNA synthesis was determined as in Figure 1.

•-•, Control; o-o, 0.75 μg/ml; □-□, 1.5 μg/ml; △-△, 3.0 μg/ml; ▽-▽, 6.0 μg/ml.

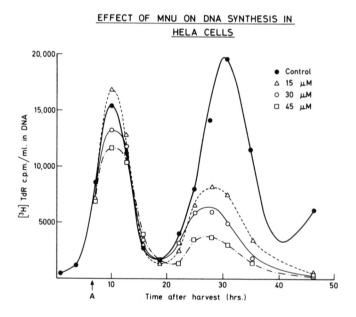

Fig 7. The effect of treatment with MNU during the G_1 phase of the cell cycle on DNA synthesis in synchronous populations of HeLa cells.

Replicate cultures were treated with MNU 6 hours after mitosis (arrowed A).

•, Control; △, 15 μM; o, 30 μM, □, 45 μM.

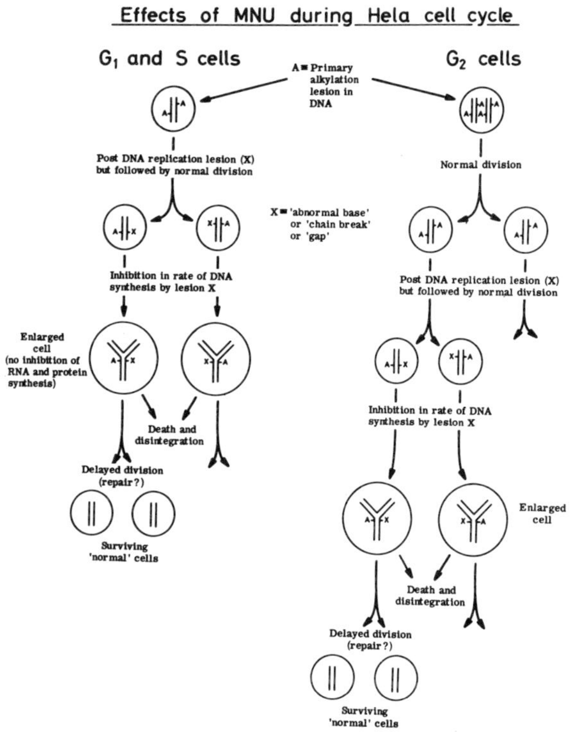

Fig 8. Scheme showing the effect of alkylation of HeLa cells with MNU during different phases of the cell cycle.

gap in the template DNA. Such gaps could be subsequently repaired by the insertion of bases or by a mechanism akin to recombination (24).

Synchronous populations of hamster cells were similarly treated with either mustard gas, half mustard gas or MNU. As was the case for HeLa cells, mustard gas and half mustard gas introduced lesions into hamster cell DNA which constituted an immediate block to DNA synthesis (Fig 9). Both cell lines are equally affected by these two agents and therefore it must be presumed that they possess similar repair potential towards these particular lesions (22). This probably requires elimination of a cross-link in the case of mustard gas or a "pseudo" cross-link in the case of half mustard gas (by virtue of its additional -OH group which could be involved in hydrogen bonding) by a "cut and patch" mechanism.

In contrast to these agents MNU is far less toxic towards hamster cells than towards HeLa cells. At equitoxic doses hamster DNA is alkylated 20 times that of HeLa DNA. Cell death following treatment of hamster cells with MNU also probably results from lesions in DNA introduced during DNA replication in one cycle blocking DNA synthesis in the next. This implies that hamster cells more readily can repair DNA damaged by MNU than HeLa cells. As it was argued earlier that replication of MNU-alkylated DNA produces gaps, then it follows that the ability to bridge these gaps differs in the two cell

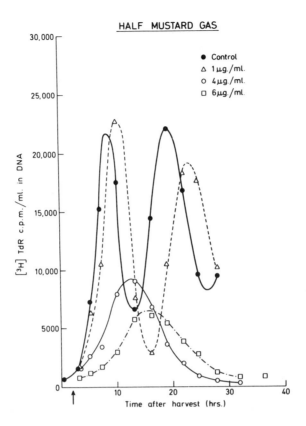

Fig 9. The effect of treatment with half mustard gas during the G_1 phase of the cell cycle on DNA synthesis in Chinese hamster V79-379A cells. Replicate cultures were treated 2 hours after mitosis (arrowed). ●, Control; △, 1 μg/ml; ○, 4 μg/ml; □, 6 μg/ml.

lines. There is one aspect in which the response to alkylation of hamster cells differs markedly from that of HeLa cells. In the former we observed a dose-dependent delay in the onset of DNA synthesis of G_1-treated cells (Fig 10). Conceivably, therefore, this delay period permits repair of these gaps in DNA before their effects are manifest in the following cell cycle.

Support for the existence of an additional repair mechanism other than "cut and patch" repair has come from an examination of the effects of caffeine on the survival of MNU-treated cells and its effect on repair replication. While the sensitivity of hamster cells towards MNU was increased by caffeine no depression in the extent of "repair synthesis" could be detected (23). This suggests that a repair mechanism not requiring nonsemiconservative DNA synthesis is being affected by this agent.

In summary, therefore, there is evidence that mammalian cells in culture recover from the otherwise lethal effects of alkylation by at least two mechanisms. In the one, alkyl groups are eliminated from DNA and the "breaks" so produced are probably repaired

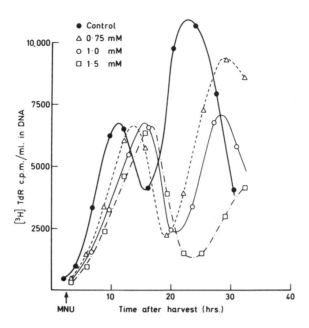

Fig 10. The effect of treatment with MNU during the G_1 phase of the cell cycle on DNA synthesis in synchronous populations of Chinese hamster V79-379A cells. Replicate cultures were treated 2 hours after mitosis (arrowed). •, Control; △, 0.75 mM; ○, 1.0 mM; □, 1.5 mM.

by nonsemiconservative or "repair" synthesis. However, since the sensitivity of cells to various agents cannot be explained in terms of differences in this mechanism of repair, another mechanism probably exists in mammalian cells for repairing DNA. This is possibly analogous to that postulated for the repair of UV-induced thymine dimers which involves the bypassing of DNA lesions during DNA synthesis and the subsequent filling of the gaps so produced by a mechanism akin to recombination (24). Experiments with microorganisms have shown that this recombination repair is error-prone and results in a high mutation yield. Perhaps it is significant that the compounds which cause DNA lesions in mammalian cells, which, we are postulating, are repaired by a similar mechanism increase the spontaneous mutation rate in Chinese hamster cells and are potent carcinogens.

REFERENCES

1. Colburn, N. H. and Boutwell, R. K.: Cancer Res., 28:653, 1968.
2. Magee, P. N. and Barnes, J. M.: Adv. Cancer Res., 10:163, 1967.
3. Dipple, A. and Slade, T. A.: Europ. J. Cancer, 6:47, 1970.
4. Boyland, E. and Sims, P.: Biochem J., 97:7, 1965.
5. Grover, P. L., Sims, P., Huberman, E., Marquardt, H., Kuroki, T. and Heidelberger, C.: P.N.A.S. 68:1098, 1971.
6. Miller, E. C. and Miller, J. A.: Pharmacol. Rev., 18:805, 1966.

7. Crathorn, A. R. and Roberts, J. J.: Nature, 211:150, 1966.
8. Roberts, J. J., Brent, T. P. and Crathorn, A. R.: Europ. J. Cancer., 7:515, 1971.
9. Reid, B. D. and Walker, I. G.: Biochim. Biophys. Acta, 179:179, 1969.
10. Lawley, P. D.: Progr. Nucl. Acid Res., 5:89, 1968.
11. Roberts, J. J., Crathorn, A. R. and Brent, T. P.: Nature, 218:970, 1968.
12. Ayad, S. R., Fox, M. and Fox, B. W.: Mutat. Res., 8:639, 1969.
13. Loveless, A. and Hampton, C. L.: Mutat. Res., 7:1, 1969.
14. Loveless, A.: Nature, 223:206, 1969.
15. Roberts, J. J., Pascoe, J. M., Plant, J. E., Sturrock, J. E. and Crathorn, A. R.: Chem. Biol. Interact., 3:29, 1971.
16. Roberts, J. J., Pascoe, J. M., Smith, B. and Crathorn, A. R.: Chem. Biol. Interact., 3:49, 1971.
17. Crathorn, A. R., Smith, B. and Roberts, J. J.: Unpublished result.
18. Howard-Flanders, P.: Ann. Rev. Biochem., 37:175, 1968.
19. Painter, R. B. and Cleaver, J. E.: Nature, 216:369, 1967.
20. Ball, C. R. and Roberts, J. J.: Chem. Biol. Interact., 2:321, 1970.
21. Plant, J. E. and Roberts, J. J.: Chem. Biol. Interact., 3:337, 1971.
22. Plant, J. E. and Roberts, J. J.: Chem. Biol. Interact., 3:343, 1971.
23. Roberts, J. J. and Ward, K.: Unpublished results.
24. Rupp, W. D. and Howard-Flanders, P.: J. Molec. Biol., 31:291, 1968.

RADIATION AND CHEMICAL MUTAGENESIS AND REPAIR IN MICE[1]

W. L. Russell

Biology Division, Oak Ridge National Laboratory
Oak Ridge, Tennessee

What is a paper on mutagenesis in mice doing in a symposium on molecular biology? One answer is provided by Dr. Beers' introductory remarks. At two separate places he mentioned the Delaney amendment to the Food and Drug Act and commented on the problem of tolerance levels. Earlier, in the process of organizing the program, Dr. Beers stated that: "The thrust or theme of this Symposium is toward the correlation of the fundamental knowledge about the biological importance of repair processes and the practical problems of maximum permissible levels of exposure to toxic factors. . . ." I believe this paper is relevant to that theme.

Our work on mutagenesis in the mouse also has a more basic relevance to molecular biology which will be discussed in the next few paragraphs. In this connection, I should like to quote, for the purposes of correction and subsequent clarification, a passage from Dr. Beers' introductory remarks, a passage about which my colleagues have been teasing me:—"The extensive and extremely tedious methods of evaluation employed by the Russells and Bentley Glass, who utilized mice and drosophila, respectively, to study low levels of radiation, have reached a point of costly diminishing returns."

It should be made clear that, although we have explored the effects of low dose rates, we have never done genetic experiments at very low radiation doses. The lowest used was 50 R, and that only in females, for a cogent secondary reason. We were forced to use doses that low in females in order to have extended fertility. With the larger doses that we normally use, the females become sterile after producing only one or two litters. We have not gone down to very low doses, because these would indeed give diminishing returns for what we have had in mind in our research. It will perhaps be helpful to make a few remarks about the rationale for our experiments and to compare our approach with the techniques usually classified as molecular biology.

Our work has not, as is sometimes mistakenly believed, been concerned primarily with simple empirical answers concerning radiation-induced mutation rates in mice. We have been much more interested in the effects of various physical and biological factors on the mutation process. Our approach has been to use the classical genetic method, namely breeding, to deduce what is happening at the molecular level. It was, of course, with the use of this kind of approach that the existence of the gene was deduced almost a century before its chemistry was hooked up with DNA. In the same way we can deduce some useful information about the nature of the mutation process and repair mechanisms while we are waiting for details on their chemistry.

[1] Research jointly sponsored by the U.S. Atomic Energy Commission and the National Institute of General Medical Sciences under contract with the Union Carbide Corporation.

The first part of this paper reviews some of the deductions on the repair of radiation-induced mutational damage, showing how these were reached. Since this is an interdisciplinary symposium, technical details and supporting data, which are available in other publications, are here kept to a minimum.

An extensive set of conclusions has been reached regarding repair of mutational or premutational damage and the effect on the repair process of such physical factors as radiation dose, dose rate and dose fractionation, and of such biological factors as sex and cell stage (1-4). This body of knowledge is far ahead of anything that could even be guessed at from what is currently known at the chemical level. Since the chemistry will have to match what we have already found out (assuming our deductions are correct), our results should serve as useful guidelines to help the molecular biologists stay on the right path. This, I think, is where our findings have their major relevance to molecular biology.

The second part of this paper presents some of the results obtained on chemical mutagenesis in the mouse. Although the conclusions reached are not yet as extensive, or as definitive, as those in radiation mutagenesis, they also suggest the existence of repair mechanisms and other complexities which will have to be fitted into any valid interpretation of what is happening at the molecular level.

RADIATION MUTAGENESIS

Our first evidence for the possible existence of repair of mutational or premutational damage in the mouse came from radiation dose-rate experiments on specific-locus mutation frequencies in spermatogonia, the stem cells in the testis (5). A dose delivered over a few weeks at the rate of 0.009 R/min gave a mutation frequency of only about 30% of that produced by the same total dose delivered in a few minutes at 90 R/min.

The possibility existed that this was not necessarily a direct effect of dose rate on mutation frequency. Since large numbers of the spermatogonia were killed by the doses used, the difference in mutation frequencies could conceivably have resulted secondarily from differential cell killing, that is, from differences in the mutational sensitivity of the populations of spermatogonial cells surviving at the two dose rates. Subsequent experiments seem to have ruled out this explanation for the spermatogonia results (2,6-8), and work with females showed an even greater dose-rate effect in the oocytes at stages in which there is little or no cell killing with the doses used (8,9). Thus, the dose-rate effect appears to be a true intracellular phenomenon. It is deduced that repair of mutational or premutational damage is occurring at low dose rates, but that the repair process is either damaged or saturated at high dose rates.

We have explored extensively an alternative hypothesis which would avoid invoking any damage or saturation of the repair process. On this hypothesis, the specific-locus mutations are assumed to be predominantly a result of two independent events, such as chromosome breaks leading to a deficiency, caused by separate ionization tracks. Various pieces of evidence taken as a whole seem to argue strongly against this (1,3,4). Even the specific-locus mutations that proved to be deficiencies appear to be produced predominantly by single ionization tracks (4). On either hypothesis, of course, the dose-rate effect is explained in terms of repair.

Further exploration of the dose-rate effect in spermatogonia revealed that, as the dose rate is lowered, a plateau is soon reached, at 0.8 R/min, below which further reduction in dose rate, even to 0.001 R/min, gives no further reduction in mutation frequency (8). In oocytes, on the other hand, mutation frequency continues to drop with lowering dose rate, and at the lowest dose rate tested in females, 0.009 R/min, the mutation frequency is not significantly higher than the control value (8).

This surprising difference in response of the two sexes, with the female showing an apparently greater capacity for repair of mutational or premutational damage than the male, is not yet understood. It could have a simple biological explanation related to the fact that the spermatogonia represent a mitotically dividing cell population, while the oocytes are all in an arrested stage. Perhaps there is a stage in the mitotic cycle when repair of damage cannot occur. If so, then, since there will always be a certain proportion of the spermatogonia in that stage, the mutational damage occurring there may be the irreducible minimum mutation frequency that is observed regardless of how far the dose rate is lowered (10).

The possibility was tested that repair might occur even at high dose rates provided the total dose is small enough to avoid damaging or saturating the repair system. It was found, in females, that a dose of 50 R at the high dose rate of 90 R/min gave significantly fewer mutations than expected on a linearly proportional basis with the results from 400 R (3). Additional evidence for the conclusion that repair can occur at the 50 R level even with high-dose-rate irradiation came from another experiment with 90 R/min irradiation in which eight fractions of 50 R, spaced 75 min apart, yielded a significantly lower mutation frequency than that obtained from a single exposure of 400 R (3).

The question of whether or not the specific-locus mutations that are still observed at low dose rates in spermatogonia represent a type of mutational damage that is qualitatively incapable of being repaired was explored by looking for changes in the relative frequencies of mutations at the seven loci used in our experiments. The pattern, or spectrum, of relative frequencies does change when mutations in different germ-cell stages and types, such as spermatogonia, spermatozoa and oocytes, are compared. The changes are related to qualitative differences in the types of mutations produced. However, within the spermatogonial stage, the spectrum of relative mutation frequencies is the same at low and high dose rates, in spite of the much lower absolute mutation frequency at the low dose rates (1). This suggests that the unrepaired mutations at low dose rates are not qualitatively different from the reparable ones. It would appear that nonrepair of a mutation induced in spermatogonia at low radiation dose rate may depend on probability rather than on any uniqueness in the type of lesion involved.

In oocytes, where repair seems to be virtually complete at the lowest dose rate of gamma rays tested, it seems unlikely that there is any large class of gamma-ray induced mutations that is irreparable.

Another phenomenon observed in females may be related to repair capacity. This is the astounding drop in mutation frequency observed, even with high-dose-rate irradiation, for conceptions occurring at intervals longer than six or seven weeks after ir-radiation. The mutation frequencies are zero or near zero, and not significantly above controls, in all sets of data from these longer intervals (3,11,12). The effect could be due to mutational insensitivity of the oocyte stages from which these offspring are derived, to a greater capacity for repair in these stages, or to selective elimination of all mutation-bearing cells. The last possibility seems unlikely for various reasons; and Oakberg's find-ing (13) on the greater metabolic activity of these oocyte stages, compared with those which produce a high mutation frequency, gives some support to the view that a greater capacity for repair might be the responsible factor.

There are a few additional pieces of information that should be mentioned be-fore concluding this brief summary of what can be deduced about repair of mutational damage in the mouse. There is little or no dose-rate effect on mutations induced in spermatozoa (5). This fits in with the view that repair is more likely to take place in cells that are metabolically active: very little metabolism is going on in spermatozoa.

The findings with fission neutrons show no dose-rate effect on mutation induc-tion in spermatogonia (14). There is a statistically significant dose-rate effect in oocytes (11), but it is much smaller than that observed with X- and gamma rays. So there is some evidence for repair of neutron-induced mutations in females. The effect of the interval be-tween irradiation and conception is also very marked with neutrons (11), again indicating the possibility that repair may be operating.

In a paper presented eight years ago (1) I stated that "studies at the molecular level have not yet reached the point where predictions can be made about the effects on the mutation process of various factors such as dose rate, cell stage, radiation quality and so forth. Since the methods applicable to the mouse have revealed, and are continuing to reveal, the roles of such factors, it is clear that the results obtained by these methods should lead to deductions about the mutation process that are not yet attainable from studies at the molecular level." I concluded: "but there is, of course, a good prospect that the two approaches will meet at some points before long." This does not yet seem to have been achieved. One of the major obstacles may be the difficulty of chemically character-izing a rare event in a small number of cells. Some entirely new approaches at the chemi-cal level may be required.

It is appropriate to conclude this section on radiation mutagenesis with a re-sponse to Dr. Beers' request to apply what we have deduced about repair processes to the practical problems of maximum permissible levels of exposure. Since this has been done at considerable length in recent publications (12,15), only the major conclusions will be given here.

Results in spermatogonia argue strongly against there being, in males, a thres-hold dose rate below which no mutation would be observed. In females, there may be, if not an absolute threshold, at least an extremely low mutational response at low dose rates.

There is no obvious reason for rejecting the applicability of the mouse sperma-togonia results to man. In the female, it should be kept in mind that the mouse and human oocyte stages primarily at risk differ somewhat in cytological appearance and markedly in sensitivity to killing. However, there is no clear correlation between cell killing and mutational sensitivity in our data. Furthermore, dose rate and interval after irradiation both have a marked effect in the female mouse, and one or the other operates on oocyte stages covering a wide range of sensitivity to killing. The operation of either one of these, even without the other, in women would still give a reduced risk under most conditions of population exposure.

If the mouse results can be carried over to man, then the risk of genetic damage, at least for the types measured by the specific-locus method, appears to be considerably less, at low dose rates and small doses, than it was estimated to be when the standards were set, on the basis of results at high dose rate and large doses, for the maximum permissible levels of radiation. In the male, the reduction is to 30%; and in the female, the risk is reduced to near zero.

CHEMICAL MUTAGENESIS

Although there is little information on the chemical nature of the mutagenic effects of ionizing radiation, there is a considerable body of knowledge on what some chemical mutagens do to the DNA. This has led to predictions, based on the argument that "DNA is DNA, wherever found," that the mutagenic response of mammals to a chemical mutagen should parallel that of microorganisms, provided the active principle of the mutagen reaches the mammalian gonad. These predictions, however, were rash, as has been shown by the results of our attempts to induce specific-locus mutations in the mouse by means of alkylating agents. This work has provided some startling surprises. Three of these will be described here to show some of the complexities encountered in trying to relate chemical mutagenesis results in mammals not only to those in microorganisms, but even to results in Drosophila.

The first surprise has been reported briefly elsewhere (16,17). Four methanesulfonates, methyl (MMS), ethyl (EMS), n-propyl (PMS), and iso-propyl (IMS), and Myleran that had proved to be efficient producers of chromosome aberrations in the mouse (dominant lethals and, in some cases, translocations as well), turned out not to be effective in inducing specific-locus mutations. In fact, the low mutation frequencies obtained in spermatogonial stages with these five compounds were not significantly above control levels, whereas the dominant lethal and translocation frequencies induced by the same doses of the chemicals in postgonial stages were very high.

This finding is diametrically opposite to what was regarded as a general principle, derived from work on Drosophila, microorganisms and higher plants, namely, that EMS, and alkylating agents in general, differ from ionizing radiation in producing a relative shortage of chromosome rearrangements compared with gene mutations (18).

Our conclusion (17) that the mouse results refuted the generality of this principle was challenged by some investigators on the basis of the fact that the dominant lethal and translocation data were obtained from treated postspermatogonial cell stages, while most of the specific-locus mutation results came from treated spermatogonia. This criticism was not valid, because the specific-locus mutation data obtained from post-spermatogonial stages, although meagre, were, nevertheless, in themselves, extensive enough to show that even the upper confidence limit of the mutation frequencies was relatively low compared with the chromosome aberration frequencies.

Further support for this conclusion comes from additional data collected in our laboratory during the past year on specific-locus mutations induced by EMS in post-spermatogonial stages. A total of six presumed specific-locus mutations was observed in 10,941 offspring from cells that were in postspermatogonial stages at the time of treatment with EMS. The mutation frequency is highly statistically significantly above the spontaneous mutation frequency, showing that the chemical can produce specific-locus mutations in postspermatogonial stages. However, this induced frequency of specific-locus mutations is less than one fifth of what would have been expected if EMS had produced the same ratio of specific-locus mutations to dominant lethals that is produced by X-rays. As has already been emphasized, this departure from X-ray results is in the opposite direction to that reported for EMS in Drosophila.

A second surprise that arose from the specific-locus mutation studies with the alkylating agents was the discovery that the ratio of the mutation frequency in spermatogonia to that in postspermatogonial stages was extremely low, much lower than that observed with ionizing radiation. No precise figure can be attached to the ratio at the present time, because, as has already been mentioned, the low specific-locus mutation frequencies obtained in spermatogonial stages from the four methane sulfonates and Myleran are not statistically significantly above the control level (17). If, however, the small, and statistically insignificant, excess over the control is taken as real, the mean mutation rate for the five compounds in spermatogonia is only approximately one twentieth of the rate in postspermatogonial stages. The true value could, of course, be much lower than that, even zero. The ratio must also be very low in the results obtained with tri-ethylenemelamine (TEM) in our laboratory by Cattanach (19). Here the actual ratio is somewhat in question because the doses used were quite different for the gonial and postgonial data. However, assuming a linear response with dose, and ignoring the spontaneous mutation rate, Cattanach gives the specific-locus mutation rates as 1.59×10^{-5} and 125.98×10^{-5} per mg/kg/locus for spermatogonial and postspermatogonial stages, respectively. This is a ratio of 1 to 79. If he had subtracted the spontaneous mutation rate obtained by us over a period of years, the ratio would have been 1 to 93.

With ionizing radiation, the ratio of spermatogonial to postspermatogonial mutation frequencies is not as low, being one half for acute irradiation and approximately one sixth for chronic.

In this case, the departure of the chemical mutagenesis results from the radiation ones appears to be in the same direction as that observed in Drosophila. The Fahmys (20) and Jenkins (21) have both reported that EMS-induced mutation frequencies in premeiotic stages are very low compared with those in postmeiotic stages.

The third surprise from the specific-locus mutation studies, like the first, reveals a marked difference between mouse and Drosophila results. Since EMS in the mouse gave a low ratio of specific-locus mutations to chromosome aberrations, compared with

Drosophila, there was a tendency to jump to the conclusion that, compared to Drosophila, the mouse must be insensitive to specific-locus mutation induction by EMS. Before making any such comparison, however, one must consider the important factor of dosage. Until recently, there was no valid information for comparing dosages between the two species. Now, however, Cumming's group, in our laboratory, is measuring EMS-induced ethylations per sperm head in the mouse (22), and Sega et al have done the same in Drosophila (23). More precision will be added to the comparison as the work continues, but it is already clear that, on the basis of number of ethylations per nucleotide, the mouse is about two orders of magnitude more sensitive than Drosophila to specific-locus mutation induction by EMS in postspermatogonial stages. Another point that is clear is that the number of ethylations per gene is vastly (orders of magnitude) in excess of the mutation rate.

It should be kept in mind that the findings presented here are based on a limited number of loci, that they may apply only to certain groups of chemicals, and that they were derived from tests involving only a narrow range of doses. Nevertheless, they have uncovered some of the unexpected complexities of chemical mutagenesis in mammals, a field that was already replete with expected complexities.

It is probably too early to speculate, except at the tentative working hypothesis level, on the details of the mechanisms involved. In a broad sense, however, it would seem likely that an effective repair system may play a major role. This could account for the low, or zero, specific-locus mutation frequency observed in spermatogonia following treatment with EMS. Since these cells are apparently able to repair genetic damage from ionizing radiation delivered at low dose rate, it is not unreasonable to suppose that they can repair some chemically-induced damage.

The possibility also exists that the extremely high frequency of chromosome aberrations, relative to specific-locus mutations, induced by alkylating agents in the mouse may be an indirect result of attempted repair. Thus, Cumming and Walton (24) speculate that chromosome breakage may be due to simultaneous excision of proximate alkylations in opposite strands of the DNA double helix by excision enzymes of the mammalian repair system.

It would appear, however, that we are still a long way from elucidating the actual processes involved in mammalian mutation and repair even with simple chemicals. The results I have discussed here have emphasized that findings in microorganisms, and even in organisms as highly evolved as Drosophila, may have little predictive value as to what to expect in the mouse. Here we have been dealing not with the complexities expected at the pharmacological level, but with differences in response between mouse and nonmammalian organisms after the active chemical principle has reached the germ cells.

Again, as in radiation mutagenesis, the very fact that much of the information obtained on mammalian chemical mutagenesis was not predictable from what is known at the molecular level, should make that information useful for guiding new approaches in molecular biology.

REFERENCES

1. Russell, W. L.: Evidence from mice concerning the nature of the mutation process. In: Genetics Today, Proc. XI Int. Congr. Genet. Edited by S. J. Geerts, Pergamon Press, Oxford, pp 257-264, 1964.

2. Russell, W. L.: The nature of the dose-rate effect of radiation on mutation in mice. Suppl., Jap. J. Genet., 40:128, 1965.

3. Russell, W. L.: Repair mechanisms in radiation mutation induction in the mouse. Brookhaven Sympos. Biol., 20:179, 1968.

4. Russell, W. L.: Observed mutation frequency in mice and the chain of processes affecting it. In: Mutation as Cellular Process (Ciba Foundation Symp.). Edited by G. E. W. Wolstenholme and Maeve O'Connor. J. & A. Churchill, London, pp 216-228, 1969.

5. Russell, W. L., Russell, Liane Brauch and Kelly, Elizabeth M.: Radiation dose rate and mutation frequency. Science, 128(3338):1546, 1958.

6. Russell, W. L., Russell, Liane Brauch and Kelly, Elizabeth M.: Dependence of mutation rate on radiation intensity. (Symp. on Immediate and Low Level Effects of Ionizing Radiation, Venice, 1959). Int. J. Radiat. Biol., Suppl., 311, 1960.

7. Russell, W. L.: Effect of radiation dose rate on mutation in mice. J. Cell. Comp. Physiol., 58, Suppl. 1:183, 1961.

8. Russell, W. L.: The effect of radiation dose rate and fractionation on mutation in mice. In: Repair from Genetic Radiation Damage. Edited by F. Sobels. Pergamon Press, Oxford, pp 205-217, 1963.

9. Russell, W. L., Russell, Liane Brauch and Cupp, Mary B.: Dependence of mutation frequency on radiation dose rate in female mice. Proc. Nat. Acad. Sci. USA, 45:18, 1959.

10. Russell, W. L.: Factors that affect the radiation induction of mutations in the mouse. An. Acad. Brasileira de Ciencias, 39:65, 1967.

11. Russell, W. L.: Effect of the interval between irradiation and conception on mutation frequency in female mice. Proc. Nat. Acad. Sci. USA, 54:1552, 1965.

12. Russell, W. L.: The genetic effects of radiation. Proc. Fourth Int. Conf. on the Peaceful Uses of Atomic Energy, Geneva, Sept. 6-16, 1971. In press.

13. Oakberg, E. F.: ^{3}H-uridine labeling of mouse oocytes. Arch. Anat. Micr. Morph. Exp., 56: Suppl., p 171, 1967.

14. Russell, W. L.: Studies in mammalian radiation genetics. Nucleonics, 23:53, 1965.

15. Russell, W. L.: Mutagenesis in the mouse and its application to the estimation of the genetic hazards of radiation. Proc. IVth Int. Congr. Radiat. Res., Evian, France, June 29-July 4, 1970. In press.

16. Ehling, U. H. and Russell, W. L.: Induction of specific locus mutations by alkyl methanesulfonates in male mice. Genetics, 61:s14, 1969.

17. Russell, W. L., Huff, Sandra W. and Gottlieb, Dorma J.: The insignificant rate of induction of specific-locus mutations by five alkylating agents that produce high incidences of dominant lethality. Biol. Div. Ann. Prog. Rep., December 31, 1969, ORNL-4535, p 122.

18. Auerbach, C.: The chemical production of mutation. Science, 158:1141, 1967.

19. Cattanach, B. M.: Induction of paternal sex-chromosome losses and deletions and of autosomal gene mutations by the treatment of mouse post-meiotic germ cells with triethylenemelamine. Mutat. Res., 4:73, 1967.

20. Fahmy, O. G. and Fahmy, M. J.: Mutagenic response to the alkyl-methane-sulphonates during spermatogenesis in Drosophila melanogaster. Nature, 180:31, 1957.

21. Jenkins, J. B.: Mutagenesis at a complex locus in Drosophila with the monofunctional alkylating agent, ethyl methanesulfonate. Genetics, 57:783, 1967.

22. Walton, Marva F. and Cumming, R. B.: Quantitative measurement of EMS ethylation of mouse sperm DNA in vitro. Genetics, 68:s73, 1971.

23. Sega, G. A., Gee, Patricia A. and Lee, W. R.: Dosimetry of a chemical mutagen in terms of alkylation of DNA per gamete. Genetics, 68:s60, 1971.

24. Cumming, R. B. and Walton, Marva F.: Fate and metabolism of some mutagenic alkylating agents in the mouse. I. Ethyl methanesulfonate and methyl methanesulfonate at sublethal dose in hyrbid males. Mutat. Res., 10:365, 1970.

EFFECT OF ULTRAVIOLET LIGHT AND A POTENT CARCINOGEN, 4-NITROQUINOLINE 1-OXIDE, ON MAMMALIAN CELLS AND THEIR SENDAI VIRUS CARRIER CULTURES[1]

Nobuto Yamamoto, Osayuki Morita and Tsugio Satoh

Fels Research Institute and Department of Microbiology
Temple University School of Medicine
Philadelphia, Pennsylvania

A potent carcinogen 4-nitroquinoline 1-oxide (4NQO) inactivates bacteria and induces a prophage. We isolated many 4NQO-sensitive mutants of Salmonella typhimurium and found that all the 4NQO-sensitive mutants were extremely sensitive to ultraviolet light (UV) and subdivided into the two groups: host cell reactivation minus (hcr⁻) mutants lacking repair activity for UV-damaged infecting phage and recombination deficient (rec⁻) mutants (8). Furthermore, UV-sensitive bacterial mutants were also found to be sensitive to 4NQO (3,8). The above finding suggests that 4NQO or its metabolic intermediates reacted with bacterial genome, resulting in the damage of DNA, and that the damaged bacterial DNA was reparable by the same mechanism as UV-damaged DNA (8).

In this presentation, we described studies on DNA repair in HeLa and human osteosarcoma cell lines, and their carrier cultures containing Sendai virus. Not only cellular DNA repair but also that of herpes simplex virus as a foreign DNA was investigated.

MATERIALS AND METHODS

Mammalian Cell Cultures:

Sendai virus is a parainfluenza virus type 1 and previously designated Hemagglutinating virus of Japan (HVJ) (5). Infection of HeLa cells and human osteosarcoma with HVJ causes cytopathic effect but virus does not multiply. HeLa cells and osteosarcoma G2 cells surviving after HVJ infection have been established as carrier cultures, HeLa (HVJ) (4) and G2 (HVJ) (6), capable of releasing noninfectious hemagglutinin. The cell cultures were grown in Eagle's basal medium containing 2-fold amino acids and vitamins, supplemented with 10% calf serum (growth medium). For cell inactivation experiments, cell cultures were trypsinized, inoculated in plastic Petri dishes (60 mm diameter) at a density of 1×10^4 cells per plate and incubated at $37°C$ in 5% CO_2 incubator. After 24 hr incubation cells attached to Petri dish were washed twice with prewarmed phosphate buffered saline (PBS) and then exposed to 4NQO or UV.

[1] Supported in part by grants NIH (AI-06429) from the National Institutes of Health, U.S. Public Health Service and NSF (GB-25098) from the National Science Foundation.

Treatment of Cell Cultures with 4NQO:

The cells attached to Petri dishes were incubated in PBS containing various concentrations of 4NQO for appropriate periods at 37°C in a CO_2 incubator. The 4NQO-treated cells were washed twice with Eagle's medium and incubated further with growth medium. The number of colonies formed after seven days of incubation served as the measure of cell inactivation.

UV-Irradiation of Cell Culture and Virus:

UV-irradiation was performed with a 8-Watt discharge bulb, 12 inches long x 5/8 inch diameter. The lamp was fixed at a distance of 15 inches above the diluted suspension (10^6 PFU/ml in PBS) of a purified virus stock to be irradiated. The intensity of UV at this distance was 21 ergs/mm^2/sec. UV-irradiation on virus was carried out with shaking, in a glass dish in which the liquid level did not exceed 1.0 mm. During irradiation, 0.05 ml samples periodically were withdrawn by pipette and diluted 20-fold in Eagle's medium. Samples were diluted further, and 0.5 ml aliquots of each diluted sample were inoculated onto monolayers of HeLa and HeLa (HVJ) cells grown in Petri dishes. After 3 hrs of absorption, cells were overlaid with 1% Noble agar containing Medium-199 supplemented with 2% calf serum, and incubated in a CO_2 incubator at 37°C. On the fourth day after infection, a secondary overlay agar containing 1:30,000 neutral red was applied. The number of plaques following 24 hr incubation at 37°C served as the measure of inactivation. To determine UV-sensitivity of cells, media were discarded and 10^4 cells seeded 24 hrs previously were exposed to UV at the intensity of 2 ergs/mm^2/sec obtained by partially covering the bulb. Then growth medium was added. On the seventh day after UV-exposure the number of colonies was counted as in the case of 4NQO-treatment.

RESULTS

4 NQO-Sensitivities of HeLa and HeLa (HVJ) Cells:

When HeLa and HeLa (HVJ) cells were treated with 4NQO at a concentration of 2 x 10^{-7}M for various lengths of time at 37°C, rapid inactivation of colony-forming ability of these cells was observed. As shown in Figure 1 the inactivation of both cell types follows a first order kinetics after short lag period. The number of colonies of HeLa (HVJ) cells was consistently higher than that of HeLa cells at any given exposure period. When HeLa and HeLa (HVJ) cells were incubated with various concentrations of 4NQO for 1 hr at 37°C, it was observed that colony-forming ability decreased as 4NQO concentration increased and HeLa cells were more sensitive to 4NQO than HeLa (HVJ) cells (Fig 2). Since the 4NQO-damaged bacterial DNA is reparable by the same mechanism as UV-damaged DNA (8), HeLa (HVJ) cells may carry more repair activity of 4NQO-damaged genome than HeLa cells.

Mammalian (7) and bacterial (2) cells contain an activating enzyme, namely diaphorase, which converts 4NQO to 4-hydroxylaminoquinoline 1-oxide (4HAQO). 4HAQO damages naked DNA and inactivates bacteriophage genomes, whereas 4NQO does not. Thus, 4NQO-sensitivity of cells may depend on diaphorase activity levels in cell

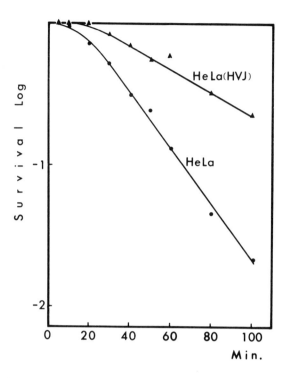

Fig 1. Inactivation kinetics of HeLa and HeLa (HVJ) cells by 4NQO at a concentration of 2×10^{-7}M.

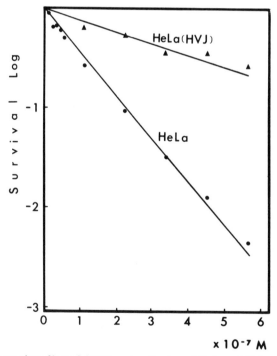

Fig 2. Concentration effect of 4NQO on inactivation of HeLa and HeLa (HVJ) cells.

cultures. However, we found no difference in diaphorase activity in both HeLa and HeLa (HVJ) cell cultures. Furthermore, we found that 4HAQO-sensitivity of these cell cultures was similar to their 4NQO-sensitivity: HeLa (HVJ) was more resistant to 4HAQO than HeLa. This observation may support the hypothesis that HeLa (HVJ) cells are more active in repairing the damaged genomes than HeLa cells.

UV-Sensitivities of HeLa and HeLa (HVJ) Cells:

UV-sensitivity of the cells was investigated in order to eliminate the possibility that permeability might be a rate-limiting factor for inactivation by 4NQO. As shown in Figure 3, HeLa cells are far more sensitive to UV than HeLa (HVJ) cells proving that HeLa (HVJ) cells contain higher repair activity than HeLa cells. From the results shown in Figure 3, HeLa (HVJ) cells are calculated to be about three times more resistant than HeLa cells.

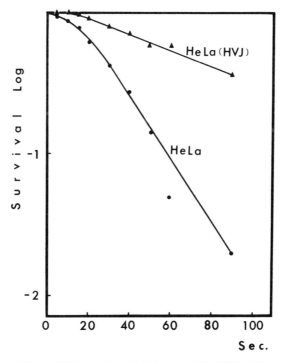

Fig 3. UV-inactivation of HeLa and HeLa (HVJ) cells.

Inactivation Kinetics of Herpes Simplex Virus by Ultraviolet Light and Repair by Host Cells:

It is of interest to test reparability of damaged foreign DNA in these cells. When UV-treated herpes simplex virus was assayed simultaneously on HeLa and HeLa (HVJ) cells, survivors of herpes simplex virus observed by plaque formation on HeLa (HVJ) cells were much higher than those on HeLa cells (Fig 4). Thus, this is a crucial evidence that HeLa (HVJ) cells carry more repair activity than HeLa cells.

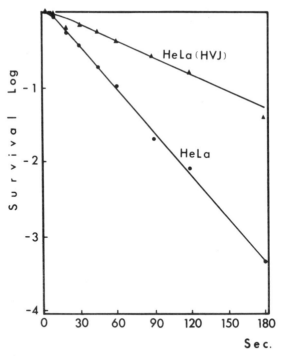

Fig 4. UV-inactivation kinetics of herpes simplex virus observed by plaque formation on HeLa and HeLa (HVJ) cell cultures.

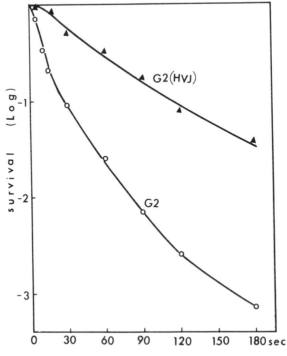

Fig 5. UV-inactivation kinetics of herpes simplex virus observed by plaque formation on a human osteosarcoma cell culture G2 and its carrier culture G2 (HVJ).

We extended this type of study to a human osteosarcoma cell culture G2 and its carrier culture G2 (HVJ). As shown in Figure 5, G2 (HVJ) cells were more active in repairing UV-damaged herpes simplex virus than G2 cells (6).

DISCUSSION

Since UV-damaged herpes simplex virus as a foreign DNA is repaired more efficiently by the carrier cultures than by parent wild type cell cultures, it is evident that the mammalian cells carry the DNA repair mechanism. However, since Sendai virus is an RNA virus, there is no suggestive mechanism for the enhancement of DNA repair activity by establishment of the carrier culture.

Herpes simplex viral DNA replicates in nucleus whereas vaccinia virus replicates in cytoplasm. When vaccinia virus was exposed to UV and assayed simultaneously on HeLa and HeLa (HVJ) cultures, no significant difference in inactivation kinetics curves on these cell cultures was observed. Thus, the enhanced DNA repair activity seems to be located in nucleus.

From the data presented in this paper, the evidence is clear that the repair mechanism of mammalian cells can repair both UV- and 4NQO-damaged DNA. This is a situation analogous to the finding that the bacterial dark repair mechanism for UV-damaged genome can also repair 4NQO-damaged genome (8).

REFERENCES

1. Endo, H., Ishizawa, M. and Kamiya, T.: Induction of bacteriophage formation in lysogenic bacteria by a potent carcinogen, 4-nitroquinoline 1-oxide and its derivatives. Nature, 198:195-196, 1963.
2. Fukuda, S. and Yamamoto, N.: Search for activating enzymes for proximal carcinogens using microbial assay systems. Proceedings of the American Association for Cancer Research, 12:42, 1971.
3. Kondo, S. and Kato, T.: Photoreactivation of mutation and killing in Escherichia coli. Advances Biol. Med. Phys., 12:283-298, 1968.
4. Maeno, K., Yoshii, S., Nagata, I. and Matsumoto, T.: Growth of Newcastle disease virus in a HVJ carrier culture of HeLa cells. Virology, 29:255-263, 1966.
5. Matsumoto, T., Yamamoto, N. and Maeno, K.: Effect of egg passage on the reaction between HVJ (haemagglutinating virus of Japan) and chicken erythrocytes. J. Immunol., 87:590-598, 1961.
6. Hatano, M., Morita, O., Satoh, T. and Yamamoto, N.: Repair of UV-damaged foreign DNA in mammalian cells, and their carrier culture. In preparation.
7. Sugimura, T., Okabe, K. and Nagao, M.: The metabolism of 4-nitroquinoline 1-oxide, a carcinogen. III. An enzyme catalizing the conversion of 4-nitroquinoline 1-oxide to 4-hydroxyaminoquinoline 1-oxide in rat liver and hepatomas. Cancer Res., 26:1717-1721, 1966.
8. Yamamoto, N., Fukuda, S. and Takebe, H.: Effect of a potent carcinogen, 4-nitroquinoline 1-oxide, and its reduced form, 4-hydroxylaminoquinoline 1-oxide, on bacterial and bacteriophage genomes. Cancer Res., 30:2532-2537, 1970.

THE ISOLATION AND PARTIAL CHARACTERIZATION OF AGE-CORRELATED OLIGO-DEOXYRIBO-RIBO-NUCLEOTIDES WITH COVALENTLY LINKED ASPARTYL-GLUTAMYL POLYPEPTIDES

P. V. N. Acharya

Bjorksten Research Foundation
Madison, Wisconsin

INTRODUCTION

In response to a variety of damages to DNA, existing repair processes may become operative. In many cases these processes seem adequate to repair the damage. However, one condition that appears to elude all known repair mechanisms is apparent damage from natural aging. Quite likely such damage, interalia, may explain the fundamental cause of aging. Just as aging is an irreversible phenomenon, so the damage to DNA due to aging becomes irreparable. Our interest is to study this irreparable damage and correlate it with the phenomenon of aging.

Since age-damaged DNA molecules have eluded all repair mechanisms, they may tend to accumulate in the cells, with increasing age. In order to trace such molecules we tritiated mother rats and examined some vital organs of their offspring at different age levels.

METHODOLOGY

Two mother rats were fed tritium in the form of 40 mc of ^{3}H-sodium acetate and 8 mc of ^{3}H-Lysine respectively.

The liver and brain of two of the offspring (621-day-old male rat A and 493-day-old male rat B) of the former, and the liver of one of the offspring (363-day-old female rat C) of the latter were examined. Their tissues were thoroughly extracted with 0.9% saline solution, acetone, $CHCl_3$:MeOH, treated with pronase, trypsin and pepsin, and the residues subjected to three successive degradations with 0.6N $HClO_4$ in cold 0.3N KOH at 37°C for 1 hour and 0.3N KOH at 37°C for 5 hours, according to the procedure of Fleck and Begg (1).

The detailed procedures concerning purification and analysis will be published elsewhere (2). The paper deals with the same class of compounds obtained by acid treatment of the residues remaining after the alkali treatment discussed in this paper. However, the procedures of purification and analysis are identical.

RESULTS

All the three steps of the Fleck and Begg degradative procedure yielded mixtures of oligo-nucleo-peptides and peptides of both high and low molecular weight. However, in the case of the brain of 493-day-old rat B and the liver of 621-day-old rat A, the oligo-nucleo-peptides were of both high molecular weight and low molecular weight, whereas in the case of the liver of 363-day-old rat C, only low molecular weight oligo-nucleo-peptides were obtained. The high molecular weight fractions in this case were only peptides.

The DEAE-cellulose column chromatography further resolved these high molecular and low molecular weight fractions into oligo-nucleo-peptides and peptides in their respective molecular weight categories (Fig 1).

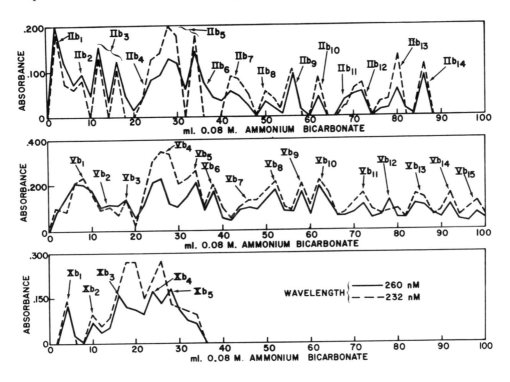

Fig 1. DEAE-Cellulose anion exchange column chromatography of low molecular weight fraction obtained from the insoluble residues of the brain of rat B, the liver of rat A, and the liver of 363-day-old rat C, by treatment with 0.3N KOH at 37°C for 1 hour. Peaks IIb_1, IIb_2, IIb_3, IIb_4, IIb_5, IIb_6, IIb_9, IIb_{11}, IIb_{12}, IIb_{14} represent low molecular weight oligo-nucleo-peptides, and peaks IIb_7, IIb_8, IIb_{10}, IIb_{13} represent low molecular peptides from rat B. Peaks Vb_1, Vb_2, Vb_3, Vb_5, Vb_6, Vb_7 ... Vb_{15} represent low molecular weight oligo-nucleo-peptides, and peak Vb_4 represents a low molecular weight peptide from the liver of rat A. Peaks Xb_1, Xb_2, Xb_3, Xb_5 represent low molecular weight oligo-nucleo-peptides, and Xb_4 a low molecular weight peptide, from the organ of rat C.

Figure 2 shows that the low mol wt fraction obtained from the brain of 493-day-old rat B after treatment with 0.3N KOH at 37°C for 1 hour was resolved into 10 oligo-nucleo-peptides and 4 peptides. An almost identical pattern of resolution emerged for the low mol wt fraction obtained from the liver of 621-day-old rat A, consisting of 14 oligo-nucleo-peptides and one peptide. The low mol wt fraction obtained from the liver of

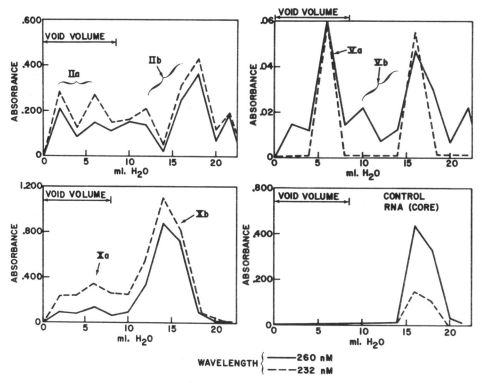

Fig 2. Gel filtration on Seph. G-75 of the substances obtained by treatment of the insoluble sub-stances (remaining insoluble after treatment with cold 0.6N $HClO_4$) from the brain of 493-day-old rat B, liver of 621-day-old rat A, and the liver of 363-day-old rat C, with 0.3N KOH at 37°C for 1 hour. Peaks IIa and Va represent mixtures of high molecular oligo-nucleo-peptides and peptides from rats B and A respectively, while peak Xa represents a mixture of high molecular weight peptides from rat C. Peaks IIb, Vb and Xb represent mixtures of low molecular weight oligo-nucleo-peptides and peptides from rats B, A, and C respectively. Oligo-ribo-nucleotides obtained from RNA (Core) using this procedure were only of low molecular weight as can be seen from the peak at bottom right of the figure.

363-day-old rat C resolved into no more than 4 oligo-nucleo-peptides and one peptide. This shows that with an increase in age, the oligo-nucleo-peptides in question not only in-crease in molecular size as observed earlier, but also increase in their quantity.

As for the homogeniety of the oligo-nucleo-peptide fractions, we have only three cases of evidence. When adsorbed on activated charcoal and eluted on a cellulose column there was no separation. When subjected to paper electrophoresis all moved towards anode as single large spots. On paper chromatography, too, they moved as single spots.

The ultraviolet spectra of some of these oligo-nucleo-peptides are seen in Figure 3, which shows that they share the characteristics of both oligo-nucleotides and peptides.

In Table I we see ribose, deoxyribose, and amino acids. Of the eight high mol wt fractions examined from older animals, five revealed aspartic and glutamic acids (three

TABLE I

Composition of Some Oligo-Nucleo-Peptides Obtained From the Organs of Rats of Different Age Levels: Expressed in nM

TABLE I

Composition of Some Oligo-Nucleo-Peptides Obtained From the
Organs of Rats of Different Age Levels: Expressed in nM

Code	Oligo-Nucleo-Peptide	$\frac{\text{A 232 nm}}{\text{A 260 nm}}$ at pH 6.5	Bases	Deoxy-ribose	Ribose	Phos-phorus	Asp. acid	Glut. acid	Neutral amino-acids
	Obtained by cold 0.6N HClO$_4$								
Ia$_1$	High mol. wt. fraction: Brain of 493 day old rat	1.3	322	225	483	288	nil	nil	Too low to be determined
Ia$_2$	High mol. wt. fraction: Brain of 493 day old rat	1.2	805	1016	357	188	nil	140	"
Ib$_1$	Low mol. wt. fraction: Brain of 493 day old rat	1.03	712	1479	638	456	89	30	"
IVa$_1$	High mol. wt. fraction: Liver of 621 day old rat	0.4	309	242	448	317	nil	nil	"
IVb$_4$	Low mol. wt. fraction: Liver of 621 day old rat	0.65	718	747	1116	312	72	111	"
IVb$_6$	Low mol. wt. fraction: Liver of 621 day old rat	1.1	152	485	1089	353	53	53	"
IXb$_3$	Low mol. wt. fraction: Liver of 363 day old rat	1.08	823	570	957	395	135	137	"
	Obtained by 0.3N KOH, 37°C, 1 hour								
IIa$_1$	High mol. wt. fraction: Brain of 493 day old rat	0.89	563	1681	560	300	74	30	"
IIb$_{14}$	Low mol. wt. fraction: Brain of 493 day old rat	1.2	28	404	350	108	nil	nil	"
Va$_1$	High mol. wt. fraction: Liver of 621 day old rat	0.69	700	364	520	390	nil	nil	"
Vb$_3$	Low mol. wt. fraction: Liver of 621 day old rat	0.9	154	404	560	235	nil	nil	"
Vb$_4$	Low mol. wt. fraction: Liver of 621 day old rat	0.7	47	175	315	180	nil	nil	"
Xb$_1$	Low mol. wt. fraction: Liver of 363 day old rat	0.64	382	0	323	190	nil	57	"
	Obtained by 0.3N KOH, 37°C, 5 hours								
IIIa$_1$	High mol. wt. fraction: Brain of 493 day old rat	0.56	213	323	273	377	nil	133	"
IIIa$_2$	High mol. wt. fraction: Brain of 493 day old rat	0.5	1000	349	476	400	43	78	"
IIIb$_2$	Low mol. wt. fraction: Brain of 493 day old rat	1.2	277	396	238	190	38	96	"
VIa$_3$	High mol. wt. fraction: Liver of 621 day old rat	1.2	160	109	130	169	58	51	"
VIb$_6$	Low mol. wt. fraction: Liver of 621 day old rat	1.2	124	214	147	84	nil	150	"
XIb$_1$	Low mol. wt. fraction: Liver of 363 day old rat	0.9	258	466	352	233	nil	nil	"
XIb$_2$	Low mol. wt. fraction: Liver of 363 day old rat	0.7	563	213	393	301	nil	nil	"

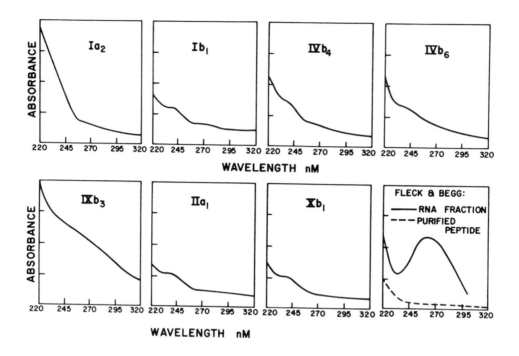

Fig 3. U.V. absorption spectra of some of the oligo-nucleo-peptides, from 320 nm to 220 nm as read on a Beckman Spectrophotometer at pH 1. Spectra for RNA and peptide as reported by Fleck and Begg have been presented for comparison. The spectra of the oligo-nucleo-peptides share the characteristics of both the RNA fraction and the peptide. Ia_2, Ib_1 are the high and low molecular weight fractions from the brain of 493-day-old rat B obtained by treatment with cold 0.6N $HClO_4$; IIa_1 is the high molecular weight fraction from the same tissue obtained by treatment with 0.3N KOH at $37^{\circ}C$ for 1 hour. IVb_4, IVb_6 are the low molecular weight fractions obtained from the liver of 621-day-old rat A by treatment with cold 0.6N $HClO_4$ and IXb_3 and Xb_1 are the low molecular weight fractions obtained from the liver of 363-day-old rat C by treatment with cold 0.6N $HClO_4$ and 0.3N KOH at $37^{\circ}C$ for 1 hour respectively. Even though fraction Xb_1 has no aspartic and glutamic acids, its spectrum is similar to others (e.g.) IIa_1, Ib_1 which contain these amino acids. This indicates that there were other neutral amino acids in this fraction which we did not isolate.

revealed both and two only glutamic acid). In contrast, of the 4 low mol wt fractions studied from the youngest animal, only one had both amino acids, and one had glutamic acid. Amino acids, especially aspartic and glutamic acids, apparently play important roles in progressive linking of DNA to RNA with increasing age.

We see in Table II that the ratios of deoxyribose to ribose in the fractions of older animals range from 0.6 to 3 (particularly so in high mol wt fractions) and in the case of the youngest animal, these ratios range from 0.54 to 1.32. In one of these fractions there was no deoxyribose at all. This implies that with the increase in age more and more DNA becomes linked with RNA and the molecules thus formed increase in size.

TABLE II

Molar Ratios of the Components in the Oligo-Nucleic-Peptides Obtained From the Rats of Different Age Levels and Their Tritium Activity

TABLE II

Molar Ratios of the Components in the Oligo-Nucleic-Peptides Obtained
From the Rats of Different Age Levels and Their Tritium Activity

Code	Oligo-Nucleo-Peptide	Deoxyribose to ribose	Total sugars to bases	Phosphorus to bases	Total sugars to amino-acids	DPM
	Obtained by cold 0.5N HClO$_4$					
Ia$_1$	High mol. wt. fraction: Brain of 493 day old rat	0.47	2.2	0.90	--	110
Ia$_2$	High mol. wt. fraction: Brain of 493 day old rat	2.8	1.7	0.23	9.8	115
Ib$_1$	Low mol. wt. fraction: Brain of 493 day old rat	2.3	3.0	0.44	17.8	--
IVa$_1$	High mol. wt. fraction: Liver of 621 day old rat	0.54	2.2	1.02	--	75
IVb$_4$	Low mol. wt. fraction: Liver of 621 day old rat	0.67	2.6	0.43	10.2	125
IVb$_6$	Low mol. wt. fraction: Liver of 621 day old rat	0.45	10.4	2.3	14.8	20
IXb$_3$	Low mol. wt. fraction: Liver of 363 day old rat	0.60	1.9	0.48	5.6	170
	Obtained by 0.3N KOH, 37°C, 1 hour					
IIa$_1$	High mol. wt. fraction: Brain of 493 day old rat	3.0	4.0	0.53	21.5	60
IIb$_{14}$	High mol. wt. fraction: Brain of 493 day old rat	1.1	27	3.9	--	80
Va$_1$	High mol. wt. fraction: Liver of 621 day old rat	0.7	1.3	0.56	--	125
Vb$_3$	Low mol. wt. fraction: Liver of 621 day old rat	0.70	6.2	1.5	--	--
Vb$_4$	Low mol. wt. fraction: Liver of 621 day old rat	0.55	10.4	3.8	--	--
Xb$_1$	Low mol. wt. fraction: Liver of 363 day old rat	--	0.9	0.5	--	75
	Obtained by 0.3N KOH, 37°C, 5 hours					
IIIa$_1$	High mol. wt. fraction: Brain of 493 day old rat	1.2	2.8	1.7	4.5	--
IIIa$_2$	High mol. wt. fraction: Brain of 493 day old rat	0.73	0.82	0.4	6.8	40
IIIb$_2$	Low mol. wt. fraction: Brain of 493 day old rat	1.7	2.3	0.69	4.7	--
VIa$_3$	High mol. wt. fraction: Liver of 621 day old rat	0.84	1.5	1.0	2.2	--
VIb$_6$	Low mol. wt. fraction: Liver of 621 day old rat	1.45	2.9	0.68	2.4	15
XIb$_1$	Low mol. wt. fraction: Liver of 363 day old rat	1.32	3.2	0.9	--	120
XIb$_2$	Low mol. wt. fraction: Liver of 363 day old rat	0.54	1.1	0.53	--	20

CONCLUSIONS

The above results, though preliminary, indicate:

A. That there is a strong correlation between aging of mammalian cells and the formation of oligo-deoxyribo-ribo-nucleo-peptides which increase not only quantitatively but also in their molecular size as aging progresses.

B. As judged from their sugar to base ratios and base to phosphorus ratios (which deviate widely from unity) these molecular aggregates represent not merely a stock of "DNA-strand breaks" (3), but structurally modified strands of DNA bound to RNA through peptide bridges consisting mainly of aspartic and glutamic acids. The linking of DNA strands to RNA through this mechanism increases as aging progresses.

C. Since these substances carry at least some tritium activity, they have remained fixed in the cells from birth, having survived a lifetime of cellular metabolic processes, and are apparently immune to known repair processes.

D. Such age-induced damage to DNA apparently also immobilizes RNA. It may be that the concept of molecular repair, so far as it concerns the age-damaged cells, may have to undergo some modification.

E. The question of exact linkages involved in these compounds is a matter for further investigation. A good guess at this stage is that the peptide bridges have serine at both ends and form stable phospho-serine bonds at oligo-ribo-nucleotides on one end and oligo-deoxyribo-nucleotides on the other end.

ACKNOWLEDGMENTS

The author acknowledges the valuable technical assistance of Mr. Steve Ashman and the financial support rendered by Dr. John Bjorksten, President of Bjorksten Research Foundation.

REFERENCES

1. Fleck, A. and Begg, D.: The estimation of ribonucleic acid using ultra violet absorption measurements. Biochemica et Biophysica Acta, 108:333-339, 1965.
2. Acharya, P. V. M., Ashman, S. M. and Bjorksten, J.: Isolation and partial characterization of age-correlated oligo-deoxyribo-ribo-nucleo-peptides. Finska Kemists. Medd. In press.
3. Price, Gerald B., Modak, S. P. and Makindon, T.: Age associated changes in the DNA of mouse tissue. Science, 171:917-920, (March), 1971.

DISCUSSION

Dr. Howard-
Flanders

I'd like to ask Dr. John Roberts about the alkylation by the various agents that he was using in HeLa cells and other cell lines. Is the principal product in every case the methylguaninoadenine? How many products are there per event? Is it likely that other more complex products are responsible for any lethal effects that are observed?

Dr. Roberts

That is a very complicated area. The major products of alkylation with whatever agent one looks at is always 7-alkylguanine. It is becoming increasingly apparent that there are a large number of other minor products, which are being identified almost weekly. These can differ between two closely related products. It is now thought that the proportion of the minor part, 0,6-methylguanine, is greater in the case of nitrosmethylurea and nitrosomethyl nitroguanidine than it is with MNS. Loveless, on the basis of his mutagenic effects on T-2 phage, would argue that since he gets more mutations with MNU than he does with MNS, the mutagenic lesion in this case is the 0,6 moiety. I think we might even have to consider that this extra lesion is vital to the understanding of what I was talking about in mammalian cells, because the difference between methylating agents is more marked for those compounds which produce this 0,6 lesion. This repair mechanism would, therefore, seem to recognize this different lesion. This is the really essential point. But I think there are many other products being identified. The situation as far as alkylating products is concerned is getting complicated. The answer I gave applies only to the type of agent I was talking about. Other alkylating agents don't necessarily react predominately with the N-7 and this is true with bromomethyl-methylbenzanthracene product which I mentioned.

Dr. Howard-
Flanders

Is it then the case that 7-methylguanine, for example, is very well tolerated and in large numbers in cells which appear to be oblivious to its existence?

Dr. Roberts

I think this is true. Now to the second part of your question, the number of lethal events. We need to put in, it seems, 100 methyl groups to have the same cytotoxic effect as one crosslink. That gives one a measure of the relative effectiveness of the lesion, if it is an agent which reacts predominately to give the 7-methylguanine. This is true in the hamster cell; it is not true in the case of particularly sensitive HeLa cells. The methylation is much, much more effective. The difference between mustard gas and nitrosomethyl nitroguanine is less marked. This might well be due to the fact that the 0,6 lesion in these cells is not as effectively repaired as in the hamster cell.

Dr. Russell   I ran out of time and did not give the figures on the amount of ethylation in the Drosophila sperm and mouse sperm. For the mouse it works out, with the kind of dose we're using for our mutagenic studies, about .4 ethylations in the sperm heads for every 1,000 nucleotides. These rates are astronomically higher than the mutation rates with EMS. So that if you look at it in terms of ethylations, EMS is a fantastically ineffective mutagen. In other words, either there's a fantastic repair of the ethylations, or they are not involved in the mutation process. I wonder if you would care to comment on that.

Dr. Roberts   I would agree with that. I ran some calculations on the number. The absolute numbers of alkylations are in the hundreds of thousands. It's an innocuous event.

Dr. Beers   Dr. Russell was referring to the difficulties of correlating his approaches with those of the molecular biologist. In this field it seems to me as a result of discussions, particularly today, that there is a difficult problem even amongst those within molecular biology itself, regarding the test system organisms that are used to compare with other people's results. It seems to be coming out repeatedly that in trying to get some kind of uniform picture, hypothesis, or model of one or more repair mechanisms you are always up against the dilemma of knowing whether you can compare peanuts with apricots. I wonder if you care to comment on how this might be resolved, or if you think it may be resolved in the future.

Dr. Russell   It seems to me that we need some new approaches entirely at the molecular level. I would like to have some answer at the molecular level to account for this vast difference we get within the oocytes, between the oocytes in the early follicule stages and those in later. These are all in one cytologically identified stage. Yet, they change from extreme sensitivity to killing to extreme resistance to killing. At the same time, they make a reverse charge in mutation sensitivity. They go from extreme resistance to mutation induction, nothing above control levels, to sensitivity greater than that of male. This is all within one cell stage. I can't see any approach with the present techniques to resolving this at the molecular level. It seems to me that we need entirely new kinds of development in the field.

Dr. Beers   Is this a problem either of discovering or developing a suitable test system or a suitable indicator or signal to tell you what is happening which is directly related to the events that you are observing, as opposed to something which might be two or three stages removed? The most obvious example, of course, is the use of cell death as an indicator of radiation effects, and this is probably the worst thing you could take in many instances. You need to look for other intermediate parameters, whether you're dealing with excision repair or recombination repair.

Dr. Roberts   I think that this is the big problem. As soon as one gets away from perfectly simple systems of cells in culture, it is very difficult to measure the parameters we are looking at, to measure the true rates of loss of alkyl groups or rate of repair replication. For example, colleagues of mine are looking at the DNA synthesis in a folic acid stimulated kidney. They can measure DNA synthesis in this kidney. If they inject an animal with an alkylating agent, they can inhibit this process. If they increase the time between the injection of an alkylating agent and the stimulation by the folic acid, they get a decreased inhibition. So one could argue that this is indicative of a repair situation occurring in vivo, of which one would like obviously to have examples. It is an extremely difficult situation to measure the types of things we have talked about at this meeting but I think it has to be done; this is the next stage, to find examples which are indications of repair in vivo.

Dr. Warwick has given a carcinogen which is not normally a hepato-carcinogen, but if he carries out a partial hepatectomy to stimulate division in the liver, this will produce tumors in urethane-injected animals. There is a certain finite time between carrying out the partial hepatectomy and the onset of DNA synthesis. If he varies the time of injection of the agent between this period, he gets a different yield of tumors. There is an 18-hour gap before the onset of synthesis. If he injects at the beginning of this time there is a lower yield than if he injects prior to this period. This could easily be interpreted, like effects on DNA synthesis in a synchronous population of cells, as indicative of repair analogous to a G-1 period where repair is occurring before damage is fixed during DNA synthesis.

Dr. P. C. Huang,   A number of papers presented at this symposium deal with
Baltimore   eukarotic cells. We know very well that eukarotic chromosomes, unlike the prokarotic, have proteins and RNA attached to the DNA. I wonder whether the panel would enlighten us by telling us whether the effect you see is a primary one or a secondary one. In other words, what kind of role do the proteins play in terms of these radiation levels, sensitivities, differences between G-1, G-2, S phase, and so forth?

Dr. Howard-   It seems to me that although the understanding of repair in
Flanders   higher cells is far from complete, at the moment it is more striking that the repair processes are essentially similar than essentially dissimilar. It may very well prove yet that there are differences in time scale, there are differences in whether synthesis is going on, but that the underlying principles are remarkably similar, that they function in the same environment as nucleases, polymerases and other enzymes, and that we should look to the same principles. At least at this time, I think there are no principles that have emerged from mammalian cells, at least in biochemical terms, that were not already worked on in bacteria. So the answer to your question would be, I think, that the effects of the nuclear protein itself are perhaps secondary.

Dr. Huang

Have you considered the correlation that can be drawn between the S phase and G phase in terms of tertiary structure of chromosomes, because the qualitative and quantitative ratio of protein to DNA is different in these stages? For instance, the sensitivity in relation to the S phase could very well be explained by lack of protection by proteins.

Dr. Howard-Flanders

There are, of course, other differences, namely as to whether the cell is about to undergo DNA synthesis or not, whether there is a lot of delay for enzymatic changes to take place prior to the inhibition, so that it is rather difficult to separate any particular parameter.

Dr. Roberts

I think in the case of the alkylating agents one would not readily invoke reactions with the protein simply on the basis of the target theory. The levels of reaction with which we are dealing are so low that one is only reacting one molecule of protein in something like 2,000. But I think we might be cautious with monofunctional compounds where one needs a high level of alkylization to inactivate the cell. One could be having other effects.

Dr. Bernard Strauss,

I would like to point out the difference between repair of MNS damage by prokarotes and eukarotes, and end by asking Dr. Roberts a question. In prokarotes, in a 40-minute generation time, there seems to be no methyl excision, no loss of methyl groups. They're stable. There is no repair replication measurable easily. Still you see some sort of recovery. In eukarotes you see methyl excision, although over a period of hours rather than minutes, so it is easy to demonstrate repair replication. Furthermore, in prokarotes, the fundamental difference seems to be between mono- and bifunctional agents. Yet in Dr. Roberts' experiments, it looked as though the fundamental differences were between methylating agents and others, because the monofunctional mustards behaved very differently from the monofunctional methylating agents. In prokarotes and bacteria, the monofunctionals all behave more or less alike. I wonder if you would comment on that.

Dr. Roberts

I'll take the last point first. There is this remarkable difference between the monofunctional methylating agents and half mustard gas, which as you rightly point out is similar qualitatively in all its effects to that of mustard gas. It requires about five times the level of alkylation at equitoxic doses to produce these effects. We think of it as almost a pseudodifunctional compound in our system. There is probably hydrogen bonding on the other OH group. I think we can rule out any possibility of contamination of the difunctional compound, so there is a remarkable difference.

Dr. Albert Kelner, (Waltham, Mass.)

I'd like to carry forward a point which I believe Dr. Russell was making. While he was showing his slides he pointed out that the permissible radiation dose standards were very much higher than the doses which were mutagenic in mice. And I gathered that the implication was that one of the lessons of DNA repair was that at very low dose rates there was so much repair that these radiations were relatively ineffective. And I wonder whether that is the only lesson we have from DNA repair. We know that without repair DNA is very much more sensitive than was ever realized and that in the human population there must be a spectrum of repair efficiencies, due perhaps to inhibitors or other normal and abnormal states. So I would like to ask him and the panel whether in their opinion the results of DNA repair knowledge in the last few years would lead us to change the permissible radiation dose for the population, to make them higher, lower, or just the same.

Dr. Russell   I think it is inappropraite for me to make a specific recommendation for raising or lowering since I am presently serving on committees that are considering this. I would be jumping the gun on the committees to come out with such a figure. I think that there is no reason for raising the levels to allow more radiation unless there is a compelling need for economic or other reasons to do this. The original levels were set, theoretically of course, on a benefit-risk basis, but the geneticists at that time, in 1956, knew they were not even estimating the risks very accurately and we felt that nobody could estimate in any kind of quantitative fashion the benefits of nuclear energy. So the levels were set partly as ones that they thought society could live with and that did not seem to be particularly hazardous. Along with the setting of a level was a very strong enjoinder to stay as far below as possible; in other words, the idea was not to set a permissible level like the minimum butterfat content of milk, where everybody would hew exactly to the line, but that industry and government would try to keep the levels as low as possible. And I think in spite of all the loss of credibility that the Atomic Energy Commission, for one, has had in recent years that a pretty good job was done of insuring that nuclear power development, in particular, would not only not go up to these levels, but would stay well below them. So I see no reason for raising the permissible levels, allowing more radiation, just because our estimates of the risk may be less. As far as the estimates of risk are concerned, I should emphasize that the data that I have been presenting are only one way of estimating the risk. We provided data back in '56 to indicate what the mouse mutation rate was, and this was used as a best guess for human mutation rates. But there are other ways of estimating the risks, such as computing the doubling dose in the mouse, the amount of radiation that would double the spontaneous rate. That would give us the mouse spontaneous mutation frequency; then take the spontaneous rate in man, and use that approach. Another approach was to look at the empirical results in Hiroshima and Nagasaki, and other bits of data on exposure of humans, and see if one could come up with any sort of upper confidence limits on those estimates. So there are various ways of estimating what the hazards would be, and ours is just one of them. Also, there is the qualification that mouse data may not be carried over to man with a great deal of confidence.

Dr. Ronald
Cole,
(New Haven)

I address my question to John Roberts. You observed the release of alkylated bases from DNA in cells. It is also known that alkylated bases in DNA are spontaneously released and an apurinic site is left; how would the rates of the two processes compare?

Dr. Roberts

We know that the alkyl groups are lost in DNA, and this occurs at a rate which is not dissimilar from that which we are observing in whole cells. The repair replication which we observe could follow as a consequence of either the enzymatic excision of alkyl groups for formation of apurinic sites, which then leads to a chain break, degradation, followed by repair replication. I don't think at this stage we can distinguish between the two possibilities.

Dr. Beers

In behalf of Dr. Herriott and myself, I want to thank the speakers for the hard work they have put in in the last two days in making this, I think, a very successful symposium. We certainly owe a debt of gratitude to our host, the Miles Laboratories, in particular to Dr. O'Donovan, who has been the coordinator of this program.

INDEX

Colophon for Beers/Herriott, MOLECULAR AND CELLULAR REPAIR PROCESSES

THE JOHNS HOPKINS UNIVERSITY PRESS

This book was composed in Press Roman Medium text,
printed on 60-lb. Matte Offset, and bound in Interlaken
Matte cloth by LithoCrafters, Inc.